Plant and Insect Mycoplasma Techniques

EDITED BY M.J. DANIELS AND P.G. MARKHAM

A HALSTED PRESS BOOK

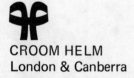

CROOM HELM
London & Canberra

JOHN WILEY & SONS
New York · Toronto

©1982 M.J. Daniels and P.G. Markham
Croom Helm Ltd, 2-10 St John's Road, London SW11

British Library Cataloguing in Publication Data

Plant and insect mycoplasma techniques.
    1. Mycoplasmatales
    I. Daniels, M.J.
    II. Markham, P.G.
    589.9   QR352

ISBN 0-7099-0272-7

Published in the U.S.A. and Canada
by Halsted Press, a Division of
John Wiley & Sons, Inc., New York

Library of Congress Cataloging in Publication Data
Main entry under title:

Plant and insect mycoplasma techniques.

    "A Halsted Press book."
    Includes index.
    1. Mycoplasmatales.   2. Mycoplasma diseases of
plants.   3. Insects—Microbiology.   I. Daniels,
M. J.   II. Markham, P. G.
QR352.P56   632'.32   81-13142   AACR2

ISBN 0-470-27262-7

Printed and bound in Great Britain by
Biddles Ltd, Guildford and King's Lynn

CONTENTS

Preface

PREFACE

Only 14 years have passed since the first publication appeared which implicated mycoplasmas as agents of plant disease. The diseases themselves have been known for much longer; indeed clover phyllody, a typical example, was described in the seventeenth century, well before any animal mycoplasma diseases had been documented. The early history of plant mycoplasmas is described in Chapter 2 and one obvious conclusion to be drawn from the frustrating experiences of the earlier workers is that the experimental methods at their disposal were simply inadequate for the task. Progress in science depends critically upon the development of new methods. Although important advances have been made in plant and insect mycoplasmology, notably in the discovery of spiroplasmas, many intractable problems remain. Most plant mycoplasmas cannot yet be cultured *in vitro*, and their natural plant habitat, the phloem, is one of the most difficult plant tissues for the experimenter to handle, placing severe restrictions on the type of experiments which can be performed *in vivo*. It is clear that radically new methods may be required to solve these problems.

A survey of the progress which has been made shows that application of techniques from a wide range of disciplines has been necessary. A successful individual or group of workers must possess the skills of a plant pathologist, a plantsman, a plant physiologist, a light- and electron microscopist, a bacteriologist, a biochemist, an immunologist, an entomologist, a virologist and a molecular geneticist. There must be few who could claim to possess practical expertise in all these fields, but some familiarity with the scope and limitations of each is essential. The editors hope that this book will serve as an introduction for those wishing to undertake research in this specialised area of mycoplasmology. We felt that a general discussion of techniques would be more useful than a detailed laboratory manual; to have included full experimental details in each chapter would have increased greatly the size and cost of the book. The details can of course be found in original papers cited, but it is rare for a method to be taken from the literature and applied without modification to a new system.

Plant and insect mycoplasmology is an expanding field, as is evidenced by the increasing number of contributions at mycoplasma meetings. Already important ramifications into human and animal mycoplasmology are developing and we can look forward to exciting scientific discoveries in the coming years.

M. J. Daniels
P. G. Markham

1 THE BIOLOGY OF MYCOPLASMAS

D. B. Archer and M. J. Daniels

1. The Class Mollicutes

A. Introduction

Mycoplasma is the trivial name given to all members of the class Mollicutes. Minimal standards for the description of new species of Mollicutes have been set by the International Committee on Systematic Bacteriology, Subcommittee on the Taxonomy of Mollicutes (1979). These standards distinguish mycoplasmas from other prokaryotes and subdivide the class into three families within the order Mycoplasmatales.

Mycoplasmas are distinguished from bacteria by their lack of peptidoglycan, and consequent resistance to penicillin, cycloserine and other antibiotics which inhibit bacterial cell wall biosynthesis. Recently it was shown that unlike bacteria and derived L-forms, mycoplasmas lack penicillin-binding proteins (Martin *et al.*, 1980). Growth of mycoplasmas may be inhibited by very high penicillin concentrations but in no case has the reason for the inhibition been established. Even *M. neurolyticum*, which is regarded as a penicillin-sensitive mycoplasma, is unaffected by cycloserine. Reversion of mycoplasmas to walled forms has never been observed under any circumstances, in contrast to the reversion of wall-less L-phase variants of bacteria to walled forms. Thus, mycoplasmas are limited by the plasma membrane, their only membrane, and although some species may have extra-membranous material this does not contain peptidoglycan.

Lack of rigidity gave rise to the name Mollicutes and explains the ability of mycoplasmas to pass through pores as small as 220 nm even though the diameter of a viable organism is greater than 300 nm. Despite their small size, mycoplasmas are capable of growth in synthetic media though they may have stringent nutritional requirements. Such requirements may have prevented the cultivation of some organisms which appear to be mycoplasmas by other criteria, so it is unclear whether Mollicutes should include organisms presently considered obligate parasites. Morphological examination by light and electron microscopy confirms their size and lack of a cell wall. Most mycoplasmas are pleomorphic although some species are characterised by particular shapes which are discussed in greater detail below. Growth conditions can affect morphology and apart from their appearance in liquid culture, colonial morphology of mycoplasmas on solid media is characteristic as most mycoplasma colonies on agar show a typical 'fried-egg' morphology in which the central zone represents growth in the medium.

Apart from the major criteria mentioned so far, other characteristics distinguish mycoplasmas from bacteria. These include a range of values of guanine-plus-cytosine content of DNA of 23 to 41 mole per cent, being at the low end of the range of values found in bacteria. Serological cross-reactivity between mycoplasmas and bacteria has been reported (Smith, 1971; Neimark, 1974), but no significant DNA homology between mycoplasmas and bacteria has been found. Bacteria do not require sterol for growth, but with the exception of *Acholeplasma* species and one *Anaeroplasma*, mycoplasmas have an absolute dependence on sterol for growth.

The current status of the taxonomic divisions within the class Mollicutes is shown in Table 1.1. One order, Mycoplasmatales, is recognised and there are three families within the order. Mycoplasma is the trivial name given to all Mollicutes, but spiroplasma will be used throughout the volume to include all mycoplasmas having a helical morphology at some stage of their growth. Presently, only one *Spiroplasma* species is recognised but the large and growing number of helical mycoplasma isolates warrants the use of a trivial name to include them all. Variants of *S. citri* need not be helical (Townsend *et al.*, 1977b) to be still considered spiroplasmas although helicity remains the simplest feature for distinguishing spiroplasmas from other mycoplasmas.

Sterol requirement is of prime importance in the taxonomic divisions (Table 1.1). Many tests determine sterol dependence, including sensitivity to digitonin or polyene antibiotics. Genome size and intracellular localisation of NADH oxidase are the other properties of major

Table 1.1: Taxonomy of the Mycoplasmas

Class: Mollicutes, Order: Mycoplasmatales

    Family I: *Mycoplasmataceae*

      1. Sterol required for growth

      2. Genome size about 5.0×10^8 daltons

      3. NADH oxidase localised in cytoplasm

      Genus I: *Mycoplasma* (about 50 species current)

        1. Do not hydrolyse urea

      Genus II: *Ureaplasma* (single species with serotypes)

        1. Hydrolyses urea

    Family II: *Acholeplasmataceae*

      1. Sterol not required for growth

      2. Genome size about 1.0×10^9 daltons

      3. NADH oxidase localised in membrane

      Genus I: *Acholeplasma* (6 species current)

    Family III: *Spiroplasmataceae*

      1. Helical organisms during some phase of growth

      2. Sterol required for growth

      3. Genome size about 1.0×10^9 daltons

      4. NADH oxidase localised in cytoplasm

      Genus I: *Spiroplasma* (1 species current)

Genera of uncertain taxonomic position

    Thermoplasma (single species)

    Anaeroplasma (two species)

Source: Tully (1978a).

importance used in the taxonomy of Mollicutes. Spiroplasmas have a genome size comparable to the acholeplasmas but unlike the acholeplasmas, spiroplasmas have a sterol growth requirement. Superoxide dismutase activity has been found in all *Acholeplasma* species but not in *Mycoplasma* species (Lee and Kenny, 1980; Lynch and Cole, 1980). *Ureaplasma* is distinguished from *Mycoplasma* species by its ability to hydrolyse urea. *Thermoplasma* and *Anaeroplasma* are of uncertain taxonomic position. *Thermoplasma acidophilum* is a wall-less prokaryote growing optimally at 59°C and pH 2 (Darland *et al.*, 1970) and having a functional flagellum (Black *et al.*, 1979). Its membrane lipids are characterised by the presence of lipopolysaccharide (Mayberry-Carson *et al.*, 1974) and ether-linked alkylglycerol (Langworthy *et al.*, 1972; Langworthy, 1979). These properties and 16S rRNA oligonucleotide catalogues distinguish *T. acidophilum* from other mycoplasmas and this organism is better regarded as belonging to the Archaebacteria than Mollicutes (Woese *et al.*, 1980). Mycoplasmas are regarded as facultative anaerobes, but *Anaeroplasma* is necessarily anaerobic and includes strains which do, and others which do not, require sterol (Robinson and Allison, 1975; Robinson *et al.*, 1975).

There are a variety of other serological and chemical criteria which distinguish mycoplasmas. Those relating specifically to spiroplasmas are discussed in detail in this book while others have been described by the Subcommittee on Taxonomy of Mollicutes (1979) and in *The Mycoplasmas* (Barile *et al.*, 1979). Differences in morphology, membrane composition, genomes and metabolic capabilities are discussed below.

B. Cytology

The resolution of the light microscope is too low to give a highly detailed picture of mycoplasma morphology but it has the advantage over the electron microscope that viable cells can be examined and so no artifactual forms, produced as a result of fixation or staining, exist. Thus, much information is gained by viewing mycoplasmas by phase-contrast or dark-field microscopy. Mycoplasmas normally appear either as spherical cells with diameters between 0.3 and 1.0 μm or as filaments. Filamentous growth can either be as mono-nucleate cells or long multi-nucleate filaments and most, if not all, mycoplasmas grow in a filamentous form under appropriate growth conditions (Rodwell and Mitchell, 1979). The morphology of *M. mycoides* subsp. *mycoides* is markedly affected by the fatty acid composition of the growth medium (Rodwell and Peterson, 1971). Rapid growth rate or supplementation of the medium with unsaturated fatty acid favours filament formation in *M. hominis* (Razin, 1978), *A. laidlawii* (Razin *et al.*, 1966, 1967; Maniloff, 1970) and *M. gallisepticum* (Razin and Cosenza, 1966). *M. gallisepticum* is, however, normally pear-shaped with a characteristic terminal bleb structure (Maniloff *et al.*, 1965). *M. pneumoniae* is a filamentous organism which has a specialised terminal structure (Biberfeld and Biberfeld, 1970). These two organisms and *M. pulmonis*, which possesses a stalk, adhere to surfaces at their specialised structures and exhibit a gliding motility (Bredt, 1973, 1974). This will be discussed in more detail in subsequent sections. Fine detail of the specialised terminal structures of some mycoplasmas has only been revealed by electron microscopy and a dense central core has been observed in the tip structures of *M. pneumoniae* (Wilson and Collier, 1976) and *M. alvi* (Gourlay *et al.*, 1977). Growth of some strains of *M. mycoides* in a defined medium favours growth in the rho form (Peterson *et al.*, 1973; Rodwell *et al.*, 1973), a form characterised by an intracellular axial fibre composed of only one protein and a cellular polarity with a specialised terminal structure at one pole (Rodwell *et al.*, 1975). The fine structures of *M. pneumoniae* and the rho form of *M. mycoides* are shown in Figure 1.1. However, unlike *M. pneumoniae*, no surface adhesion or motility of *M. mycoides* has been demonstrated.

Spiroplasmas are characterised by a helical morphology which is easily seen by light microscopy or by electron microscopy. The helices have a polarity with one pointed and one blunt end (Cole *et al.*, 1973). These helical organisms are motile (Davis and Worley, 1973) although helicity and motility are lost in ageing cultures (Cole *et al.*, 1973; Razin *et al.*, 1973). There is little information on what determines the characteristic shape of *M. gallisepticum* or *M. pneumoniae*, but it seems probable that intracellular filaments seen in spiroplasmas are responsible for their helicity (Williamson, 1974). Fibrils 3.6 nm in diameter with a 9 nm repeat are relased from cells lysed with sodium deoxycholate (Williamson, 1974). Fibrils with similar dimensions have been isolated and purified from the honey-bee spiroplasma (Clark, 1977) by Townsend *et al.* (1980). These fibrils were isolated after lysis of the cells in Triton X-100, and shown to be composed of protein subunits with a molecular weight of 55,000 (Figure 1.1). The non-helical variant of *S. citri* (Townsend *et al.*, 1977b) also contained fibrils but lacked one membrane protein which, it has been speculated, may be involved in attachment of the fibrils to the cell membrane.

Electron microscopy has revealed the presence of a chromosome, ribosomes and granular material in mycoplasmas (Maniloff and Morowitz, 1972; Razin, 1978). Apart from the plasma membrane there are no other membranes present within the cell. The possible occurrence of plasmids in mycoplasmas has been suggested on the basis of electron microscopy and satellite bands of DNA found in density gradients (Maniloff and Morowitz, 1972; Zouzias *et al.*, 1973). Until recently there has been very little characterisation of the extrachromosomal DNA and the possibilities remained that it represented non-viral plasmid material or viral DNA present in a carrier state. However, in *S. citri* the presence of plasmid DNA has now been established (Ranhand *et al.*, 1980). Viruses infect *Acholeplasma* (Gourlay, 1970) and *Spiroplasma* (Cole *et al.*, 1973) and, recently, unequivocal demonstration of a *Mycoplasma* virus was made (Howard *et al.*, 1980).

Extramembranous material has been described in many mycoplasmas.

Figure 1.1: Fibrillar Structure in Mycoplasmas. (a) rho fibre of *Mycoplasma mycoides* showing characteristic terminal structure. Bar represents 250 nm. (Courtesy of J.E. Peterson and A.W. Rodwell.) (b) Rod-like terminal structure of *Mycoplasma pneumoniae*. Bar represents 100 nm. (Courtesy of U. Göbel.) (c) Lysed cell preparation of *Spiroplasma citri* clearly showing flexuous fibrils within the cell. Bar represents 200 nm. (Courtesy of R. Townsend and K. Plaskitt.) (d) Purified fibrils from *Spiroplasma citri*. Bar represents 100 nm. (Courtesy of R. Townsend and K. Plaskitt.)

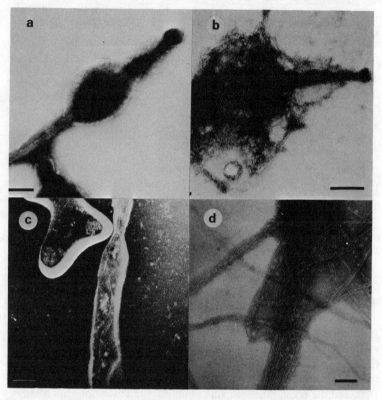

M. mycoides subsp. *mycoides* elaborates a galactan (Gourlay and Thrower, 1968) while subsp. *capri* synthesises a glucan (Jones *et al.*, 1965). A hexosamine polymer is associated with the *A. laidlawii* membrane (Gilliam and Morowitz, 1972; Terry and Zupnik, 1973.) Electron microscopy has suggested the presence of extracellular material in a number of mycoplasmas and some of these stain with ruthenium red (Razin, 1978). Ruthenium red binds to a range of high molecular weight anions and although it is quite likely that the binding to mycoplasmas is to acid polysaccharides, the exact nature of the material remains to be established. Anionic sites are also visualised by binding polycationic ferritin (Schiefer *et al.*, 1976) and surface carbohydrate binds lectins (Schiefer *et al.*, 1974. Kahane and Tully, 1976; Kahane *et al.*, 1977) but detailed characterisation of the carbohydrate-containing moieties is lacking. Ruthenium red is known to bind to the acid polysaccharide of glycoproteins and does bind to *M. pneumoniae* (Wilson and Collier, 1976) which contains a glycoprotein (Kahane and Brunner, 1977), but it is premature to equate ruthenium red binding with presence of glycoproteins in other mycoplasmas.

C. The Cell Membrane

The mycoplasma cell membrane has been described in a number of recent reviews (Rottem, 1979; Razin, 1979; Archer, 1981). The cell membrane has received considerable research interest, not only because of its central role in the functions of these wall-less organisms, but also because it is the only membrane in the cell and is relatively easy to isolate free from cytoplasmic contamination so that it is an ideal system for the study of biomembrane structure and function.

The chemical composition of mycoplasma membranes varies with species but generally falls within the range 50-60 per cent protein, 30-40 per cent lipid and 1-3 per cent carbohydrate with RNA and DNA considered as cytoplasmic contaminants (Razin, 1975). Acholeplasmas are distinguished from other mycoplasmas by their ability to grow in the absence of sterol and by the presence of terpenes and lipopolysaccharides in the membrane. The sterol requirement of mycoplasmas is met by all sterols with a 3β-hydroxyl and a relatively planar nucleus. The fatty acids in *Mycoplasma* and *Spiroplasma* species are incorporated unmodified into complex lipids, whereas *Acholeplasma* species can synthesise straight-chain saturated fatty acids from acetate and can elongate medium-chain length unsaturated fatty acids (Razin, 1975; Bové and Saillard, 1979). This means that acholeplasmas differ from other mycoplasmas in the ways in which they maintain the membrane in a state of suitable fluidity under certain constraints. This subject has been fully discussed elsewhere (Rottem, 1979; Archer, 1981). A range of complex lipids is found in mycoplasmas, the phospholipids being mainly phosphatidylglycerol and diphosphatidylglycerol. Phosphatidylcholine (PC) and phosphatidylethanolamine (PE) have been encountered but, in the main, have been absorbed from the medium although PC in *M. gallisepticum* is synthesised by incorporation of a fatty acid into medium-derived lyso-PC (Rottem and Markowitz, 1979) and PE may be synthesised by *Ureaplasma* (Romano *et al.*, 1972). A sphingolipid has been described in *A. axanthum* (Plackett *et al.*, 1970; Mayberry *et al.*, 1973) and plasmalogens have been detected in *Anaeroplasma* (Langworthy *et al.*, 1975). Glycolipids are also major constituents of mycoplasma membranes, comprising more than 50 per cent of the total lipids in *A. laidlawii*. Lectin binding studies have indicated that carbohydrate residues are solely in the exterior half of the bilayer, although in *A. laidlawii* some carbohydrate-containing lipids are present in the inner half of the bilayer (Razin, 1978; Gross and Rottem, 1979). Phospholipids are also distributed asymmetrically in the two halves of the bilayer, as determined by phospholipase action (Bevers *et al.*, 1977a, 1978) and radioiodination (Gross and Rottem 1979). Cholesterol is distributed equally in resting cells of *M. gallisepticum* (Bittman and Rottem, 1976; Rottem *et al.*, 1978) but its distribution in *M. capricolum* is known to be affected by cell growth (Clejan *et al.*, 1978).

Mycoplasma membrane proteins include those removed by mild treatments (peripheral proteins) and those that are solubilised only by complete membrane disruption (integral proteins) (Razin, 1975). Two groups of peripheral membrane proteins have been recognised in *A. laidlawii* (Archer *et al.*, 1978). Group I peripheral proteins were removed from the membrane at low ionic strength and faced the cell interior whereas group II peripheral proteins were removed by EDTA and faced the cell exterior. Asymmetry of mycoplasma membrane proteins has been demonstrated by freeze-etching and by chemical labelling techniques and more protein faces the cell interior than the exterior (Razin, 1979; Archer, 1981).

There is undoubtedly much carbohydrate on the surface of mycoplasmas and this forms part of glycoproteins, glycolipids, lipopolysaccharide (lipoglycan) and polysaccharide. Glycoproteins have been purified from *M. pneumoniae* (Kahane and Brunner, 1977) and *M. gallisepticum* (Goel and Lemcke, 1975), two motile organisms with characteristic shapes which adhere to surfaces. A glycoprotein has also been isolated from *T. acidophilum* (Yang and Haug, 1979). However, the evidence for a glycoprotein in *M. gallisepticum* has been questioned (Razin, 1978; Archer, 1981) and although there is some support for glycoproteins in many other mycoplasmas, including *S. citri* (Kahane *et al.*, 1977) this topic remains one which requires much more thorough examination. In eukaryotic cells glycoproteins are often exported, or involved in cell-cell recognition and have their carbohydrate exterior to the cell membrane (Rothman and Lenard, 1977). It would be of great interest if the glycoprotein found in *M. pneumoniae* (Kahane and Brunner, 1977) is the protein responsible for attachment of the organisms to host tracheal cells (Hu *et al.*, 1977).

A number of enzymic activities and transport processes are known to be associated with mycoplasma membranes (Maniloff and Morowitz, 1972; Razin, 1975). ATPase is membrane-associated in all mycoplasmas examined including *S. citri* (Mudd *et al.*, 1977) whereas NADH oxidase is membrane-associated only in acholeplasmas. ATPase activity is dependent upon membrane lipids (de Kruyff *et al.*, 1973; Rottem *et al.*, 1973; Bevers *et al.*, 1977b). The phosphoenolpyruvate-dependent sugar phosphotransferase system is present in *Mycoplasma* but absent from *Acholeplasma* species (Razin, 1975). A major non-enzymic membrane protein of *S. citri* has been purified and called spiralin (Wróblewski *et al.*, 1977). Spiralin is an integral membrane protein of approximate molecular weight 26,000 and represents about 22 per cent of the membrane protein. Spiralin, by itself, is not responsible for helicity as a non-helical variant of *S. citri* also contains spiralin (Townsend *et al.*, 1977b) but some role in shape determination and motility seems likely.

Adherence to surfaces and gliding motility are properties of *M. pulmonis, M. pneumoniae* and *M. gallisepticum* (Bredt, 1973, 1974). Motility has been observed only on a surface, and a non-motile variant of *M. pneumoniae*, which was avirulent, also had reduced capacity to adsorb to glass (Bredt, 1974). The mechanism of motility in these organisms is unknown although there is evidence for an actin-like protein synthesised by *M. pneumoniae* (Neimark, 1977; Meng and Pfister, 1980). Many mycoplasmas are known to contain proteins with some solubility properties and molecular weights similar to eukaryotic muscle actin (Rodwell *et al.*, 1978; Maniloff and Chaudhuri, 1979; R. Townsend, unpublished observations) but only in *M. pneumoniae* has it been reported that filaments which became 'decorated' with heavy meromyosin could form (Neimark, 1977). Filament formation should facilitate purification of the protein so that comparison with eukaryotic actins could be made but this has not yet been done. No *M. pneumoniae* protein of molecular weight 42,000 has an isoelectric point similar to rabbit muscle actin (Rodwell *et al.*, 1978) whereas eukaryotic actins from a variety of sources have remarkable sequence homology (Korn, 1978). Antiserum to eukaryotic actin binds to the external membrane surface of *S. citri* (Williamson *et al.*, 1979) and

specifically recognises one *S. citri* protein (Mouches *et al.*, 1980)
The relationship, if any, of mycoplasma actin-like proteins to the
prokaryotic elongation factor EF-Tu must be elucidated and it seems
premature to ascribe a role in motility to the mycoplasma actin-like
proteins. The presence of a contractile system in mycoplasmas is not
in doubt but the molecular basis of shape changes, cell division and
motility remains unclear.

D. The Genome

Mycoplasmas, in their smallest non-filamentous forms, have a single
chromosome which consists of double-stranded circular DNA
(Maniloff and Morowitz, 1972; Razin, 1978). With the exception of
T. acidophilum (Searcy, 1975) there are no known associated proteins.
As indicated earlier there is a range of guanine-plus-cytosine (GC)
values for mycoplasmas between 23 and 41 mole per cent which is
at the low end of the range found in other prokaryotes. *Mycoplasma*
and *Ureaplasma* species have a haploid genome size of about 5×10^8
daltons whereas in *Acholeplasma* and *Spiroplasma* species it is
approximately twice as large. Methylation of bases has been reported
in four *Mycoplasma* and one *Acholeplasma* species (Razin and Razin,
1980).

Replication of the mycoplasma genome is semi-conservative (Smith,
1969; Maniloff and Morowitz, 1972) and in two mycoplasmas examined
(*M. orale* and *M. hyorhinis*) one DNA polymerase was detected in each
organism (Mills *et al.*, 1977) whereas in *S. citri* two DNA polymerases
have been found (Charron *et al.*, 1979). Although mycoplasmas generally
reproduce by binary fission, cell division often lags behind genome
replication and multinucleate filaments are produced as a result.
Filamentation is a common event and it is known that lipid, protein
and DNA synthesis are not necessarily co-ordinated in *M. mycoides*
(Rodwell *et al.*, 1972). Fragmentation or budding of filaments to
produce mono-nucleate cells are modes of reproduction in addition to
binary fission, but all three modes involve semi-conservative replication
of the genome followed by cell division. The only difference between
their modes of reproduction is the degree of synchrony at the level of
individual cells between DNA replication and cell division, and all
three may occur side by side in the same culture (Rodwell and Mitchell,
1979). The DNA growing-point appears to be membrane-associated in
M. gallisepticum and the bleb structure of this organism is probably
the site of the DNA replication complex (Quinlan and Maniloff, 1972,
1973; Maniloff and Quinlan, 1974). The DNA growing-point is also

membrane-associated in *A. laidlawii* (Smith, 1969; Smith and Hanawalt, 1969).

There are two mechanisms of repair of ultra-violet-induced DNA damage in *A. laidlawii* (Maniloff and Morowitz, 1972). Not only is there an ultra-violet-induced repair mechanism but also a separate dark repair mechanism. However, neither repair mechanism was found in *M. gallisepticum* (Ghosh *et al.*, 1977), a finding unprecedented in prokaryotes. If there is a total lack of DNA repair after irradiation in *M. gallisepticum* it remains to be explained how the organism accommodates DNA damage or whether it is normally largely protected from irradiation damage.

E. Ribosomes and Transfer RNAs

Mycoplasma ribosomes have a sedimentation coefficient of 70S, and three ribosomal RNA species with sedimentation coefficients of 22S, 16S and 5S (Maniloff and Morowitz, 1972; Stanbridge and Reff, 1979). The rRNA has a GC content between 43 and 48 per cent which, although higher and less variable than mycoplasma DNA, is low in comparison with the values reported for bacterial rRNA. A number of modified nucleosides have been detected in *M. hominis* rRNA (Johnson and Horowitz, 1971) and Maniloff and Morowitz (1972) concluded that the compositions of mycoplasma rRNAs are not too dissimilar to *E. coli* rRNA. However, Reff *et al.* (1977) showed by mobility on polyacrylamide gels that mycoplasma 16S rRNA was shorter than eubacterial rRNA by about 37 nucleotides. In addition, the mycoplasma 22S rRNA must be slightly different from the bacterial 23S rRNA. Ribosomal proteins in mycoplasmas have not been examined in any detail apart from gel electrophoresis in one dimension (Johnson and Horowitz, 1971). Resistance to ribosome-active antibiotics in mycoplasmas was shown to be due to reduced membrane permeability rather than alteration to ribosomal proteins (Fratterigo and Perlman, 1971; Schwarz and Perlman, 1972) but this is to be expected, particularly with clinical isolates. Ribosomal modification by mutation could also account for antibiotic resistance but remains to be demonstrated. GC contents of mycoplasma transfer RNAs are high compared to DNA and are comparable with levels in *E. coli* (Maniloff and Morowitz, 1972). Available data indicate that mycoplasma tRNAs have a similar secondary structure to *E. coli* tRNAs, but that the mycoplasma tRNAs contain fewer modified bases (Kimball *et al.*, 1974; Kimball and Söll, 1974; Walker and RajBhandary, 1975, 1978). The high GC values reported for rRNAs and tRNAs compared to mycoplasma DNA suggest that there are regions of DNA with high GC, but that there would be relatively few of them. This in turn indicates that few isoaccepting tRNAs would be transcribed. Experiments confirm these suppositions in that only 44 tRNA cistrons were found in *M. capricolum* (Maniloff and Morowitz, 1972) and in the same organism only one tRNA^{Phe} was detected (Kimball *et al.*, 1974) although some isoaccepting tRNAs are known (Maniloff and Morowitz, 1972). Similar findings for other tRNAs are known (Maniloff and Morowitz, 1972), and details of other tRNAs in *M. mycoides* subsp. *capri* have been summarised by Razin (1978)who also points out that in acholeplasmas, and presumably spiroplasmas, which have larger genomes, more isoaccepting tRNAs might be expected.

F. Metabolic Activities

Only *Acholeplasma* has NADH oxidase located in the membrane whereas this activity is cytoplasmic in other mycoplasmas (see Section A). Even in *A. laidlawii*, however, the NADH oxidase is simple (Jinks and Matz, 1976a, b) and although flavins are associated, no quinones or cytochromes have been detected (Razin, 1978). Of all the mycoplasmas only *T. acidophilum* (Belly *et al.*, 1973; Holländer *et al.*, 1977) has a complex respiratory chain. Holländer *et al.* (1977) could detect no cytochromes in *M. arthritidis* even though this organism was previously supposed to be capable of oxidative phosphorylation (Van Demark and Smith, 1964). On the basis of their energy-yielding mechanisms, mycoplasmas are divided into fermentative and non-fermentative species.

Fermentative mycoplasmas produce ATP via fermentation of glucose or some other hexoses and polymers such as starch or glycogen to lactate. Pyruvate may also be oxidatively decarboxylated to acetyl-CoA which can be metabolised to acetate, yielding ATP by phosphoacetyltransferase and acetate kinase (Kahane *et al*, 1978). Anaerobically, however, lactate is the major end product of glucose metabolism resulting in acidification of the growth medium. Aeration of cultures may result in production of H_2O_2 either from glycerol oxidation or flavin-terminated oxidation of NADH (Rodwell and Mitchell, 1979). Phosphoacetyltransferase and acetate kinase are present in fermentative and non-fermentative species (Kahane *et al.*, 1978), but the energy-yielding mechanisms of non-fermentative species are not well understood. *M. arthritidis* can oxidise short-chain fatty acids and metabolise other short-chain carbon compounds, and *M. hominis* may derive ATP from the phosphoacetyltransferase-acetate kinase system (Rodwell and

Mitchell, 1979). The arginine dihydrolase pathway is a possible energy-yielding mechanism and most non-fermentative species possess arginine deiminase (Tully and Razin, 1977). Arginine certainly stimulates the growth of non-fermentative species (Schimke *et al.*, 1966; Fenske and Kenny, 1976) but whether the arginine dihydrolase pathway is the major energy-yielding mechanism in all non-fermentative strains has been questioned (Fenske and Kenny, 1976) as in *M. hominis* induction of arginine deiminase occurred only in the late logarithmic phase of growth. *S. citri* ferments glucose and catabolises arginine, but arginine utilisation made only a limited contribution to the energy requirements of the organism which grew poorly when arginine was the sole energy source (Townsend, 1976).

The energy source for *Ureaplasma* is unknown. Even the supposed urea requirement for growth (Ford and McDonald, 1967; Kenny and Cartwright, 1977) has been questioned (Masover *et al.*, 1974, 1977). The growth requirements of *Ureaplasma* and the possibility that urea may act as an energy source have been discussed by Rodwell and Mitchell (1979).

Knowledge of the nutritional requirements of mycoplasmas is of enormous benefit towards an understanding of their metabolic capabilities. Growth requirements of mycoplasmas are exacting and only *M. mycoides* and *A. laidlawii* have been grown in defined media (Rodwell and Mitchell, 1979). For this reason most information on metabolism in mycoplasmas is with these organisms and these results have been fully discussed elsewhere (Rodwell, 1969, 1977; Rodwell and Mitchell, 1979).

G. Mycoplasmas and the Minimal Cell Concept

Mycoplasmas are small in comparison with all other free-living organisms. They have limited genetic material and, though free-living, are nutritionally exacting. This had led to much discussion and theory as to whether it is possible for organisms smaller than mycoplasmas to be free-living (Maniloff and Morowitz, 1972; Pirie, 1973). Such analysis has led towards an appreciation of what might be essential in a minimal cell and mycoplasmas are nearer to that concept than any other group of organisms.

The diameter of a theoretical minimal cell has been estimated as 150 nm, less than half that of a mycoplasma, by Maniloff and Morowitz (1972) although, owing to their plasticity, mycoplasmas can pass through filters with pore sizes less than the cell diameter. The same authors calculate that the mycoplasma genome would occupy a sphere of roughly 150 nm diameter, so viable mycoplasmas less than about 200 nm are unlikely and have not been observed. Smaller bodies have been observed but were not viable and so were probably anucleate. The genomes of mycoplasmas could code for between 700 and 1,400 polypeptides depending on the genome size (Morowitz, 1969; Morowitz and Wallace, 1973). High resolution two-dimensional gel electrophoresis of mycoplasma proteins (Archer *et al.*, 1978; Rodwell and Rodwell, 1978; Mouches *et al.*, 1979) has resolved about 350 polypeptides from a number of species. Whether some of the spots on the electrophoretograms contained more than one polypeptide is unknown. Isofunctional proteins, from different cell types, such as eukaryotic actins (Korn, 1978) or cytochrome c (Barlow and Margoliash, 1966) have regions of conserved sequence although the extent of sequence homology is variable. The isoelectric points and molecular weights of such isofunctional proteins are remarkably constant, however, reflecting sequence homology of the polar residues and it is unlikely that such proteins would be distinguished by two-dimensional gel electrophoresis as described by Archer *et al.* (1978). Indeed, Garrels and Gibson (1976) separated *a*, *β* and *γ* actins by isoelectric focussing only by using long gels and shallow pH gradients. When comparing related mycoplasma strains by two-dimensional protein patterns it therefore seems possible that polypeptides with identical mobilities may in fact have many sequence differences although functionally they may be identical. However, actin and cytochrome c are possibly unusually well-conserved molecules in eukaryotes and although polypeptide sequence conservation may be high among strains of one species, between different species this need not be so as evidenced by the difficulty in matching groups of spots on two-dimensional gels from different mycoplasma species (A.W. Rodwell, E.S. Rodwell and D.B. Archer, unpublished observations).

2. Ecology of Mycoplasmas

A. Mycoplasma Habitats

An author addressing himself to this topic a mere twelve years ago could have confined his discussion to the distribution of mycoplasmas in animal hosts, with a brief mention of the apparently saprophytic acholeplasmas. We now realise that wall-free prokaryotes may have a very wide distribution in nature, but there are still many questions to be answered, particularly concerning primary habitats of many mycoplasmas.

(1) Vertebrate Animals. The first mycoplasmas to be isolated were animal pathogens and today the list of vertebrates known to harbour mycoplasmas is long and constantly increasing (Table 1.2). It must be remembered that only a minority of mycoplasmas have been shown to be pathogens, so that it follows that animals harbour a normal flora of 'harmless' mycoplasmas. An intriguing possibility is that some mycoplasmas may benefit the host, but to our knowledge there is no published work germane to this matter.

Table 1.2: Animals from Which Mycoplasmas Have Been Isolated

Man	Pig
Non-human primates:	Puma
African green monkey	Sheep
Baboon	Laboratory animals:
Bush baby	Chinese hamster
Chimpanzee	Guinea pig
Gorilla	Lemming
Grivet monkey	Mouse
Irus macaque	Rabbit
Marmoset	Rat
Orangutan	Tortoise
Patas	Wild animals:
Rhesus monkey	Bighorn sheep
Squirrel monkey	Chamois
Domestic and zoo animals:	Fieldmouse
Camel	Fox
Cat	Ground squirrel
Cattle	Hedgehog
Dog	Shrew
Egyptian buffalo	Vole
Elephant	Birds:
Goat	Chicken
Horse	Duck
Leopard	Goose
Lion	Turkey
Lynx	Wild birds belonging to at least 13 orders

Razin (1978) has emphasised that animal mycoplasmas can in general be regarded as 'membrane parasites', meaning that they are generally found in close association with the epithelial lining of infected organs and tissues. The commonest sites for mycoplasma colonisation are the respiratory and genito-urinary tracts, but isolations have been made from many other sites including the oral cavity and alimentary tract (anaeroplasmas have been found only in the rumen), the mammary gland and milk therefrom, eggs (embryos) of birds, joints, lymph nodes, eyes, liver, kidney, spleen, heart, brain (and CSF), parotid gland and serum. In addition there are some reports of isolations from human clinical material (leukaemic bone marrow, wounds and burns) (Somerson and Cole, 1979).

An additional 'animal' habitat of mycoplasmas which is largely artificial in character but which has received a great deal of attention is the laboratory tissue culture. A large proportion of cell cultures have been found to be contaminated with mycoplasmas, and the contamination can drastically affect the results of experiments with the cells (Barile, 1979). Cultures seem to become contaminated either because of poor technique (e.g. mouth pipetting or using procedures which generate aerosols), or because of contamination by mycoplasmas of commercial sera used in culture media.

(2) Plants. The rapid growth of information on mycoplasmas associated with plants provides the *raison d'être* of this volume, and since most aspects are treated exhaustively in subsequent chapters we shall confine ourselves here to pointing out that plants appear to offer three distinct niches for mycoplasmas. The most extensively studied is the interior of phloem sieve tubes, wherein are found the presumptive mycoplasma pathogens of yellows diseases. Secondly, following the discovery that honeybees feeding on spring-flowering trees became infected with spiroplasmas (Clark, 1977), a search was made for these organisms in the nectar of flowers, and a number of isolates have now been made, not only of spiroplasmas but also of non-helical mycoplasmas, both sterol-dependent and independent. Thirdly, there is now good evidence that acholeplasmas may be secondary saprophytic invaders of diseased plant tissues. Earlier sporadic reports of isolation from plants may perhaps be reinterpreted in the light of the finding that lethal-yellowing diseased coconut tissue frequently harbours acholeplasmas, particularly *A. axanthum* (Eden-Green, 1978 and Chapter 7 of this volume).

(3) Arthropods. The mycoplasma flora of arthropods (particularly leafhoppers) has been studied in recent years concurrently with work on plants. The reason of course is that mycoplasma diseases of plants

had for many years been known to be spread by phloem-feeding leafhoppers, and there was evidence that the plant pathogens could multiply and, in some cases, cause disease in the insect vectors (cf. Chapter 2). The availability of cultivable plant/insect spiroplasmas has facilitated experiments on the natural infection cycles, and information is now beginning to emerge on factors leading to acquisition of spiroplasmas by feeding insects, and on growth and localisation within the insect tissues (Chapter 10). Until very recently there was a tendency to view insect mycoplasmology as merely another facet of plant work, but the field has burgeoned with the discovery of spiroplasmas pathogenic to bees, to fruit flies, and with the recognition that some tick-derived agents which can cause experimental disease in mammals are spiroplasmas. In addition there are some reports of presumed mycoplasma symbionts of insects (see Saglio and Whitcomb, 1979).

An interesting difference between animal mycoplasmas on the one hand and plant and insect associates on the other is that the former, although often found in intimate contact with the host cell membrane, are never found within the cells in a topological sense, i.e. bathed by soluble cytoplasmic components. Plant pathogenic mycoplasmas are always found in phloem tissue, and while it may be a matter for debate whether the lumen of a mature sieve tube element can reasonably be considered an intracellular environment, there are cases where mycoplasmas in companion cells and immature sieve cells are indisputably intracytoplasmic (Figure 1.2). Similarly mycoplasmas have been shown to be not only present but also replicating inside leafhopper gut epithelial cells (Maillet and Gouranton, 1971). Further work is needed to determine whether plant/insect mycoplasma surfaces have special properties which enable them to penetrate host cell membranes without causing detectable disruption of the cell.

(4) Other Hosts. There are claims in the literature that mycoplasma-like organisms may be found in molluscs and in fungi, but, as Saglio and Whitcomb (1979) have pointed out, these tantalising reports contain insufficient information to justify the conclusion that wall-free prokaryotes are present in the host cells.

(5) Free-living Mycoplasmas. *Acholeplasma laidlawii* was isolated from sewage by Laidlaw and Elford (1936) and from soil and compost by Seiffert (1937), and since the organism differed from other known mycoplasmas by its ability to grow at room temperature, and by not requiring serum or sterol for growth, it was considered to be a saprophyte for many years. It has however been isolated from many animals, from serum and from some plants. In view of the ability of some

Figure 1.2: Electron Micrograph of a Section through Immature Phloem Tissue in a Petiole of a Mycoplasma-infected Siberian Wall-flower Plant. The cytoplasm of the cell is packed with mycoplasmas. (Bar = 1μm.)

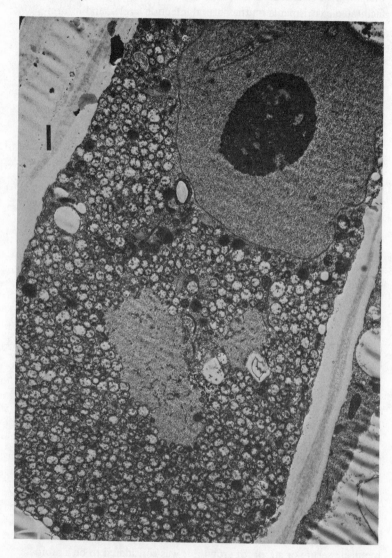

acholeplasmas to survive and multiply in insects and the recent finding of acholeplasmas as secondary invaders of diseased plant tissue (see

Tully, 1979), the feeling is developing that insects may be a principal reservoir for these organisms, and contamination by visiting insects may account for their apparently wide distribution. The thermoplasmas are unquestionably free-living, being found only in coal refuse piles at 60° and pH 2. We leave to others the question of whether thermoplasmas should be regarded as Mollicutes or Archaebacteria (Woese *et al.*, 1980).

A single report (in abstract form) described a mycoplasma from the sea which had a requirement for salt (Praznik, 1974). Unfortunately no further information has been published about this organism.

B. Host Range and Diversity of Mycoplasmas

Most named species of mycoplasmas have each been isolated from single animal species and until recently it was thought that mycoplasmas had very restricted host ranges, so that the first edition of the recommended minimal standards for designation of new species (International Committee on Systematic Bacteriology, Subcommittee on the Taxonomy of Mycoplasmatales, 1972) suggested that new isolates need only be compared with all known species from the same habitat. However, since then many cases have occurred of mycoplasma species isolated from a range of hosts, so that the latest edition of the document (Subcommittee, 1979) requires comparison with all previously named species. It must be realised that any consideration of host range is constrained by published details of isolations, which may well be fortuitous since few workers are in a position to carry out comprehensive surveys. Figure 1.3, based on data taken from Appendix 1 of the Report of Consultations of the Board of the WHO/FAO Programme on Comparative Mycoplasmology (1978), gives some idea of the extent of known host relationships of animal mycoplasmas. It is clear that: (1) most species have been isolated from a single animal host; (2) about one-third have been isolated from two or three hosts; and (3) two species, *A. laidlawii* and *M. arginini*, have a very wide host range. A caveat must be entered here: most of the animals studied are domesticated or kept in zoos or laboratories and may have been contaminated with alien mycoplasmas. Relatively few surveys have been made of wild animals. The ubiquity of *A. laidlawii* may be connected with the possibility mentioned earlier that insects may be an important reservoir of this mycoplasma and so may act as vectors to animals or to vegetation with which animals may have contact. Studies of the host range of plant mycoplasmas are in their infancy, but already important facts have emerged suggesting that host ranges may be

Figure 1.3: Host Range of Animal Mycoplasmas. The hatching indicates from which combinations of animal hosts mycoplasmas have been recovered. All species not mentioned in the final column (about 42) have been isolated from only one host group.

Number of Host Groups	Man	Other Primates	Laboratory Animals	Cats	Dogs	Horses	Cattle	Sheep and Goats	Pigs	Wild Animals	Birds	Mycoplasma Species
7	▨	▨						▨	▨			A. laidlawii
6			▨	▨			▨		▨	▨		M. arginini
4			▨	▨	▨		▨					M. bovigenitalium
3		▨	▨						▨			M. salivarium
3		▨	▨						▨			M. buccale
3				▨	▨		▨					M. gatae
3							▨	▨		▨		M. conjunctivae
2	▨	▨										M. faucium M. fermentans M. hominis M. orale M. lipophilum M. primatum
2		▨	▨									M. arthritidis
2			▨		▨							M. canis
2			▨			▨						M. pulmonis A. equifetale
2				▨	▨							M. feliminutum
2				▨		▨						M. felis
2						▨	▨					M. equirhinis
2							▨	▨				A. granularum A. oculi
2							▨		▨			M. bovis M. mycoides An. abactoclasticum
2									▨	▨		A. axanthum A. modicum
2										▨	▨	M. gallinarum M. gall.septicum
1												about 42

quite wide. Spiroplasmas indistinguishable from *S. citri* have been recovered in the field from diseased plants belonging to more than fifteen families, and from several leaf-hopper species. Corn stunt spiroplasma has been found naturally in four monocotyledonous hosts, but the spiroplasmas can be transmitted experimentally to dicotyledons (Markham *et al.*, 1977). The details of the flower-insect group of spiroplasmas have yet to be unravelled.

C. Interaction of Mycoplasmas with their Environment

Temperature. Animal mycoplasmas have an optimum growth temperature around 37°C, and most are unable to grow at 22°C. Ability to grow at lower temperatures was mentioned above as a property pointing to the classification of *A. laidlawii* as a saprophyte. It might be expected that an ability to grow over a large temperature range would be a charateristic of plant and insect mycoplasmas but the limited data available do not entirely support this notion. *S. citri* grows well only over a limited temperature range (c. 27-35°C), although some spiroplasmas from plant nectar may be less restricted by temperature. Thermoplasmas have an optimum temperature for growth of $59°C$, and a permissible range for growth of $45-62°C$. Langworthy (1979) has summarised available information on the biochemical properties of these organisms.

pH. Optimal growth of most mycoplasmas takes place between pH 7 and pH 8 and deviations of one pH unit are usually inhibitory to the organisms. Exceptions to the rule are the thermoplasmas (optimum pH 2.0, range 0.5-4.0) and ureaplasmas (optimum pH 6-6.5). For ureaplasmas and arginine-metabolising mycoplasmas expediency dictates the use of an acid pH value for the culture medium because ammonia production by the cells rapidly drives the pH up to lethal levels.

Osmotic Pressure. Most mycoplasma culture media have an osmotic pressure of around 7 atm., although the spiroplasmas from plants are usually grown in a medium of higher OP (c. 14 atm.) designed to simulate the contents of sieve tubes. Animal mycoplamas cannot usually grow in the OP exceeds 14 atm., but many can survive in media which are too dilute to maintain the integrity of bacterial protoplasts. To explain this it has been suggested that the mycoplasma membrane has unusual mechanical strength or that the cytoplasmic contents have a lower osmotic pressure than bacterial protoplasts. What is not often realised, however, is that for small cells like mycoplasmas immersed in an aqueous medium elementary theory predicts that surface tension will generate an excess pressure within the cell of the order of 10 atm., so that *ad hoc* hypotheses to explain the relative lack of osmotic fragility of mycoplasmas are unnecessary.

Atmospheric Conditions. The majority of mycoplasmas are facultative anaerobes. Growth on agar is frequently enhanced in an atmosphere containing higher levels of CO_2. Only the anaeroplasmas are strict anaerobes in the sense that oxygen is toxic to them. Some mycoplasmas can use oxygen as a terminal electron acceptor but there is still much to be learned about energy-yielding pathways of these organisms (Pollack, 1979).

Specific Chemical Substances. The nutritional requirements of mycoplasmas are highly complex and chemically-defined media capable of supporting growth have been devised for only two mycoplasmas (*M. mycoides* and *A. laidlawii*). In general a wide range of amino acids, vitamins, some coenzymes, nucleic acid precursors, inorganic ions and an energy source are required. A characteristic requirement of mycoplasmas is for lipids — a sterol (except for acholeplasmas) and fatty acids. The need to add these water-insoluble substances raises problems because in the free state they may cause cell lysis. The solution usually adopted is to add them as non-toxic protein complexes, either in the form of animal serum components or as artificial mixtures made up with protein, non-ionic surfactants or phosphomannan.

In common with other microorganisms the growth of mycoplasmas is inhibited by accumulated products of metabolism, for example lactic acid, hydrogen peroxide, and ammonia.

Other Organisms. The majority of mycoplasma species are not pathogenic to their hosts and can probably be regarded as commensals. For example, of the dozen species isolated from humans, only *M. pneumoniae* and *U. urealyticum* are pathogens, although other species such as *M. hominis* may be opportunists in abnormal situations, for example in patients with impaired immune function whose bacterial flora has been suppressed with antibiotics.

The spiroplasmas of plant and insect origin present an interesting picture. The known plant pathogens (*S. citri* and the corn stunt organism) may also be pathogenic to certain of their leafhopper vectors (Whitcomb *et al.*, 1974). Spiroplasmas from flower nectar can also be pathogenic to insects, as are the spiroplasmas isolated from bees. Certain flower isolates seem to be closely related to bee isolates. So far there is no information concerning possible pathogenicity of bee or flower spiroplasmas to plants (e.g. after inoculation into the phloem by leafhoppers). The tick spiroplasmas are capable of inducing experimental disease in newborn rodents (Tully *et al.*, 1977), although there are no reports of natural disease in animals caused by spiroplasmas, and it is not known whether ticks could act as vectors. The possibility that there may be spiroplasmas pathogenic to humans has been considered by Tully (1978b). Sera from patients with neurological disorders of unknown aetiology were tested for complement-fixing antibody to the suckling mouse cataract agent (a spiroplasma from ticks), and in some cases small but significant responses were found. We may therefore be witnessing the opening of a new chapter in human infectious diseases.

Little is known about pathogenic mechanisms of mycoplasmas. *M. neurolyticum* induces the characteristic 'rolling disease' in mice, and Tully (1974) has described the partial purification of a high molecular weight exotoxin from cultures which induces disease symptoms following injection into animals. *M. gallisepticum* can also induce neurotoxic symptoms in turkeys but no extracellular neurotoxin could be detected in cultures and viable cells were necessary to demonstrate the effect (Thomas, 1967). Killed cells or membranes from *M. fermentans* can kill mice if injected in large quantities, suggesting that an endotoxin is present (Gabridge *et al.*, 1972) although little is known about the properties of the agent. An extracellular galactan produced by *M. mycoides* subsp. *mycoides* is believed to contribute to symptom expression in infected animals (Lloyd *et al.*, 1971). *S. citri* has been shown to produce low molecular weight phytotoxins which may be responsible for some of the symptoms of diseased plants (Daniels and Meddins, 1974; Daniels, 1979). It has been suggested that products of mycoplasma intermediary metabolism such as ammonia and hydrogen peroxide may accumulate locally to cytotoxic levels in animals, and that deprivation of cells of arginine may result from mycoplasma utilisation. There is evidence that many animal mycoplasma diseases involve autoimmune phenomena, although the detailed causes of these conditions are obscure.

An example of mycoplasma antagonism was noted by Nakamura (1976), who found that *M. salivarium* and a few other species produced an antibiotic or bacteriocin inhibitory to *M. pneumoniae*.

As will be discussed in detail in Chapter 11, mycoplasmas are themselves subject to parasitism by viruses. Suggestions have sometimes been made that virus infection may modify the effect of the mycoplasma on its own host, but no concrete facts have yet emerged to support the notion. On the other side of the coin, the environment of the mycoplasma may influence virus infection, an example being provided by *S. citri* (Townsend *et al.*, 1977a). In cultured spiroplasmas the virus SVC-2 is difficult to detect inside cells by electron microscopy, but when spiroplasmas colonising insect salivary glands are examined, virus particles are abundantly visible.

The manner in which animal hosts defend themselves against mycoplasma infections has been recently reviewed by Fernald (1979). In contrast the defensive responses of plants have not been studied at all. Little evidence of hypersensitivity is usually seen and the question of whether plant mycoplasmas elicit phytoalexin production is unanswered.

References

Archer, D.B. (1981). The structure and functions of the mycoplasma membrane. *International Review of Cytology 69*, 1–43.
Archer, D.B., Rodwell, A.W. and Rodwell, E.S. (1978). The nature and location of *Acholeplasma laidlawii* membrane proteins investigated by two-dimensional

gel electrophoresis. *Biochimica et biophysica Acta 513* 268-83.
Barile, M.F. (1979). Mycoplasma-tissue cell interactions. In *The Mycoplasmas*, Vol. 2., pp. 425-74, J.G. Tully and R.F. Whitcomb (eds). New York: Academic Press.
Barile, M.F., Razin, S., Tully, J.G. and Whitcomb, R.F. (eds) (1979). *The Mycoplasmas*, New York: Academic Press.
Barlow, G.H. and Margoliash, E. (1966). Electrophoretic behaviour of mammalian-type cytochromes c. *Journal of Biological Chemistry 241*, 1473-7.
Belly, R.T., Bohlool, B.B. and Brock, T.D. (1973). The genus *Thermoplasma*. *Annals of the New York Academy of Sciences 225*, 94-107.
Bevers, E.M., Op Den Kamp, J.A.F. and Van Deenen, L.L.M. (1978). Physicochemical properties of phosphatidyl glycerol in membranes of *Acholeplasma laidlawii*: a study with phospholipase A_2. *European Journal of Biochemistry 84*, 35-42.
Bevers, E.M., Singal, S.A., Op den Kamp, J.A.F. and Van Deenen, L.L.M. (1977a). Recognition of different pools of phosphatidylglycerol in intact cells and isolated membranes of *Acholeplasma laidlawii* by phospholipase A2. *Biochemistry 16* 1290-5.
Bevers, E.M., Snoek, G.T., Op den Kamp, J.A.F. and Van Deenen, L.L.M. (1977b). Phospholipid requirement of the membrane-bound Mg^{2+}-dependent adenosinetriphosphatase in *Acholeplasma laidlawii*. *Biochimica et biophysica Acta 467*, 346-56.
Biberfeld, G. and Biberfeld, P. (1970). Ultrastructural features of *Mycoplasma pneumoniae*. *Journal of Bacteriology 102*, 855-61.
Bittman, R. and Rottem, S. (1976). Distribution of cholesterol between the outer and inner halves of the lipid bilayer of mycoplasma cell membranes. *Biochemical and Biophysical Research Communications 71*, 318-24.
Black, F.T., Freundt, E.A., Vinther, O. and Christiansen, C. (1979). Flagellation and swimming motility of *Thermoplasma acidophilum*. *Journal of Bacteriology 137*, 456-60.
Bové, J.M. and Saillard, C. (1979). Cell biology of spiroplasmas. In *The Mycoplasmas*, Vol. 3, pp. 83-153, R.F. Whitcomb and J.G. Tully (eds). New York: Academic Press.
Bredt, W. (1973). Motility of Mycoplasmas. *Annals of the New York Academy of Sciences 225*, 246-50.
— (1974). Structure and motility. *Les Mycoplasmes/Mycoplasmas. Les Colloques de l'Institut National de la Santé et de la Recherche Médicale 33*, 47-52.
Charron, A., Bebear, C., Brun, G., Yot, P., Latrille, J. and Bové, J.M. (1979). Separation and partial characterization of two deoxyribonucleic acid polymerases from *Spiroplasma citri*. *Journal of Bacteriogy 140*, 763-8.
Clark, T.B. (1977). Spiroplasma sp., a new pathogen of honey bees. *Journal of Invertebrate Pathology 29*, 112-13.
Clejan, S., Bittman, R. and Rottem, S. (1978). Uptake, transbilayer distribution, and movement of cholesterol in growing *Mycoplasma capricolum* cells. *Biochemistry 17*, 4579-83.
Cole, R.M., Tully, J.G., Popkin, T.J. and Bové, J.M. (1973). Morphology, ultrastructure and bacteriophage infection of the helical mycoplasma-like organism (*Spiroplasma citri* gen. nov., sp. nov.) cultured from 'stubborn' disease of citrus. *Journal of Bacteriology 115*, 367-86.
Daniels, M.J. (1979). A simple technique for assaying certain microbial phytotoxins and its application to the study of toxins produced by *Spiroplasma citri*. *Journal of General Microbiology 114*, 323-8.
Daniels, M.J. and Meddins, B.M. (1974). The pathogenicity of *Spiroplasma citri*. *Les Mycoplasmes/Mycoplasmas. Les Colloques de l'Institut National de la*

Santé et de la Recherche Médicale 33 , 195–200.

Darland, G., Brock, T.D., Samsonoff, E.W. and Conti, S.F. (1970). A thermophilic, acidophilic mycoplasma isolated from a coal refuse pile. *Science 170*, 1416–18.

Davis, R.E. and Worley, J.F. (1973). Spiroplasma: motile, helical microorganism associated with corn stunt disease. *Phytopathology 63*, 403–8.

de Kruyff, B., Van Dijck, P.W.M., Goldbach, R.W., Demel, R.A. and Van Deenen, L.L.M. (1973). Influence of fatty acid and sterol composition on the lipid phase trasition and activity of membrane-bound enzymes in *Acholeplasma laidlawii*. *Biochimica et biophysica Acta 330*, 269–82.

Eden-Green, S.J. (1978). Isolation of acholeplasmas from coconut palms affected by lethal yellowing disease in Jamaica. *Zentralblatt für Bakteriologie, Parsitenkunde, Infectionskrankheiten und Hygiene, Erste Abteilung Originale 241*, 226.

Fenske, J.D. and Kenny, G.E. (1976). Role of arginine deiminase in growth of *Mycoplasma hominis*. *Journal of Bacteriology 126*, 501–10.

Fernald, G.W. (1979). Humoral and cellular immune responses to mycoplasmas. In *The Mycoplasmas*, Vol. 2, pp. 399–423, J.G. Tully and R.F. Whitcomb (eds). New York: Academic Press.

Ford, D.K. and MacDonald, J. (1967). Influence of urea on the growth of T strain mycoplasmas. *Journal of Bacteriology 93*, 1509–12.

Fratterigo, C.C. and Perlman, D. (1971). Tetracycline inhibition of mycoplasma ribosomal protein synthesis. *Journal of Antibiotics (Tokyo) 24*, 185–8.

Gabridge, M.G., Abrams, G.D. and Murphy, W.H. (1972). Lethal toxicity of *Mycoplasma fermentans* for mice. *Journal of Infectious Diseases 125*, 153–60.

Garrels, J.I. and Gibson, W. (1976). Identification and characterization of multiple forms of actin. *Cell 9*, 793–805.

Ghosh, A., Das, J. and Maniloff, J. (1977). Lack of repair of ultraviolet light damage in *Mycoplasma gallisepticum*. *Journal of Molecular Biology 116*, 337–44.

Gilliam, J.M. and Morowitz, H.J. (1972). Characterization of the plasma membrane of *Mycoplasma laidlawii*: IX. Isolation and characterization of the membrane polyhexosamine. *Biochimica et biophysica Acta 274*, 353–63.

Goel, M.C. and Lemcke, R.M. (1975). Dissociation of *Mycoplasma gallisepticum* membranes with lithium diidosalicylate and isolation of a glycoprotein. *Annales de Microbiologie Collection des Annales de l'Institut Pasteur 126B*, 299–312.

Gourlay, R.N. (1970). Isolation of a virus infecting a strain of *Mycoplasma laidlawii*. *Nature 225*, 1165.

Gourlay, R.N. and Thrower, K.J. (1968). Morphology of *Mycoplasma mycoides* thread phase growth. *Journal of General Microbiology 54*, 155–9.

Gourlay, R.N., Wild, S.G. and Leach, R.H. (1977). *Mycoplasma alvi*, a new species from bovine intestinal and urogenital tracts. *International Journal of Systematic Bacteriology 27*, 86–96.

Gross, Z. and Rottem, S. (1979). Lipid distribution in *Acholeplasma laidlawii* membrane. A study using the lactoperoxidase-mediated iodination. *Biochimica et biophysica Acta 555*, 547–52.

Holländer, R., Wolf, G. and Mannheim, W. (1977). Lipoquinones of some bacteria and mycoplasmas, with considerations on their functional significance. *Antonie van Leeuwenhoek, Journal of Microbiology and Serology 43*, 177–85.

Howard, C.J., Gourlay, R.N. and Wyld, S.G. (1980). Isolation of a virus, MVBr 1, from *Mycoplasma bovirhinis*. FEMS Microbiology Letters 7, 163–5.

Hu, P.C., Collier, A.M. and Baseman, J.B. (1977). Surface parasitism by

Mycoplasma pneumoniae of respiratory epithelium. *Journal of Experimental Medicine 145*, 1328–43.

International Committee on Systematic Bacteriology, Subcommittee on the Taxonomy of Mycoplasmatales (1972). Proposal for minimal standards for descriptions of new species of the order Mycoplasmatales. *International Journal of Systematic Bacteriology 22*, 184–8.

—— (1979). Proposal for minimal standards for description of new species of the class Mollicutes. *International Journal of Systematic Bacteriology 29*, 172–80.

Jinks, D.C. and Matz, L.L. (1976a). The reduced nicotinamide adenine dinucleotide 'oxidase' of *Acholeplasma laidlawii* membranes. *Biochimica et biophysica Acta 430*, 71–82.

—— (1976b). Purification of the reduced nicotinamide adenine dinucleotide dehydrogenase from membranes of *Acholeplasma laidlawii*. *Biochimica et biophysica Acta 452*, 30–41.

Johnson, J.D. and Horowitz, J. (1971). Characterization of ribosomes and RNAs from *Mycoplasma hominis*. *Biochimica et biophysica Acta 247*, 262–79.

Jones, A.S., Tittensor, J.R. and Walker, R.T. (1965). The chemical composition of the nucleic acids and other macromolecular constituents of *Mycoplasma mycoides* var. *capri*. *Journal of General Microbiology 40*, 405–11.

Kahane, I. and Brunner, H. (1977). Isolation of a glycoprotein from *Mycoplasma pneumoniae* membranes. *Infection and Immunity 18*, 273–7.

Kahane, I., Greenstein, S. and Razin, S. (1977). Carbohydrate content and enzymic activities in the membrane of *Spiroplasma citri*. *Journal of General Microbiology 101*, 173–6.

Kahane, I., Muhlrad, A. and Razin, S. (1978). Possible role of acetate kinase in ATP generation in *Mycoplasma hominis* and *Acholeplasma laidlawii*. *FEMS Microbiology Letters 3*, 143–5.

Kahane, I. and Tully, J.G. (1976). Binding of plant lectins to mycoplasma cells and membranes. *Journal of Bacteriology 128*, 1–7.

Kenny, G.E. and Cartwright, F.D. (1977). Effect of urea concentration on growth of *Ureaplasma urealyticum* (T-strain mycoplasma). *Journal of Bacteriology 132*, 144–58.

Kimball, M.E. and Söll, D. (1974). The phenylalanine tRNA from *Mycoplasma* sp. (kid): a tRNA lacking hypermodified nucleosides functional in protein synthesis. *Nucleic Acids Research 1*, 1713–20.

Kimball, M.E., Szeto, K.S. and Söll, D. (1974). The nucleotide sequence of phenylalanine tRNA from *Mycoplasma* sp. (kid). *Nucleic Acids Research 1*, 1721–32.

Korn, E.D. (1978). Biochemistry of actomyosin-dependent cell motility (a review). *Proceedings of the National Academy of Sciences, United States of America 75*, 588–9.

Laidlaw, P.P. and Elford, W.J. (1936). A new group of filterable organisms. *Proceedings of the Royal Society Series B 120*, 292–303.

Langworthy, T.A. (1979). Special features of thermoplasmas. In *The Mycoplasmas*, Vol 1, pp. 495–513, M.F. Barile and S. Razin (eds). New York: Academic Press.

Langworthy, T.A., Mayberry, W.R., Smith, P.F. and Robinson, I.M. (1975). Plasmalogen composition of *Anaeroplasma*. *Journal of Bacteriology 122*, 785–7.

Langworthy, T.A., Smith, P.F. and Mayberry, W.R. (1972). Lipids of *Thermoplasma acidophilum*. *Journal of Bacteriology 112*, 1193–1200.

Lee, G.Y. and Kenny, G.E. (1980). Electrophoretic and immunologic heterogeneity of the superoxide dismutases in the *Acholeplasmataceae*. *Abstracts of the Third Conference of the International Organization for Mycoplasmology,*

Custer, South Dakota, p. 39.

Lloyd, L.C., Buttery, S.H. and Hudson, J.R. (1971). The effect of the galactan and other antigens of *Mycoplasma mycoides* var. *mycoides* on experimental infections with that organism in cattle. *Journal of Medical Microbiology 4,* 425–39.

Lynch, R.E. and Cole, B.C. (1980). *Mycoplasma pneumoniae:* a prokaryote which consumes oxygen and generates superoxide but which lacks superoxide dismutase. *Biochemical and Biophysical Research Communications 96,* 98–105.

Maillet, P.L. and Gouranton, J. (1971). Etude du cycle biologique du mycoplasme de la phyllodie du trèfle dans l'insecte vecteur *Euscelis lineolatus* Brullé (Homoptera, Jassidae). *Journal de Microscopie 11,* 143–62.

Maniloff, J. (1970). Ultrastructure of *Mycoplasma laidlawii* during culture development. *Journal of Bacteriology 102,* 561–72.

Maniloff, J. and Chaudhuri, U. (1979). Gliding mycoplasmas are inhibited by cytochalasin B and contain a polymerizable protein fraction. *Journal of Supramolecular Structure 12,* 299–304.

Maniloff, J. and Morowitz, H.J. (1972). Cell biology of the mycoplasmas. *Bacteriological Reviews 36,* 263–90.

Maniloff, J., Morowitz, H.J. and Barrnett, R.J. (1965). Ultrastructure and ribosomes of *Mycoplasma gallisepticum. Journal of Bacteriology 90,* 193–204.

Maniloff, J. and Quinlan, D.C. (1974). Partial purification of a membrane-associated deoxyribonucleic acid complex from *Mycoplasma gallisepticum. Journal of Bacteriology 120,* 495–501.

Markham, P.G., Townsend, R., Plaskitt, K. and Saglio, P. (1977). Transmission of corn stunt to dicotyledonous plants. *Plant Disease Reporter 61,* 342–5.

Martin, H.H., Schilf, W. and Schiefer, H.-G. (1980). Differentiation of Mycoplasmatales from bacterial protoplast L-forms by assay for penicillin binding proteins. *Archives of Microbiology 127,* 297–9.

Masover, G.K., Benson, J.R. and Hayflick, L. (1974). Growth of T -strain mycoplasmas in medium without added urea: effect of trace amounts of urea and of a urease inhibitor. *Journal of Bacteriology 117,* 765–74.

Masover, G.K., Razin, S. and Hayflick, L. (1977). Effects of carbon dioxide, urea, and ammonia on growth of *Ureaplasma urealyticum* (T -strain mycoplasma). *Journal of Bacteriology 130,* 292–6.

Mayberry, W.R., Smith, P.F., Langworthy, T.A. and Plackett, P. (1973). Identification of the amide-linked fatty acids of *Acholeplasma axanthum* S743 as D(-)3-hydroxyhexadecanoate and its homologues. *Journal of Bacteriology 116,* 1091–5.

Mayberry-Carson, K.J., Langworthy, T.A., Mayberry, W.R. and Smith, P.F. (1974). A new class of lipopolysaccharide from *Thermoplasma acidophilum. Biochimica et biophysica Acta 360,* 217-29.

Meng, K.E. and Pfister, R.M. (1980). Intracellular structures of *Mycoplasma pneumoniae* revealed after membrane removal. *Journal of Bacteriology 144,* 390–9.

Mills, L.B., Stanbridge, E.J., Sedwick, W. D. and Korn, D. (1977). Purification and partial characterization of the principal deoxyribonucleic acid polymerase from Mycoplasmatales. *Journal of Bacteriology 132,* 641–9.

Morowitz, H.J. (1969). The genome of mycoplasmas. In *The Mycoplasmatales and the L-phase of Bacteria,* pp. 405-12, L. Hayflick (ed), New York: Appleton-Century-Crofts.

Morowitz, H.J. and Wallace, D.C. (1973). Genome size and life cycle of the mycoplasma. *Annals of the New York Academy of Sciences 225,* 62–73.

Mouches, C., Menara, A., Geny, B., Charlemagne, D. and Bové, J.M. (1980).

S. citri synthesizes a protein which is specifically recognized by rabbit immunoglobulins against rabbit actin. *Abstracts of the Third Conference of the International Organization for Mycoplasmology, Custer, South Dakota*, p. 100.

Mouches, C., Vignault, J.C., Tully, J.G., Whitcomb, R.F. and Bové, J.M. (1979). Characterization of spiroplasmas by one- and two-dimensional protein analysis on polyacrylamide slab gels. *Current Microbiology 2*, 69-74.

Mudd, J.B., Ittig, M., Roy, B., Latrille, J. and Bové, J.M. (1977). Composition and enzyme activities of *Spiroplasma citri* membranes. *Journal of Bacteriology 129*, 1250-6.

Nakamura, M. (1976). Mycoplasma growth inhibitory substance (Mycoplasmacin) derived from mycoplasmas. *Proceedings of the Society for General Microbiology 3*, 173.

Neimark, H.C. (1974). Implications of the phylogenetic relationship between acholeplasmas and lactic acid bacteria. *Les Mycoplasmes/Mycoplasmas. Les Colloques de l'Institut National de la Santé et de la Recherche Médicale 33*, 71-8.

— (1977). Extraction of an actin-like protein from the prokaryote *Mycoplasma pneumoniae. Proceedings of the National Academy of Sciences, United States of America 74*, 4041-5.

Peterson, J.E., Rodwell, A.W. and Rodwell, E.S. (1973). Occurrence and ultrastructure of a variant (rho) form of *Mycoplasma. Journal of Bacteriology 115*, 411-25.

Pirie, N. (1973). On being the right size. *Annual Review of Microbiology 27*, 119-32.

Plackett, P., Smith, P.F. and Mayberry, W.R. (1970). Lipids of a sterol-non-requiring mycoplasma. *Journal of Bacteriology 104*, 798-807.

Pollack, J.D. (1979). Respiratory pathways and energy-yielding mechanisms. In *The Mycoplasmas*, Vol 1, pp. 187-211, M.F. Barile and S. Razin (eds). New York: Academic Press

Praznik, J. (1974). Marine water, reservoir of mycoplasma-like organisms. *Abstracts of the International Congress on Mycoplasmas of Man, Animals, Plants and Insects, Bordeaux*, p. 35.

Quinlan, D.C. and Maniloff, J. (1972). Membrane association of the deoxyribonucleic acid growing-point region in *Mycoplasma gallisepticum. Journal of Bacteriology 112*, 1375-9.

— (1973). Deoxyribonucleic acid synthesis in synchronously growing *Mycoplasma gallisepticum. Journal of Bacteriology 115*, 117-20.

Ranhand, J.M., Mitchell, W.O., Popkin, T.J. and Cole, R.M. (1980). Covalently-closed circular deoxyribonucleic acids in spiroplasmas. *Journal of Bacteriology 143*, 1194-9.

Razin, A. and Razin, S. (1980). Methylated bases in mycoplasmal DNA. *Nucleic Acids Research 8*, 1383-90.

Razin, S. (1975). The mycoplasma membrane. *Progress in Surface and Membrane Science 9*, 257-312.

— (1978). The Mycoplasmas. *Microbiological Reviews 42*, 414-70.

— (1979). Membrane proteins. In *The Mycoplasmas*, Vol. 1, pp. 289-322, M.F. Barile and S. Razin (eds). New York: Academic Press.

Razin, S. and Cosenza, B.J. (1966). Growth phases of mycoplasma in liquid media observed with phase-contrast microscope. *Journal of Bacteriology 91*, 858-69.

Razin, S., Cosenza, B.J. and Tourtellotte, M.E. (1966). Variations in mycoplasma morphology induced by long chain fatty acids. *Journal of General Microbiology 42*, 139-45.

— (1967). Filamentous growth of mycoplasma. *Annals of the New York*

Academy of Sciences 143, 66–72.

Razin, S., Hasin, M., Ne'eman, Z. and Rottem, S. (1973). Isolation, chemical composition and ultrastructural features of the cell membrane of the mycoplasma-like organism *Spiroplasma citri. Journal of Bacteriology 116*, 1421–35.

Reff, M.E., Stanbridge, E.J. and Schneider, E.L. (1977). Phylogenetic relationships between mycoplasmas and other procaryotes based upon the electrophoretic behaviour of their ribosomal ribonucleic acids. *International Journal of Systematic Bacteriology 27*, 185–93.

Robinson, I.M. and Allison, M.J. (1975). Transfer of *Acholeplasma bactoclasticum* Robinson and Hungate to the genus *Anaeroplasma* (*Anaeroplasma bactoclasticum* Robinson and Hungate comb. nov.): amended description of the species. *International Journal of Systematic Bacteriology 25*, 182–6.

Robinson, I.M., Allison, M.J. and Hartman, P.A. (1975). *Anaeroplasma abactoclasticum* gen. nov., sp. nov.: an obligatory anaerobic mycoplasma from the rumen. *International Journal of Systematic Bacteriology 25*, 173–81.

Rodwell, A.W. (1969). Nutrition and metabolism of mycoplasmas. In *The Mycoplasmatales and the L-phase of bacteria*, pp. 413–50, L. Hayflick (ed). New York: Appleton-Century-Crofts.

Rodwell, A.W. (1977). Qualitative requirements and utilization of nutrients: Mycoplasma *CRC Handbook series in Nutrition and Food Section D: Nutritional Requirements*, Vol. 1, pp. 57–65. Cleveland, Ohio: CRC Press Inc.

Rodwell, A.W. and Mitchell, A. (1979). Nutrition, growth and reproduction. In *The Mycoplasmas*, Vol. 1, pp. 103–39, M.F. Barile and S. Razin (eds). New York: Academic Press.

Rodwell, A.W. and Peterson, J.E. (1971). The effect of straight chain saturated, monoenoic and branched chain fatty acids on growth and fatty acid composition of Mycoplasma strain Y. *Journal of General Microbiology 68*, 173–86.

Rodwell, A.W., Peterson, J.E. and Rodwell, E.S. (1972). Macromolecular synthesis and growth of mycoplasmas. In *Pathogenic Mycoplasmas. Ciba Foundation Symposium.* pp. 123–39, K. Elliott and J. Birch (eds). London: Associated Scientific Publishers.

— (1973). Nature of striated structures in mycoplasmas. *Annals of the New York Academy of Sciences 225*, 190–200.

— (1975). Striated fibers of the *rho* form of *Mycoplasma. In vitro* reassembly composition and structure. *Journal of Bacteriology 122*, 1216–29.

Rodwell, A.W. and Rodwell, E.S. (1978). Phylogenetic relationships between strains of *Mycoplasma mycoides* subspp. *mycoides* and *capri* studied by two-dimensional gel electrophoresis of cell proteins. *Journal of General Microbiology 109*, 259–63.

Rodwell, A.W., Rodwell, E.S. and Archer, D.B. (1978). Mycoplasmas lack a protein which closely rembles α-actin. *FEMS Microbiology Letters 5*, 235–8.

Romano, N., Smith, P.F. and Mayberry, W.R. (1972). Lipids of a T-strain of *Mycoplasma. Journal of Bacteriology 109*, 565–9.

Rothman, J.E. and Lenard, J. (1977). Membrane asymmetry. *Science 195*, 743–53.

Rottem, S. (1979). Molecular organization of membrane lipids. In *The Mycoplasmas*, Vol. 1, pp. 259–88, M.F. Barile and S. Razin (eds). New York: Academic Press.

Rottem, S., Cirillo, V.P., De Kruyff, B., Shinitzky, M. and Razin, S. (1973). Cholesterol in mycoplasma membranes. Correlation of enzymic and transport activities with physical state of lipid in membranes of *Mycoplasma mycoides* var. *capri* adapted to grow with low cholesterol concentrations. *Biochimica et biophysica Acta 323*, 509–19.

Rottem, S. and Markowitz, O. (1979). Membrane lipids of *Mycoplasma galli-septicum*: a disaturated phosphatidylcholine and a phosphatidylglycerol with an unusual positional distribution of fatty acids. *Biochemistry 18*, 2930–5.

Rottem, S., Slutzky, G.M. and Bittman, R. (1978). Cholesterol distribution and movement in the *Mycoplasma gallisepticum* cell membrane. *Biochemistry 17*, 2723–6.

Saglio, P.H.M. and Whitcomb, R.F. (1979). Diversity of wall-less prokaryotes in plant vascular tissue, fungi, and invertebrate animals. In *The Mycoplasmas*, Vol. 3, pp. 1–36, R.F. Whitcomb and J.G. Tully (eds). New York: Academic Press.

Schiefer, H.-G., Gerhardt, U., Brunner, H. and Krüpe, M. (1974). Studies with lectins on the surface carbohydrate structures of mycoplasma membranes. *Journal of Bacteriology 120*, 81–8.

Schiefer, H.-G., Krauss, H., Brunner, H. and Gerhardt, U. (1976). Ultrastructural visualization of anionic sites on mycoplasma membranes by polycationic ferritin. *Journal of Bacteriology 127*, 461–8.

Schimke, R.T., Berlin, C.M., Sweeney, E.W. and Carroll, W.R. (1966). The generation of energy by the arginine dihydrolase pathway in *Mycoplasma hominis* 07. *Journal of Biological Chemistry 241*, 2228–36.

Schwarz, J.L. and Perlman, D. (1972). Antibiotic resistance mechanism in mycoplasma species. *Journal of Antibiotics (Tokyo) 24*, 575–82.

Searcy, D.G. (1975). Histone-like protein in the prokaryote *Thermoplasma acidophilum*. *Biochimica et biophysica Acta 395*, 535–47.

Seiffert, G. (1937). Uber des Vorkommen filtrabler Mikroorganismen in die Natur und ihre Zuchtbarkeit. *Zentralblatt für Bakteriologie, Parasitenkunde, Infectionskrankheiten und Hygiene. Erste Abteilung Originale 139*, 337–42.

Smith, D.W. (1969). DNA replication in *Mycoplasma laidlawii* B. *Biochimica et biophysica Acta 179*, 408–21.

Smith, D.W. and Hanawalt, P.C. (1969). Repair replication of DNA in ultra-violet irradiated *Mycoplasma laidlawii* B. *Journal of Molecular Biology 46*, 57–72.

Smith, P.F. (1971). *The Biology of Mycoplasmas*. New York: Academic Press.

Somerson, N.L. and Cole, B.C. (1979). The mycoplasma flora of human and non-human primates. In *The Mycoplasmas*, Vol. 2, pp. 191–216, J.G. Tully and R.F. Whitcomb (eds). New York: Academic Press.

Stanbridge, E.J. and Reff, M.E. (1979). The molecular biology of mycoplasmas. In *The Mycoplasmas*, Vol. 1, pp. 157–85, M.F. Barile and S. Razin (eds). New York: Academic Press.

Terry, T.M. and Zupnik, J.S. (1973). Weak association of glucosamine-containing polymer with the *Acholeplasma laidlawii* membrane. *Biochimica et biophysica Acta 291*, 144–8.

Thomas, L. (1967). The neurotoxins of *M. neurolyticum* and *M. gallisepticum*. *Annals of the New York Academy of Sciences 143*, 218–24.

Townsend, R. (1976). Arginine metabolism by *Spiroplasma citri*. *Journal of General Microbiology 94*, 417–20.

Townsend, R., Archer, D.B. and Plaskitt, K.A. (1980). Purification and pre-liminary characterization of spiroplasma fibrils. *Journal of Bacteriology 142*, 694–700.

Townsend, R., Markham, P.G. and Plaskitt, K. (1977a). Multiplication and morphology of *Spiroplasma citri* in the leafhopper *Euscelis plebejus*. *Annals of Applied Biology 87*, 307–13.

Townsend, R., Markham, P.G., Plaskitt, K.A. and Daniels, M.J. (1977b).

Isolation and characterization of a non-helical strain of *Spiroplasma citri. Journal of General Microbiology 100*, 15-21.

Tully, J.G. (1974). Mycoplasma neurotoxins: partial purification of the toxin from *Mycoplasma neurolyticum. Les Mycoplasmes/Mycoplasmas. Les Colloques de l'Institut National de la Santé et de la Recherche Médicale 33*, 317-24.

— (1978a). Biology of the Mycoplasmas. In *Mycoplasma Infection of Cell Cultures*, pp. 1-33, G.J. McGarrity, D.G. Murphy and W.W. Nichols (eds). New York: Plenum Publishing Corporation.

— (1978b). The interaction of spiroplasmas with vertebrates. *Zentralblatt für Bakteriologie, Parasitenkunde Infectionskrankheiten und Hygiene. Erste Abteilung Originale 241*, 191.

— (1979). Special features of the acholeplasmas. In *The Mycoplasmas*, Vol. 1, pp. 431-49, M.F. Barile and S. Razin (eds). New York: Academic Press.

Tully, J.G. and Razin, S. (1977). The Mollicutes (mycoplasmas). In *CRC Handbook of Microbiology*, 2nd ed., Vol. 1, pp. 405-59, A.J. Larkin and H. Lechevalier (eds). Cleveland, Ohio: CRC Press.

Tully, J.G., Whitcomb, R.F., Clark, H.F. and Williamson, D.L. (1977). Pathogenic mycoplasmas: cultivation and vertebrate pathogenicity of a new spiroplasma. *Science 195*, 892-4.

Van Demark, P.J. and Smith, P.F. (1964). Evidence for a tricarboxylic acid cycle in *Mycoplasma hominis. Journal of Bacteriology 88*, 1602-7.

Walker, R.T. and RajBhandary, U.L. (1975). Formylatable methionine transfer RNA from mycoplasma: purification and comparison of partial nucleotide sequences with those of other prokaryotic initiator tRNAs. *Nucleic Acids Research 2*, 61-78.

— (1978). The nucleotide sequence of formylmethionine tRNA from *Mycoplasma mycoides* sp. *capri. Nucleic Acids Research 5*, 57-70.

Whitcomb, R.F., Williamson, D.L., Rosen, J. and Coan, M. (1974). Relationship of infection and pathogenicity in the infection of insects by wall-free prokaryotes. *Les Mycoplasmes/Mycoplasmas. Les Colloques de l'Institut National de la Santé et de la Recherche Médicale 33*, 275-82.

Williamson, D.L. (1974). Unusual fibrils from the spirochete-like sex ratio organism. *Journal of Bacteriology 117*, 904-6.

Williamson, D.L., Blaustein, D.I., Levine, R.J.C. and Elfvin, M.J. (1979). Anti-actin-peroxidase staining of the helical wall-free prokaryote *Spiroplasma citri. Current Microbiology 2*, 143-5.

Wilson, M.H. and Collier, A.M. (1976). Ultrastructural study of *Mycoplasma pneumoniae* in organ culture. *Journal of Bacteriology 125*, 332-9.

Woese, C.R., Maniloff, J. and Zablen, L.B. (1980). Phylogenetic analysis of the mycoplasmas. *Proceedings of the National Academy of Sciences, United States of America 77*, 494-8.

Wróblewski, H., Johansson, K.-E. and Hjertén, S. (1977). Purification and characterization of spiralin, the main protein of the *Spiroplasma citri* membrane. *Biochimica et biophysica Acta 465*, 275-89.

Yang, L.L. and Haug, A. (1979). Purification and partial characterization of a prokaryotic glycoprotein from the plasma membrane of *Thermoplasma acidophilum. Biochimica et biophysica Acta 556*, 265-77.

Zouzias, D., Mazaitis, A.J., Simberkoff, M. and Rush, M. (1973). Extrachromosomal DNA of *Mycoplasma hominis. Biochimica et biophysica Acta 312*, 484-91.

2 PLANT AND ARTHROPOD MYCOPLASMAS: A HISTORICAL PERSPECTIVE

R.F. Whitcomb and L.M. Black

1. Introduction

The existence of plant and insect mycoplasmas first became evident as the result of plant diseases that they cause. Indeed, Daniels (1979) has noted that as early as 1666 Merrett described clover phyllody as *Trifolium album umbella siliquosa*. Peach yellows was first noted (Smith, 1888) in the latter part of the eighteenth century, and, as it spread, became a serious limitation on peach production. Over the years, fifty or more plant diseases of the yellows type have been recognised. Some of them, such as coconut lethal yellowing (Tsai, 1979b), are economically devastating. The serious study of the etiological agents of such diseases began during the latter part of the nineteenth century, when the classical studies of Anton de Bary (1853, 1861) and Robert Koch (1877) began to change the perception of infectious disease. After the discovery of filterable viruses by Ivanowski (1892), Beijerinck (1898), and Loeffler and Frosch (1898), it was natural to classify the agents of diseases caused by mycoplasma-like organisms as viruses (Smith, 1902; Kunkel, 1926; Whitcomb *et al.*, 1968a, b) since the infectious agents were filterable and not visible by light microscopy. Also, the syndromes that they caused in plants were similar in some respects to those induced by viruses.

Mycoplasmas were first recognised as a result of contagious pleuro-pneumonia, a highly contagious lung disease of bovine animals (reviewed by Hayflick, 1969). Although the disease may have been recognised as early as 1713, it was not until 1898 that Nocard and colleagues at the Pasteur Institute cultivated the causal agent in collodion sacs in the peritoneal cavity of rabbits. This initial discovery led to the cultivation of the organisms in serum enriched broth *in vitro* and, eventually, to growth on solid media (Dujardin-Beaumetz, 1900). The morphologies of the organisms were described later (Bordet, 1910; Borrel *et al.*, 1910). Because the organisms passed through filters with small pore sizes (Elford, 1929) they were regarded by many workers as viruses. In these early years, it was not clear, of course, that viruses are incapable of growth *in vitro*.

Recognition of the intrinsic differences between viruses and other small filterable agents did not occur until the 1950s, when it was discovered that virus multiplication in cells was a replicative process that required cellular machinery (Hershey and Chase, 1952). More complex nonviral agents, such as chlamydiae (Moulder, 1966), rickettsiae (Weiss, 1968), or mycoplasmas (Klieneberger-Nobel, 1962), whether intracellular or extracellular in their parasitic residence, were cells in their own right that eventually proved able to harbour viruses of their own (Gourlay, 1970). Viruses were eventually perceived to consist of a nucleic acid genome capable of coding for proteins necessary for protection and replication (Gierer and Schramm, 1956). Finally, in the late 1960s it was discovered that certain nucleic acids were naturally infectious without protein protection; these were the viroids (Diener and Raymer, 1967).

Viruses in general, including those that infect plants and insects, proved to be astonishingly diverse. Indeed, given the simplicity of their chemical constitution, the structural diversity of viruses in these habitats appeared to be about as great as possible (Whitcomb and Davis, 1970). Given this situation, the existence of wall-less prokaryotes among a vast array of uncharacterised 'viruses' went unnoticed until 1967, when Doi and his colleagues (Doi *et al.*, 1967; Ishiie *et al.*, 1967) published papers in the *Annals of the Phytopathological Society of Japan* reporting that mycoplasma-like organisms might cause plant disease.

As we have written this chapter, it has been natural for us to reflect and reminisce on our own experiences and efforts, particularly as they

were influenced by the rapidly unfolding events in medical microbiology, virology and plant pathology. A large part of these efforts has
been concerned with the agent of aster yellows (AY) disease. Since the
classical studies of L.O. Kunkel at the Boyce Thompson Institute in
1926, this disease had been considered to be representative of a large
group of agents — the 'yellows diseases' — that were responsible for
inducing virescence and proliferation in plants.

In the late 1950s, when RFW was a graduate student in the laboratory of LMB in the Botany Department at the University of Illinois,
intensive focus was placed on the purification of the 'aster yellows
virus'. One of the very first experiments in this effort was one in which
we attempted to use antibiotics to improve the survival of injected
leafhopper vectors of the disease. In this unpublished experiment, we
observed that when streptomycin was added to an inoculum prepared
from infected insects, AY infectivity was destroyed. We can recall
speculating that the AY agent — and its relatives — might not be viral,
and thought of rickettsiae as possibilities. On balance, however, it
seemed to us that it was more likely (perhaps quite correctly) that
streptomycin was merely acting upon the surface of the pathogen,
and was not exerting a specific antibiotic effect.

At that time, all indications appeared to favour a viral hypothesis
for AY etiology. After all, three very dissimilar viruses, wound tumour
(Brakke *et al.*, 1954), potato yellow dwarf (Brakke, 1953), and tomato
spotted wilt (Black *et al.*, 1963) had only recently been isolated by the
newly developed technique of density gradient centrifugation. Also,
earlier work on properties of the AY agent (Black, 1943) had indicated
that the agent passed with difficulty through filters that retained small
bacteria; also, it was sedimented by centrifugation at a top speed of
30,000 rpm for 1 minute. The agent was unstable, but could be studied
in extracts of infected plants or insects by the methods of virology.
These methods offered a means of 'tracking' the agent through purification procedures such as density gradient centrifugation and electrophoresis (Brakke *et al.*, 1954).

Thus it was that we began a lengthy series of experiments, with all
the experience provided by the successful purification of wound
tumour, potato yellow dwarf and tomato spotted wilt viruses. Our
unpublished results indicated that the AY agent, in contrast to these
viruses, did not occur in sharp zonal patterns after centrifugation;
instead, it was found throughout the tubes after either rate zonal or
quasi-equilibrium density gradient centrifugation. Today, as we leaf
back through our notes, it is still possible to feel the frustration that

we experienced upon analysing the results of experiment after experiment, all of which indicated that infectivity could be found from meniscus to pellet of the gradient tubes. But even now, it is difficult to see how we might have tested (and discarded) the hypothesis that the AY agent was a virus with special ionic requirements for solubility. For example, such had proved to be the case for the tomato spotted wilt virus (Black *et al.*, 1963). In any case, as results on AY continued to be disheartening, we gradually turned our attention to the viruses — wound tumour and potato yellow dwarf — whose purification had opened new doors for the study of disease biology.

Efforts to purify the presumed viruses of plant mycoplasma diseases were subsequently renewed when RFW joined the laboratory of D.D. Jensen in the University of California in Berkeley in the early 1960s to work on the western X-disease agent. This agent (Gilmer and Blodgett, 1976), like the AY pathogen, was leafhopper-borne (Wolfe *et al.*, 1951) and caused yellowing in plants. Unlike AY, the WX pathogen did not cause conspicuous proliferation or virescence, so it seemed reasonable to hope that the agent would prove to be significantly different from the aster yellows agent and, hopefully, more amenable to purification. However, attempts to purify the WX agent met with similar difficulties; infectivity after density gradient centrifugation appeared to be associated with many fractions (Whitcomb *et al.*, 1968a). Eventually, the possibility that WX, AY and their allies might not be viruses at all had to be considered. In the early 1960s, however, the clearest example of a prokaryote misidentified as a virus was the 'psittacosis virus', which was known to be susceptible to various antibiotics (Weiss, 1950; Gogolak and Weiss, 1950). We (RFW and DDJ) were sufficiently frustrated by our purification attempts to decide, taking psittacosis as a precedent, that the day had come for testing the effects of antibiotics on the WX agent. So we prepared solutions of penicillin, streptomycin, chloramphenicol and tetracycline, and evaluated their effect on the vector insects in preparation for testing against the WX agent. Three of these antibiotics eventually *were* tested against the agent, and the results, as well as the effect of all four antibiotics on the insects, were published (Jensen *et al.*, 1967). However, the day for testing tetracycline never came. We knew, after all, that tetracycline was active against certain 'viruses', as well as bacteria and chlamydiae, so it did not seem to us that we would obtain any particular taxonomic insight by using this antibiotic. Those workers whose memory extends to those days will, of course, recall that among the 'viruses' affected by tetracycline was the agent of primary atypical

human pneumonia shown (Chanock *et al.*, 1962) to be caused by
Mycoplasma pneumoniae!

There is no assurance, of course, that we would have discovered the
nature of the pathogen if we had employed tetracycline. In retrospect, the discovery that MLOs are associated with X-disease could
have been made in another, simpler manner. During the years of
failure to isolate the causative agent, we had discovered a distinctive
pattern of pathology in the insect vector (Whitcomb *et al.*, 1968b)
that accounted for the premature death of the insects that had been
noted by Jensen (1959). Light microscopy showed that cells of many
tissues of the insect contained accumulations of basophilic material
that often involved the entire cell. The intracellular pathological areas
were considered to be too extensive to consist of the pathogen. Instead,
we believed we were observing cellular necrosis induced by viral infection.
Later, it turned out that the pathological areas were simply areas in
which MLOs had accumulated (Nasu *et al.*, 1970). And so the microbial
identity of the western X-disease pathogen escaped us.

During these years, electron microscopic techniques for visualisation of plant and insect viruses *in vivo* were beginning to be explored
by Shikata and Granados in Maramorosch's laboratory at the Boyce
Thompson Institute (Shikata and Maramorosch, 1965; Granados *et
al.*, 1967). A general feeling developed that electron microscopy
would eventually yield important clues to the nature of the AY pathogen.
We now know that the agents were actually envisioned in several laboratories but were not recognised. Instead, they were thought to be
'vesicles'. Actually, without careful analysis, this mistake is easy to
make, as is the reverse mistake of identifying vesicles induced by
viruses as mycoplasmas (de Zoeten *et al.*, 1972) or as normal vesicles
in certain stages of development of certain cells.

In 1966, a team was assembled at Beltsville, Maryland by R.L. Steere
to concentrate on the isolation of the AY pathogen. One of us (RFW)
joined the team and was soon followed by R.E. Davis. The team worked
for a year applying the prevalent techniques for virus purification –
charcoal and celite adsorption, density gradient centrifugation and
electrophoresis and agar gel chromatography – but succeeded only in
duplicating the unfortunate experience of the previous ten years.
Simply, the AY pathogen was either a virus with extremely peculiar
properties in extracts or a large, pleomorphic agent with a mean
sedimentation coefficient similar to that of vaccinia virus which
existed as an infectious agent with a range of densities. Thus it was
that when the report of Doi *et al.*, (1967) appeared we compared, with

mycoplasmologists, the behaviour of mycoplasmas as infectious agents in extracts; we (RFW and RED) soon recognised that a new epoch of plant and invertebrate pathology had begun.

It is easy today to look back over these years of frustration and see that certain of our misfortunes were brought about by prevailing attitudes in plant pathology. An open-mindedness about the nature of disease agents that prevailed in the early part of the twentieth century had given way to the assumption that still unidentified pathogens would surely turn out (when proper methods were finally made available for their study) to be representative of taxa already known to cause plant disease. Perhaps among some workers there had even been a decline of interest in the pathogens *per se*, induced perhaps by the extreme difficulty experienced in searching for the agents not visible by light microscopy.

L.O. Kunkel, trained as a biologist and possessed of an acutely perceptive eye for nature, recognised the extreme importance of iden-tification of the pathogens, and, when director of plant research at the Rockefeller Institute, was instrumental in bringing to the institute a young chemist to attempt to define the chemical nature of viruses. The chemist, Wendell Stanley, subsequently purified and characterised tobacco mosaic virus (Stanley, 1935). However, even after this dis-covery and other subsequent advances of virology, the 'virus' of aster yellows remained a mystery, awaiting the report of Doi *et al.* (1967).

The elucidation of etiology is difficult — perhaps as difficult as any study that one might undertake. However, when the answer becomes available, it is of great importance that others be able readily to repeat the key observations. It is probably fitting in this regard to note that the first repetition of Doi and Ishiie's report was performed by a junior high school student, Sandra Weikel. Sandra wrote one of us (RFW) a letter very shortly after publication of the Japanese work, for suggestions about testing the possibility that a 'plant virus' might be susceptible to an antibiotic. Using plants carrying AY that were mailed to her and tetracyclines prescribed for them by the family physician, she showed that leaves of plants sprayed with antibiotic became green again and that the plants developed normal flowers; untreated plants experienced no symptomatic remission and failed to flower. A brief description of her work, with pictures of treated and control plants, appeared in the Elizabethton, Tennessee *Star* of 18 February 1968 and was presented (Weikel, 1968) to the Southern Appalachian Science Fair, Knoxville, Tennessee, March 1968.

2. Taxonomy of Plant and Arthropod Mycoplasmas

Some comments on the taxonomy of mycoplasmas (Freundt and Edward, 1979) will be necessary, not only for our discussion of historical perspectives, but also for understanding the contemporary literature. The class Mollicutes (trivial term: mycoplasma) was erected by Edward and Freundt (1967) for wall-less prokaryotes. One group of these organisms required sterol for growth, but another did not. This fundamental difference proved to be associated with many other fundamental differences, and the two groups were given family status reflecting sterol dependence (Mycoplasmataceae) or independence (Acholeplasmataceae) (Edward and Freundt, 1970). During the early years, mycoplasmas were considered to be associated with vertebrate animals (Freundt, 1974). However, some acholeplasmas appeared to be saprophytic, as reflected by their isolation from sewage or soil. A claim by Ozkal (1958) that a mycoplasma had been isolated from plants was overlooked or received little credence. The revelation of Doi *et al.* (1967) that wall-less prokaryotes cause disease in plants therefore came as a great surprise. In subsequent years, however, ties between medical or veterinary workers and plant and insect workers have been unusually close. This closeness was greatly enhanced by an international conference at the Ciba foundation in 1972 (Elliott and Birch, 1972), which brought workers from these disparate disciplines together in an international forum for the first time. This conference was also remarkable, in that papers presented there documented helical filaments that later proved to represent the discovery of a new mycoplasmal taxon (the spiroplasmas), and the first cultivation of a plant mycoplasma, which proved to be the type species of that taxon. As a result of the Ciba meeting, two international conferences were organised, one at the New York Academy of Sciences (Maramorosch, 1973) and a second at Bordeaux, France, in 1974, organised by J.M. Bové (Bové and Duplan, 1974). At the Bordeaux conference, the International Organisation of Mycoplasmology was founded. The third international meeting of this organisation at Custer, South Dakota, in September 1980, witnessed a broad attendance of workers from all disciplines of mycoplasmology. Thus, it seems natural today for animal, plant, insect and veterinary mycoplasmologists to sit together and discuss their common interests. Accordingly, the Subcommittee on Taxonomy of the Mollicutes (formerly of the Mycoplasmatales) (1967, 1977) has enlisted plant and insect microbiologists and has been influential in assisting plant and insect workers unfamiliar with microbial taxonomy.

The minimal standards proposed by the Subcommittee (1972, 1979) form the basis for the description of new species of Mollicutes.

Present studies in the laboratory of C. Woese at Urbana, Illinois, are of exceptional taxonomic interest. Woese's group has been applying the cataloguing of rRNA for analysis of phylogenetic relationships of the prokaryotes (Fox *et al.*, 1980). Briefly, their data show that the mycoplasmas belong to a cluster of wall-less prokaryotes that shows affinities with gram-positive bacteria (Woese *et al.*, 1980). This cluster forms the basis for the class Mollicutes.

The prokaryotes associated with plants and insects are now recognised to be taxonomically diverse. This diversity is best illustrated by the discovery of the causal agent of clover club leaf disease. This disease incites symptoms, including virescence, that are reminiscent of those caused by members of the aster yellows group. It was believed, therefore, that the clover club leaf disease was caused by a mycoplasma-like organism. However, when Windsor and Black (1973) tested sensitivity of the disease to tetracycline and included a penicillin control, they discovered that symptom remission was induced by penicillin. Electron microscopy subsequently revealed that the causal agent was a small bacterium, which is now recognised to be a member of a group of fastidious bacterial phloem pathogens.

Mycoplasmas known to be associated with plants or insects belong to several taxa (Table 2.1). Several untyped sterol-dependent, apparently non-helical organisms have been isolated from plant surfaces (Clark, 1978; Davis, 1978; McCoy *et al.*, 1979). These organisms, when typed, may be placed in the genus *Mycoplasma*.

The genus *Spiroplasma* was erected by Saglio *et al.* (1973) as the result of a team effort stemming from the 1972 Ciba Symposium. These organisms are recognised as helical, motile, wall-less prokaryotes (Davis and Worley, 1973) that lack periplasmic fibrils (*sensu* Spirochetes), but that possess a system of conspicuous fibrils (Williamson, 1974; Townsend *et al.*, 1980). The organisms have NADH oxidase localised on the cell membrane (Kahane *et al.*, 1977; Mudd *et al.*, 1977) and possess a phosphoenol pyruvate phosphotransferase system (Cirillo, 1979). Skripal (1974) proposed the erection of a family (Spiroplasmataceae) for the spiroplasmas. To date, the type species, *Spiroplasma citri*, is the only species that has been given a binomial name, but at least four other serotypes of cultivable spiroplasmas are candidates for species description (Junca *et al.*, 1980). Some members of the genus *Acholeplasma* are also apparently associated with plants. For example, in the course of efforts to elucidate the etiology

Table 2.1: Taxonomic Status of Plant and Arthropod Mycoplasmas

---

Class *Mollicutes* (wall-less prokaryotes phylogenetically related to gram-positive bacteria); order *Mycoplasmatales*.

> Family *Mycoplasmataceae* (sterol-dependent nonhelical organisms; genome size 5×10^8 daltons)
>
> > Several untyped sterol-dependent nonhelical prokaryotes from plant surfaces
>
> Family *Spiroplasmataceae* (sterol-dependent helical, motile organisms; genome size 1×10^9 daltons)
>
> Genus *Spiroplasma*
>
> > 1. *Spiroplasma citri*
> >
> > 2-5. At least four distinct serogroups other than *S. citri* are candidate species
>
> Family *Acholeplasmataceae* (sterol non-dependent, nonhelical organisms; genome size 1×10^9 daltons)
>
> Genus *Acholeplasma*
>
> > 1. *Acholeplasma oculi* ⎫ isolated from coconut in Jamaica
> > 2. *Acholeplasma axanthum* ⎭
> >
> > 3. *Acholeplasma laidlawii*, possible inhabitant of plants; requires confirmation
>
> Mycoplasma-like organisms (MLOs) (non-helical wall-less organisms that have not been cultivated)
>
> > *Yellows agents:* organisms that induce proliferation and virescence in plants, often occur intracellularly in insect hosts. Includes agents of aster yellows, clover phyllody, peach yellows, mulberry dwarf, etc.
> >
> > *Other MLOs:* agents of some diseases, e.g. coconut lethal yellowing, appear to be MLOs, but do not cause typical yellows disease.

---

of the devastating coconut lethal yellowing disease in Jamaica, S. Eden-Green discovered that several acholeplasmas were apparently associated with diseased and healthy palms. These were later identified by Eden-Green and Tully (1980) as *A. axanthum* and *A. oculi*. A third acholeplasma, *A. laidlawii*, has been isolated by several workers from plants. However, the occurrence of this species in plant associations should probably be confirmed by more extensive studies (Tully, 1979). Recent studies (Somerson *et al.*, 1980) indicate that acholeplasmas occur on some vegetables used for food; whether these organisms are epiphytes or are deposited on the plants by arthropods is unclear.

Most workers currently believe that there is at least one other group of plant and insect mycoplasmas. This is the group represented by the 'yellows agents' (Kunkel, 1926; McCoy, 1979). Although symptom expression has proved to be an inaccurate indicator of the taxon of causal agents in the past, the similarity of the classical yellows syndrome in many plant hosts has led to a widely-held assumption that these classical agents represent a single taxon. The symptoms that they induce include virescence and proliferations such as witches' broom. The pathogens are never helical, and often occur intracellularly in their insect hosts. They have so far resisted cultivation. These agents cause diseases such as aster yellows, clover phyllody, peach yellows, mulberry dwarf, etc. (reviewed by Maramorosch *et al.*, 1970). Other nonhelical MLOs cause plant diseases that cannot be readily classified. These include diseases such as rice yellow dwarf (Nasu *et al.,* 1967), pear decline (Hibino and Schneider, 1970), coconut lethal yellowing (Tsai, 1979b), and peach X-disease (Gilmer and Blodgett, 1976).

Recently it has been claimed that aster yellows (Maramorosch and Kondo, 1978), clover phyllody (Giannotti and Giannotti, 1978), western X-disease (Lowe and Raju, 1978) and pear decline (Lowe and Raju, 1978) are caused by cultivable mycoplasmas, but the taxonomic array of organisms that emerge from such studies is diverse, and the evidence is not convincing.

3. Yellows Agents: Disease Recognition and Vector Relationships

Although the pathogens of yellows agents were difficult to find and identify, this can hardly be said of the diseases. Diseases of the yellows type such as aster yellows and peach yellows have frequently caused devastating economic loss. Other diseases whose causal agents have caused severe economic losses include coconut lethal yellowing, western X-disease and pear decline. All of these diseases have been studied rather intensively from the standpoint of epidemiology and vector relations. Indeed, these aspects have led in some cases to disease control. In this section we will outline some of the history of these important diseases.

A. Aster Yellows

Although the aster yellows pathogen is known today to affect many plant hosts, the various symptoms that are induced on its diverse hosts were not originally recognised as signs of infection with a single disease agent. For this reason, initial descriptions of the disease refer to the syndrome induced on China aster (*Callistephus chinensis*), an ornamental plant that was very much in favour in the early part of the twentieth century. Perhaps the first comprehensive description of the disease in aster was that of Ralph E. Smith in 1902. His description of a disease 'caused by no fungus, insect, or other organism' as 'one of the most peculiarly obscure diseases with which any plant is affected' is reminiscent of our own bewilderment more than half a century later as we groped for the etiological agent. Smith noted the major symptoms of the disease, including the 'spindling yellow growth' of the vegetative parts of the plant and the floral symptoms. The flowers, he noted, were 'of the same greenish yellow as . . . the affected leaves'. He also noted that other diseases, such as peach yellows, had many similarities and were symptomatologically similar to aster yellows.

None of the stones available to Smith for determining the etiology of the disease was left unturned. He examined the sources of disorders known at that time – nematodes, insects, plant variety, seed source and age, cultural practices, soil characteristics, genetics and weather conditions – as possible causes. Apparently in despair he concluded that the disease was due to 'an obscure perversion or derangement of the vital functions of the plant', or alternatively that it resulted from 'an inherent constitutional weakness or misadjustment'. The 'fundamental *cause* of all this' however was 'unexplained'.

In 1926, L.O. Kunkel published the results of a three-year reinvestigation of the aster yellows disease. The thoroughness with which he pursued this work and subsequent studies on aster yellows, together with his studies on peach yellows, gives him clear priority as the founding father of plant and insect mycoplasmology. Reading through this contribution, it is difficult to believe that it was written 57 years ago, only two decades after Smith's original description. Kunkel redescribed the symptoms of the disease in elegant detail, and investigated its transmissibility by *Macrosteles fascifrons* (at that time *Cicadula sexnotata*), but not by other leafhoppers such as *Empoasca* or *Aceratagallia* species. Life history data of the vectors were obtained, some with special reference to the disease epidemiology. He also developed methods for obtaining pathogen-free insects, and recognised the importance of using an immune plant host for experimental work on the insects. Details of the transmission process such as retention and acquisition times were determined, and the efficiency of transmission was studied. By using the vector he demonstrated that the agent had a wide range of experimental plant hosts in various families.

Clearly, Kunkel's own outstanding conceptions about scientific research were aided by the fact that the time was ripe in 1926 for studies of insect transmission of plant disease. Important groundwork

had been laid by N. Takami (1901) in his studies on rice stunt, by H.H.P.
Severin (1921) in his studies on curly top disease of sugar beets, and by
H.H. Storey (1925a, b) in studies of maize streak. In addition, the exist-
ence of filterable viruses (which have proved since to induce all three of
the diseases) had been widely accepted, and failure to find visible etio-
logical agents had ceased to baffle scientists, as it had Smith in 1902.
The mechanisms of insect transmission of plant pathogens proved to be
similar, whether the etiological agents were mycoplasmas or viruses.
Thus, it was the transmissibility of the aster yellows agent that led
Kunkel to conclude that AY was an infectious agent:

> the intimate and specific relationship which has been shown to exist
> between aster yellows and its insect carrier is important evidence
> in favor of the view that the causative entity is biological rather
> than chemical. It is difficult to conceive that any agent other than a
> living organism would require an incubation period in the insect
> carrier or would be retained by the insect for long periods of time in
> the absence of susceptible host plants.

Although earlier work on insect transmission had involved other
agents, aster yellows became, in Kunkel's hands, the most important
model disease for the study of insect transmitted 'viruses'. Thus,
Kunkel (1926, 1931, 1932, 1937, 1938, 1954) defined for the first
time many distinctive features of the insect transmission process. He
found, for example, that an incubation period of at least ten days
intervened between acquisition and the first transmissions of AY by
Macrosteles fascifrons and that thereafter the insect could inoculate
plants for the remainder of its life. He was unable to find microscopic
evidence of disease in inoculative insects, and determined that the
average length of life for pathogen-bearing and pathogen-free insects
was the same. These observations were later confirmed in an extensive
study (Dobroscky, 1929).

Further, Kunkel (1937) demonstrated that inoculative leafhoppers
held at 32°C for various numbers of days were unable to inoculate
plants for some period when they were returned to 24°C. The length
of this period of inability to transmit was roughly proportional to the
length of the heat treatment. If treatment was for twelve days or more,
the insects never recovered their ability to transmit unless they were
allowed to reacquire the agent by feeding on diseased plants. Kunkel
interpreted his results on the basis of the inactivation of the pathogen
at 32°C and its renewed multiplication at 24°C. Mild strains of the

pathogen were frequently recovered after such heat treatments, indicating a direct effect of heat on the pathogen. On the other hand, he (1938) demonstrated that the leafhoppers could undergo completely normal life cycles at $35°C$. Moreover, the pathogen could be eradicated from infected *Vinca* (=*Catharanthus*) *rosea* and *Nicotiana rustica* plants by heat treatment. The plants subsequently recovered from disease and grew in a healthy condition unless re-inoculated.

In 1954, Kunkel demonstrated that, after acquisition access periods of 2 hours, 1 day, 7 days and 14 days, 13, 69, 84 and 100 per cent, respectively, of leafhoppers became inoculative. After the end of the incubation period, individual insects in the same four groups transmitted the disease to 71, 72, 75 and 78 per cent, respectively, of plants on which they were allowed one-day inoculation access. Thus, the length of the acquisition access period did not affect the inoculativity of any insect that acquired the pathogen, a result consistent with multiplication in the vector.

There had been many attempts to inoculate susceptible plants mechanically with the aster yellows agent by means of extracts from diseased plants. However, to our knowledge, not a single successful transmission was ever reported, not even a mistaken success. Using techniques modified from the early work of Storey (1925a, b), Black (1941) transmitted the pathogen by injection of leafhopper vectors with extracts from inoculative leafhoppers. These injected leafhoppers later transmitted the agent to healthy plants, in which typical disease appeared. Black used the injection technique to demonstrate that the concentration of the AY pathogen was at least 100 times greater late in the incubation period than it was at the beginning in insects that were being maintained on healthy susceptible plants. Because susceptible plants upon which these insects fed during the incubation period subsequently did not become diseased, the experiment provided strong evidence for multiplication of the agent in the insect. However, an experiment in which multiplication of a plant mycoplasma in its vector was proved definitively was published by Maramorosch (1952). After ten serial passages of the pathogen from insect to insect by injection, he determined that the final concentration in the injected insects could have been attained only by multiplication. Under the conditions of the experiment, the injected insects could not have acquired the pathogen from plants and although the cumulative dilution of the injected extracts was about 10^{40} the concentration of pathogen in the insects at the end of the series was essentially the same as that in the insects that had provided the starting inoculum.

Much of the impetus for continuing studies of multiplication in insect vectors derived from F.C. Bawden. Until 1950, Bawden remained unconvinced that plant 'viruses' multiplied in their vectors, and in the first edition of his valuable and influential textbook (Bawden, 1950) suggested alternative explanations for results of experiments designed to demonstrate multiplication. During this period, all of the pathogens studied in this connection were presumed to be viruses. Eventually his stand was reversed on the basis of an experiment with the clover club leaf pathogen (Black, 1950), which is ironic because this agent was subsequently found to be a phloem-limited bacterium. The controversy surrounding multiplication of plant disease agents in their vectors was reviewed and analysed by Black (1959).

It was during the same period that Kunkel (1952) found that several mycoplasmal pathogens could be transmitted from plant to plant by making use of dodder (*Cuscuta* sp.). The use of these parasitic plants was enhanced by his discovery that they parasitised a much wider range of host species in the greenhouse than they did in the field. This use overcame to some extent the limitation on transmission by grafting scion to stock. Usually this can be done only with species within families or even smaller taxa. The use of dodder also overcame limitations that resulted from the inability of an insect vector to feed on certain plant species. With dodder, transmissions were sometimes possible between plants that could not be grafted, even when the vector was not known; some of these transmissions were from woody to herbaceous plants. For example, Kunkel was able to transfer yellows agents to Madagascar periwinkle (*Vinca rosea*), tomato (*Lycopersicon esculentum*) and carrot (*Daucus carota*). Sometimes the distinctive or similar symptoms of two infections which occurred on different hosts in the field were readily observed on a common host. The use of *Vinca* is one of many legacies of Kunkel's pioneering research; this species is routinely used today in plant mycoplasma research.

Although Kunkel was certainly the first and foremost investigator of the aster yellows disease, other workers devoted large portions of their careers to its study and contributed greatly to its position as the classical disease of the yellows type. Kunkel's close contemporary, H.H.P. Severin of the Department of Entomology in Berkeley, divided his early efforts between curly top virus and aster yellows. In 1929, Severin showed that a yellows disease of celery was caused by an agent transmissible by *Macrosteles fascifrons* and identified the disease as aster yellows. The subsequent study of the agent in both eastern and western parts of the United States was important, because the geographical types had been found (Kunkel, 1932) to differ in several respects. For example, in the western United States the agent had a wide host range not only in plants (Frazier and Severin, 1945), but also in the leafhopper vector of the disease (Severin, 1945). Severin later found that insects feeding on diseased plants had *greater* longevities than insects feeding on healthy plants (Severin, 1945). This effect, later studied in more detail by Maramorosch and his colleagues (Orenski *et al.*, 1965) came to be thought of as a 'beneficial' effect of the agent on the vector.

The study of aster yellows begun by Severin in the twenties has continued to the present time in the Berkeley laboratory. Much of the intervening work was that of J. Freitag. Perhaps the most memorable of these studies was the demonstration of mutual suppression by various strains of aster yellows (Freitag, 1964). Kunkel (1955) had previously shown that eastern and western strains of the aster yellows pathogen interfered with each other's transmission to China aster by *Macrosteles fascifrons*. Insects that had acquired the eastern strain and were transmitting it were unable to acquire and transmit the western strain and vice versa. Similar interference also occurred in plants. Before serological techniques were available, such interference (cross protection) appeared to provide a better basis for inferring a relationship than similarity of symptoms. However, Freitag's study in 1964 showed that such concepts, while useful in a general way, greatly oversimplified the possible interactions. In particular, he showed that certain combinations of strains exhibited mutual suppression in which the normally severe symptomatic profiles induced by all known strains of aster yellows were less severe or absent.

As noted, Kunkel had been impressed in his earlier studies by the incubation period in plants inoculated by insects at the earliest stage of their inoculative period. He felt that 'the condition of the virus in the insect' was the explanation. It remained for Maramorosch (1953) to show that in reality, dosage of pathogen, rather than any postulated developmental stage of the pathogen, was responsible for such prolonged latent periods.

In the laboratory of R. Chapman, at Madison, Wisconsin, epidemiology and control of the aster yellows pathogen was emphasised (Chapman, 1974). One major contribution was the demonstration that *M. fascifrons* dispersed into northern states from south-central states, where the vector and pathogen overwintered (Drake and Chapman, 1965). Monitoring the migratory population led to more rational decisions regarding control.

Continuing studies of yellows pathogens in the western United

States and Canada have finally led to the realisation that a large complex
of pathogen strains is involved (Chiykowski, 1974). The fine details of
their transmission and the sorting of the various strains has been the
major thrust of recent work (reviewed by Tsai, 1979a). With this long
history of study of AY in North America, it is indeed ironic that the
major breakthrough in determining its etiology derived from a group
of workers in Japan.

B. Peach Yellows

Peach trees were introduced into America sometime before 1633
(E.F. Smith, 1888, p. 11) and were grown in abundance without any
evidence of yellows disease until 1791 (Smith, 1888, p. 10, 17) when
the peach yellows disease was found near Philadelphia. From there the
disease spread northward into Canada, southward (as far as North
Carolina in mountainous areas) and westward to the Mississippi. It did
not invade warmer areas of the south. Outbreaks of the disease in certain
years were devastating. For example, between 1874 and 1884 the
acreage in peaches in Berrien County, Michigan, dropped from 6,000
to 500 acres because of peach yellows (Wood, 1953, p. 8).

There were many hypotheses regarding the cause of the disease
(Smith, 1888, p. 7). Smith (1888, p. 154) reviewed the evidence that
the disease could be transmitted by grafting diseased scions (buds)
into healthy stocks (trees) and eliminated all doubt by proving such
transmission in well-controlled experiments. Although the disease agent
could not be transmitted by sap inoculations, his grafting experiments
established that yellows was a transmissible disease and eliminated from
further serious consideration many hypotheses such as soil exhaustion
or supposed degeneracy due to continued vegetative propagation.

Because Smith's proof of graft-transmissibility did not resolve the
question of how yellows spread in nature, and because of the serious
damage to the peach industry, extensive efforts were made to discover
the answer. Insect transmission was among the many possibilities
suggested and investigated. Nevertheless, 45 years were to elapse before
Kunkel demonstrated that the plum leafhopper, *Macropsis trimaculata*,
was the vector of peach yellows. The latter statement is often all that
there is room for in literature crammed with bare facts about the disease.
The fascinating story behind this discovery is only partly told in
Kunkel's paper (1933) describing his important experiment. One day in
a greenhouse of the Rockefeller Institute at Princeton, New Jersey, he
reminisced with one of us (LMB) about his work. For some years he
had made a practice of planting a small peach orchard when he moved

to a new location. After a time peach yellows would appear in these home orchards. He also made it a practice in his spare time to observe the insects on his peach trees. Kunkel came to know such insects thoroughly, but on one occasion found a cast insect skin that he realised had come from an insect he had never seen. Eventually he discovered the leafhopper that left such skins and found that it always moved to the back of the twig as he approached. It would then run down a twig or branch and hide in a crack in the bark. Kunkel observed that this leafhopper was unlike many others in several respects. It never hopped; it ran more rapidly than most and seldom took wing. His paper reports that 'the adults seldom fly when slightly disturbed' but instead 'resort to flight only when closely pressed or when they move for considerable distances in the course of their feeding and breeding activities'. However, when they did fly they moved very rapidly. Also, although occasionally found feeding on leaves, both nymphs and adults preferred twigs and large branches (old woody branches rather than succulent young shoots) and old trees rather than young.

The plum leafhopper overwinters in eggs and produces only one generation each year. Kunkel found the first adults about 15 June and numerous adults between 25 June and 10 July, but noted a sharp decline in numbers thereafter. When inserted into the bark by the female, the eggs are dormant and 'apparently require the low temperatures of winter to bring them out of that dormant condition'. This limits the time available for transmission experiments to the relatively short period when the single brood is feeding each year. He reported that *M. trimaculata* was more numerous on peach than on plum in the early part of the summer, but was more numerous on plum late in the season.

As a result of Kunkel's discovery, *M. trimaculata* was studied and described carefully by others. For example, Hartzell (1935) noted that the reddish brown colour of nymphs and adults provided protection as they fed on the bark of their hosts. Manns (1942, p. 43) also reported that 'in color, both nymphs and adults adapt themselves to the color of the host, being quite dark and sooty on most plums'.

It is usually assumed that vectors of plant diseases are common pests on their host plants. However, Kunkel (1933) was able to cite only one previous report of the leafhopper on peach, that of Stearns (1927), who listed three collections in Virginia between 17 June and 9 July. Also, *M. trimaculata* had not been reported from Delaware prior to Kunkel's 1933 paper (Manns, 1942, p. 38). Actually, *M. trimaculata* prefers plums to peaches and had been reported on plums in Colorado (Ball, 1903) and on wild plums in New York (Felt, 1906). Indeed, it had become known as the plum hopper.

An extensive survey by Manns (1934) showed that in Delaware and several adjacent states *M. trimaculata* lived primarily on plum — most abundantly on Japanese varieties (*Prunus salicina*) or on crosses between that and *P. domestica, P. americana* and *P. munsoniana*. It was found only sparingly on peach. Hartzell (1935, p. 203) considered that in comparison with other leafhoppers of economic importance *M. trimaculata* was a rare species. He reported that he had 'collected a greater number of adults of *Empoasca fabae* in the potato fields of Iowa in a half hour than of *Macropsis trimaculata* that could be collected during a whole season'.

To test the possibility that the plum hopper, despite its name, might be the answer to a peach problem that had puzzled plant pathologists for almost half a century, Kunkel carefully designed a transmission experiment. Had he been less thorough in his methods, this insect might easily have escaped detection as a vector despite being subjected to test. Kunkel found that as few as ten adults feeding on a young foot-high peach tree for only one week caused a sudden wilting of the tree which resulted in its death if the insects were not promptly removed. Older, bigger trees survived such exposure without wilting. He recognised that, although the wilt had nothing to do with yellows itself, it did limit the combination of insect numbers and exposure intervals that could be used in testing young trees. Therefore he allowed nymphs and adults collected from healthy and yellowed orchard trees to feed on yellowed peach seedlings for 2 to 21 days and then allowed colonies of 2 to 100 insects to feed for 2 to 27 days on healthy seedling trees. Although he inoculated 74 seedling trees, only 7 became diseased. However, none of 193 control trees (133 in this experiment and 60 comparable trees exposed to another insect) developed yellows.

Later investigators soon confirmed that *M. trimaculata* transmitted peach yellows but, like Kunkel, obtained only low percentages of transmission. Kunkel obtained no transmissions in tests with 14 other insect species, Hartzell obtained none in tests with 47 species of insects and mites, and Manns obtained none in tests of several species (Kunkel *et al.*, 1951).

It is obvious that *M. trimaculata* had many traits that made it difficult to identify as the vector of peach yellows. For example, Kunkel *et al.* (1951, p. 3) reported that in the field the incubation period of the disease in the plant may be as long as three years. Thus, it is likely that most inoculations by this insect would tend to produce recognisable field symptoms one, two or more years subsequent to inoculation. Also, because vector populations probably varied from year to year, the causal association could easily have been obscured. However, other factors also could have contributed to the difficulty. Because grafting of diseased buds from peach trees on plum stocks did not cause yellows in plums, Smith concluded (1888, p. 9, 167) that plums were immune — a conclusion natural enough at a time long before symptomless carriers of virus (or mycoplasmas) had been demonstrated. In fact, Manns (1932, p. 46-7) had actually begun experiments to test plum species as symptomless carriers of yellows before Kunkel reported *M. trimaculata* as the vector. First he grafted buds from peach trees with yellows to plum trees; then after a period of incubation, buds from the inoculated plums were grafted back to healthy peaches. In this way, buds from certain symptomless plums, including *Prunus myrobalan*, a species commonly used as the rootstock for plums by grafting, were found to transmit the disease to peaches. Manns (1942, p. 24) therefore suggested that plums could provide a reservoir of both vector and pathogen and supported this suggestion by field records.

Other observers had also noted important facets of the disease epidemiology. For example, as early as 1924, McCubbin (1928, p. 12-25) had begun to observe and diagram the patterns involved in the appearance of yellows in young peach orchards. The disease seemed to appear first in, and subsequently spread from, areas that were not in cultivation and that supported the growth of a diverse assemblage of native and introduced plant species. The most notable reservoir areas occurred around sinkholes — rather abrupt circular depressions that occurred in limestone regions. McCubbin identified five plant species that occurred in all of nine sinkhole areas that he studied. None of the five species was a member of the genus *Prunus*, and none is now known to play any role in peach yellows epidemiology. However, four different *Prunus* species occurred in one, two, or three of the nine areas. The significance of this observation went unrecognised at the time, even though McCubbin realised that a plant species could have disappeared from a given area before his survey was made. If any of the *Prunus* species in McCubbin's sinkholes or other centres had shown symptoms resembling peach yellows it is likely that they would have been noticed by the observant McCubbin, who was a state inspector of yellows in peach orchards. McCubbin reasoned from his observations that the wild reservoir areas might support a plant host susceptible to the peach yellows agent, or that supported large populations of an insect vector. In general terms his well-reasoned speculations came remarkably close to the truth. Yet, although Hartzell, a colleague of Kunkel at Boyce Thompson, knew of his work and visited one of his sites (McCubbin, 1928, p. 19), McCubbin's observations seem to have had no connection with Kunkel's discovery of the vector.

Understanding of the disease cycle of peach yellows led to effective control. By 1951, peach yellows was no longer considered to be a serious disease in well-kept commercial orchards if nearby plum trees were removed, diseased trees were removed as soon as detected and the vector was controlled by spraying (Kunkel *et al.*, 1951).

In retrospect, it is clear that Kunkel's conception of how he would search for an insect vector of peach yellows was of crucial importance. Although his earlier work on aster yellows (Kunkel, 1926) had provided a wealth of basic information on insect transmission of plant mycoplasmas, Kunkel was open-minded about the different situation confronting him with peach yellows. For example, if he had collected insects for testing by sweeping with a net in the conventional manner, he probably would have fared no better than other investigators. Also, the manner of testing plum hoppers was critical. It would be difficult to find a better example of the importance and execution of a well-conceived field study. Indeed, if Kunkel had not discovered the vector in 1933, one wonders how many years would have elapsed before someone discovered how the disease was spreading and how to control it.

C. Coconut Lethal Yellowing

The lethal yellowing disease was apparently first observed in Jamaica by Fawcett (1891). He noted that young plant parts were the first to be affected, including young fruits whose dropping was the first sign of disease. The disease, he opined, was 'due to an organized ferment which is able to attack the very tender tissues of the youngest parts'. The remedy was to set fire to the fibrous material at the base of the leaves; eventually all the leaves burned. New fronds developed, however, and the tree was 'at any rate for the time saved'. This procedure, of course, was 'not safe near buildings', and fruit production was delayed. Drenching of the tree with iron sulfate was recommended as a safer, although more expensive, alternative which was justified by the annual value of each tree, estimated at four shillings..For many years after the report, lethal yellowing in Jamaica was confined to the western coast. This period of epidemiological quiescence led some workers (Hansen, 1952) to conclude that the disease was the result of toxins from the saline spray of the ocean, and led others to conclude tentatively that soil or other environmental conditions might be the root of the problem (Leach, 1946; Martyn, 1945a, b, 1955). However, the advocates of an association with soil were puzzled by many anomalies of the disease epidemiology, including the apparent absence of spread by wind-borne vectors. The anomalies seemed to justify calling the malady 'the unknown disease' of coconut. In a postscript to his 1946 paper, Leach noted the presence of the unknown disease in Haiti, where its 'existence on slightly acid soils of igneous origin tends to mitigate against any theory of soil deficiency'. Further, the sudden spread of the disease to Gonaives, forty miles away from Cape Haities, where it had existed for sixty years without jump spread, was 'alarming in regard to the situation in Jamaica' where the disease had not spread from the western end of the island in forty years. In 1961, jump spread in Jamaica began, fulfilling all of Leach's worst fears. The disease took a destructive course, spreading throughout the island, and killed 200,000 palms per annum (Romney, 1972). The pattern of spread evident in this outbreak made it likely that an insect vector was transmitting the disease (Grylls and Hunt, 1971); therefore, it became clear that the disease was infectious. Because the symptoms of the disease were consistent with viral symptoms, and for other reasons, the disease was thought until 1971 to be induced by a virus. However, by that time, spurred by the discoveries of mycoplasmas in many other plant diseases, three research groups discovered mycoplasma-like organisms in diseased palms (Beakbane *et al.*, 1972; Pravsic-Banjac and Maramorosch, 1972; Heinze *et al.*, 1972).

If search for the etiological agent of the 'unknown disease' had been difficult, search for the vector was more so. The history of some of the early trials (and failures) has been detailed by Eden-Green (1979). Very recently, transmission by naturally infective insects may have been achieved by massive transfers of the fulgorid *Myndus* (= *Haplaxius*) *crudus* to screened healthy palms (Howard and Thomas, 1980).

4. Yellows Agents: Discovery of Microbial Identity

Members of the 'yellows' group of plant pathogens have not yet been assigned a microbial identity, if one means by that isolation, cultivation and characterisation. We make this statement despite recent claims to the contrary, for reasons outlined in detail in a recent review (Whitcomb, 1981). In 1967, however, groundwork was laid for eventual resolution of their taxonomic position by a group of Japanese workers who developed convincing evidence that the diseases were caused not by viruses, but by prokaryotic organisms (Doi *et al.*, 1967; Ishiie *et al.*, 1967).

In examinations of thin sections of leaves and shoots of mulberry infected with dwarf disease, Doi and his colleagues failed, as others had, to find virus particles. Instead, they consistently found 'specific pleomorphic bodies', 80–800 nm in diameter, that possessed a two-layered limiting membrane about 8 nm in thickness. The bodies were structurally simple, but contained ribosome-like granules and strands of material interpretable as prokaryotic nucleic acid. The prokaryotes were thought to be similar to mycoplasmas or chlamydiae (at that time termed psittacosis-lymphogranuloma-trachoma: PLT-group organisms). Because of the pleomorphism of the bodies they observed, they felt that the organisms most closely resembled mycoplasmas.

Observation of organisms is not, of course, proof of etiology. Doi *et al.* clearly recognised this, and indicated that cultivation of the agents and fulfilment of Koch's postulates were the obvious next steps. They also recognised that visualisation of the organisms allowed at least two interpretations, only one of which required that the observed organisms cause plant disease. The alternative explanation, that the organisms were secondary invaders, seemed unlikely to them because the characteristic bodies were not present in plants affected with known viruses.

Evidence concerning etiology was provided by the experiments of Ishiie *et al.* (1967). Tetracycline and chlortetracycline, but not kanamycin, were shown to induce remission of symptoms in infected mulberry. Although treated plants eventually relapsed, the remissions were clear-cut and electron microscopic examination showed that the bodies disappeared during the period of remission.

A further prediction, that other diseases of the 'yellows' type would prove to have similar bodies associated with them, also proved to be true. Potato plants with witches' broom, paulownia with witches' broom, and petunia with aster yellows all showed similar bodies.

As Doi *et al.* predicted, the publication of their observations led to discoveries of similar organisms in many other members of the yellows group. Today, however, thirteen years after the publication of the Japanese report, little additional information or evidence has been added to the study of yellows disease etiology. The final step, cultivation of the agents, has eluded all of the many workers who have attempted it, so elucidation of a microbial identity must await future discoveries.

5. Spiroplasmas: Disease Recognition and Vector Relationships

A. *Citrus Stubborn*

The 'stubborn' disease of citrus, it is now realised, is a condition that had been recognised under several names since 1915 (Fawcett *et al.*, 1944). The disease was given its present name by E.R. Waite, who had top-worked nonproductive orange trees in California with carefully selected buds only to see the same characteristics return in the original trees. Hence, he termed them 'stubborn'. In Israel, the disease was termed 'little leaf' (Reichert and Perlberger, 1931), and in Egypt 'safargali' (Nour-Eldin, 1959). Even in the western United States, other names such as 'crazy top' of grapefruit were applied (Fawcett *et al.*, 1944). Nevertheless, by 1956 the Egyptian and Californian diseases were suspected to be identical (Childs *et al.*, 1956); shortly thereafter, it was suggested that little leaf and stubborn were identical (Reichert, 1958; Patt, 1964; Calavan and Christiansen, 1966). By 1959 the disease had been found in Algeria, Tunisia, Lebanon, Syria, Turkey and Corsica, and was also suspected to occur in Italy and Spain (Chapot, 1959). Thus it was widespread, and proved to have a broad host range among citrus varieties (Calavan and Christiansen, 1966).

Although symptoms of leaves and fruits may appear characteristic today (Calavan and Oldfield, 1979), earlier analyses of the 'stubborn' condition confused it with other citrus diseases such as xyloporosis (Reichert, 1958) or greening (Calavan and Christiansen, 1966). Apparently, the commonest means of spread of citrus stubborn in early years was through cultural practices, a circumstance that obscured recognition of natural spread by insect vectors. In fact, discovery of vectors of the disease occurred only after discovery of its etiological agents.

Studies of the etiology of stubborn were probably not pursued intensively, judging by the sparseness of discussion in the literature. The disease was generally assumed to be viral. In 1946, because the condition could be transmitted by budding, Fawcett came 'to the definite conclusion that stubborn disease on navel orange trees is of virus origin'. It is interesting to contrast the ease with which the disease was accepted as being of viral etiology (despite the lack of evidence that any virus was present) with the intense interest of R.E. Smith and Kunkel in the elusive agent of aster yellows. In the late 1960s, however, the discoveries of Doi and his colleagues (1967) provided a stimulus for reinvestigation of the etiology of citrus stubborn. Thus, the stage was set for electron microscopic demonstration of wall-less prokaryotes in the phloem of diseased citrus plants (Igwegbe and Calavan,

1970; Laflèche and Bové, 1970) and demonstration of their *in vivo* antibiotic sensitivity (Igwegbe and Calavan, 1973).

B. Corn Stunt

The corn stunt disease, like many other plant mycoplasma diseases, was at first confused with other apparently similar diseases. In 1945, Alstatt described a disease of maize from south Texas that has since been termed corn stunt. For many years this name was used for a complex of diseases of virus, mycoplasma and spiroplasma etiology. For example, Frazier (1945) described a disease in California that was regarded by early workers as stunt but that, in retrospect, was more likely to have been a strain of sugarcane mosaic virus. The full diversity of maize viruses and mycoplasmas has only recently been recognised. For example, Nault *et al.* (1979) found maize rayado fino virus, maize stripe virus, maize dwarf mosaic virus, maize chlorotic mottle virus, and, probably maize mosaic virus, as well as the corn stunt spiroplasma and maize bushy stunt mycoplasma in Peru, where maize has been culti-vated for at least 3,000 years. Of these pathogens, maize bushy stunt mycoplasma was most often confused with corn stunt. The Mesa Central (Maramorosch, 1955) and Louisiana (Granados *et al.*, 1966) isolates were considered strains of corn stunt for many years, until Nault and his colleagues, and Mexican workers (Bascope and Galindo, 1978) recognised that the causal agent in both cases was a non-helical mycoplasma (Bradfute *et al.*, 1977; Nault, 1980) that they termed maize bushy stunt. Rio Grande corn stunt, whose causal spiroplasma was later cultivated and shown to induce typical disease (Chen and Liao, 1975; Williamson and Whitcomb, 1975), was brought into the laboratory in 1955 (Maramorosch, 1955) and is now regarded as the classical labor-atory strain.

In 1946, Kunkel began to study a disease agent from corn that he regarded as typical stunt. Although the pathogen was not preserved, his description of the symptoms it induced makes it relatively certain that he had worked with the corn stunt spiroplasma. Following up on an observation that the leafhopper *Dalbulus* (then *Baldulus*) *maidis* was abundant in California in corn fields where diseased plants had been observed, Kunkel showed that this insect transmitted the pathogen to healthy corn. In subsequent work, Kunkel (1948) studied the details of insect transmission of the agent and used it to determine the host range of the pathogen. Many plants, in various families, were found to be immune; therefore, the agent appeared to have a much narrower host range than the aster yellows agent. Furthermore, the agent, like that of aster yellows, was not vertically transmitted in plants or insects. Later, Kunkel (1948) found that the agent was transmitted efficiently, but the incubation periods in the plant and the vector were longer than those of most other pathogens. Kunkel regarded this as further evidence that plant 'viruses' multiplied in their insect vectors.

Results of Maramorosch (1958) on interactions of the Mesa Central agent (now recognised as the causal agent of maize bushy stunt mosaic) and the Rio Grande corn stunt spiroplasma are interpretable today as interference between two mycoplasma species in a common insect host. Although the Mesa Central agent was transmitted if it was acquired first, Rio Grande corn stunt eventually was the predominant organism transmitted.

The Rio Grande strain collected by Maramorosch in 1955 was preserved by continuous transfer in the maize-leafhopper cycle until 1975, when the breakthrough in its cultivation occurred (Chen and Liao, 1975; Williamson and Whitcomb, 1975). In retrospect, the particularly confusing history of the corn stunt pathogen points to a general failure of workers in plant mycoplasma research to preserve, or attempt to preserve, the agents with which they worked so painstakingly. Thus, the aster yellows and corn stunt strains that Kunkel worked with for many years have been lost. To some extent, these losses may have occurred because of a lack of technology for storage of the agents. Today, however, the availability of ultra-low temperature storage units and sophisticated lyophilisation equipment makes failure to store pathogens inexcusable. Infectivity of the agents has been preserved for at least several years after storage of frozen whole insects carrying the pathogens and/or lyophilisation of extracts of infected insects (A. Smith, 1980; Chiykowski, 1977).

6. Spiroplasmas: Discovery of Microbial Identity

In 1961, Poulson and Sakaguchi studied an infectious agent that had been found to eliminate males from progeny of certain members of the *Drosophila willistoni* species complex (Malogolowkin, 1958). Studies of the infectious agent indicated that it occurred in high concentration in the hemolymph (Malogolowkin and Poulson, 1957; Malogolowkin *et al.*, 1959). Poulson and Sakaguchi consequently examined the *Drosophila* hemolymph under phase optics and observed numerous fine filaments that appeared to be helical. They regarded the observed insects' sex ratio organisms (SROs) to be spirochetes.

Eventually, when phase optics were replaced by dark field optics, optimum visualisation of the organisms was possible.

In 1967, Pickens *et al.*, at the Rocky Mountain Laboratory in Hamilton, in the course of searches for rickettsiae in ticks, encountered a helical organism that they also identified as a spirochete. They were able to cultivate the organism (277F) not only in embryonated eggs, but also in a complex cell-free medium.

Meanwhile, another agent had been isolated from the rabbit tick (Clark, 1964). This agent proved to be pathogenic for suckling rodents, and was termed the suckling mouse cataract agent. This agent was studied mainly by H.F. Clark who, like many other workers who encountered mycoplasmas unawares, had received training that was predominantly virological. The SMCA agent proved to be filterable and could be studied by many of the contemporary techniques of virology, so the search for the structural nature of the agent was postponed.

As a consequence of the revelation of Doi and others in 1967, work on the corn stunt and citrus stubborn agents gained new focus. For example, R.R. Granados and his co-workers at the Boyce Thompson Institute began careful ultrastructural examination of plants and insects carrying the corn stunt agent. Their thin-section electron micrographs showed what appeared to be typical mycoplasma-like organisms, especially in insect material. Negatively-stained preparations of sap from corn infected with the corn stunt agent showed peculiar filamentous forms emerging from larger bodies. The filaments appeared to be uniform in calibre and were thought to be the causal organism (Granados, 1969). The identification of the organism was challenged (Wolanski and Maramorosch, 1970) but it was later conceded that the envisioned bodies were specific for the disease (Wolanski, 1973). T.A. Chen and Granados began a series of attempts to cultivate the corn stunt agent that culminated in achievement of maintenance for extended periods in primary culture (Chen and Granados, 1970). It was during this period that the corn stunt organism came under scrutiny in Beltsville. Prompted by keen observation of the micrographs of Granados, R.E. Davis and his colleagues began to search for the organism, as Poulson and Sakaguchi had done, by using phase contrast optics; preparations from plants that were being bioassayed were routinely monitored for organisms of unusual morphology. It was not long before Davis noted a few perfectly helical filaments in extracts from diseased corn. These helical filaments were associated with the corn stunt disease syndrome in plants (Davis *et al.*, 1972) and, at least at certain times, in the insect (Davis, 1974; Whitcomb and Williamson,

1975).

Meanwhile, studies on the citrus stubborn disease agent showed
that it too was a wall-less prokaryote. This work was performed simultaneously and independently in two laboratories, those of J.M. Bové in
Bordeaux and E.C. Calavan in Riverside. This agent, unlike the corn
stunt agent, yielded rather easily (in retrospect) to cultivation attempts.
However, general acceptance of the successful cultivation of *S. citri* was
delayed and made difficult for many by a plethora of claims by other
researchers that they had cultivated yellows agents. Most of these other
reports have never been confirmed (Maramorosch, 1972). There was at
that time, therefore, an atmosphere of confusion and healthy scepticism.
Nevertheless, at the Ciba meeting, the case for culture of the stubborn
organism by Saglio was articulately expressed by Bové. Saglio's careful
and extensive experiments, replete with proper controls, demonstrated
consistent association of the cultivated microorganisms with the citrus
stubborn disease syndrome. Furthermore, Bové was able to cite in his
communication work that had been underway since 1970 by
A.E.S. Fudl-Allah in E.C. Calavan's laboratory, where similar results
had been independently obtained. The ensuing discussion left animal
mycoplasmologists largely convinced, and a natural result of the inter-
change was a collaborative effort to characterise the agent according
to the Minimal Standards outlined by the Subcommittee on Taxonomy
of the Mollicutes (1972). A particularly significant segment of the
characterisation was done in the laboratory of J.G. Tully at Bethesda.
One of the very first steps in analysis of the new mycoplasma was
examination under phase and dark field optics. Tully immediately
found large numbers of helical filaments that appeared to be identical
in every respect to those he had observed in corn stunt preparations
of his Beltsville colleagues. On very nearly the same day, Takashi
Ishijima, returning to Japan after a year's stay in the Beltsville laboratory, examined organisms that had been cultured (Fudl-Allah *et al.*,
1972) in Calavan's laboratory. His excited letter to Beltsville reported
the observation of many helical filaments!

In the years since its discovery, *S. citri* has emerged as an important
model for studies on basic microbiology. For example, it was *S. citri*
in which spiroplasma viruses, now recognised to be ubiquitously present
in the helical cells, were first observed (Cole *et al.*, 1974).

Cultivation of the citrus stubborn spiroplasma led to basic discoveries about its biology. Markham *et al.* (1974), using *Euscelis*, a
leafhopper with no known connection with the disease, were able to
fulfil Koch's postulates by demonstrating disease transmission by

insects injected with the pathogen. Shortly thereafter, Rana *et al.* (1975) similarly demonstrated transmission after acquisition of the agent through membranes by *Circulifer tenellus*. This leafhopper, however, appeared to harbour the pathogen naturally (Lee *et al.*, 1973), and could transmit the agent to citrus (Oldfield *et al.*, 1976). Although another leafhopper, *Scaphytopius nitridus*, could transmit the pathogen from citrus to citrus (Oldfield *et al.*, 1977), *Circulifer* appears to be the major vector, at least in the south-western United States.

Extensive efforts were made to cultivate the corn stunt spiroplasma continuously during the years after its primary isolation. Major efforts continued to be made in T.A. Chen's laboratory, and in the Plant Virology Laboratory at Beltsville. Meanwhile, a publication from a Brazilian laboratory (Pereira and Oliveira, 1971) reported that the agent had been cultivated and that the cultured organisms produced symptoms in healthy corn after mechanical inoculation. However, the organisms were not tested serologically, their morphology was not elucidated, and they were not preserved, so there is no means by which we can now determine validity. Eventually, it began to seem that the corn stunt agent might pose an intractable cultivation problem (Davis *et al.*, 1974). However, a collaborative study was undertaken to investigate the ability of the sex ratio and corn stunt spiroplasmas to multiply in unusual hosts (Williamson and Whitcomb, 1974). The SROs fared poorly in leafhoppers, but the corn stunt spiroplasma, after a period of initial adaptation, grew well in *Drosophila*. Williamson passed the cultures monthly for nearly a year, at which time he felt that the adaptation to a new host might make them more amenable to cultivation. He therefore removed organisms from the *Drosophila* hemolymph and placed them in Schneider's *Drosophila* medium, in which they survived. They were then passed in Saglio's medium for *S. citri*. In this combined medium they did very well, and soon it was apparent that they were multiplying during serial passage. Almost to the day that success became apparent T.A. Chen telephoned one of us (RFW) to confide that he also had been successful in cultivating the agent. It was therefore agreed to publish the results side-by-side. The important components of this initial publication would involve demonstration: (1) of continuous cultivation of the agent; (2) of consistent association of the agent with the corn stunt syndrome; (3) that the cultivated agent was serologically distinct from *S. citri*; (4) of colonial structure on solid medium; and (5) that the cultured organisms could be injected into leafhoppers, and could then produce the typical corn stunt disease syndrome. It was agreed that the papers would be submitted as soon as one of the research groups had achieved all these objectives. The initial observations of successful culture were made during the early summer of 1974; by early October, both groups had achieved all five objectives. The papers appeared side-by-side in 1975 (Chen and Liao, 1975; Williamson and Whitcomb, 1975).

When one looks back over the years during which cultivation of corn stunt seemed impossibly difficult, it is not easy to identify mistakes. The two media that were ultimately used with success were, in fact, very different, both in composition and rationale. Further, Liao and Chen showed that the corn stunt agent could be isolated in a medium that was very simple from the point of view of number of constituents (Liao and Chen, 1975, 1977). Indeed, the sentence in their abstract (Liao and Chen, 1975) reporting that 'A simple medium containing horse serum, 20 ml, PPLO broth 1.5 g, sucrose 16 g, and distilled water 74 ml, meets all the nutritional and physical requirements for the isolation and cultivation of the corn stunt spiroplasma' may be the most information-laden sentence ever published in a phytopathological abstract! However, a different approach, comparing the growth of *Spiroplasma citri* and corn stunt spiroplasmas in various medium variations, suggested that growth of the corn stunt organism was stimulated by certain factors (Jones *et al.*, 1977). Also, primary isolation of the corn stunt organism was improved by the presence of each of several ingredients supplied by Schneider's Drosophila medium (phosphate, a-ketoglutaric acid, amino acids).

The study of Jones *et al.* (1977) provided a basis for further advances in spiroplasma cultivation. When J.G. Tully had examined published micrographs of the suckling mouse cataract agent, he had sensed that the agent might be a spiroplasma. Then examination of fluids from embryonated chick eggs inoculated with SMCA showed helical organisms that proved to be spiroplasmas (Tully *et al.*, 1976). However, the agent could not be cultivated in existing media. Accordingly, utilising the approach of Williamson and Jones, medium variations were prepared whose compositions were compromises between the composition of media used for vertebrate tissue cultures, and for spiroplasmas. At least two of the variations supported growth of the SMCA spiroplasma, and the cultivated organisms readily produced (Tully *et al.*, 1977) the cataract symptoms in rodents that are the pathogenic hallmark of the experimental disease (Clark and Rorke, 1979).

During these years, the 277F agent was also considered to be a spirochete. In 1975, a conference on the pathobiology of invertebrate vectors was held at the New York Academy of Sciences. At this meeting, W. Burgdorfer, who had collaborated with Pickens in 1968, listening to a presentation on spiroplasmas, recognised immediately that the 277F agent was probably not a spirochete, but a spiroplasma. Certain features of the agent had troubled him at the time; for example it had been difficult to demonstrate the typical ultrastructural features of 'spiro-chetes'. The problems were therefore put on the shelf and the workers, whose major emphasis was rickettsiae, returned to their primary work. A subsequent study of the agent, which had been carefully preserved, showed that it indeed was a spiroplasma (Brinton and Burgdorfer, 1976). Surprisingly, the agent, though it seemed to share a common host with the suckling mouse cataract spiroplasma, appeared to be serologically distinct (Stalheim *et al.*, 1978). Indeed, if initial indications of low DNA-DNA homologies with other spiroplasmas (Junca *et al.*, 1980) are confirmed, the 277F agent may be a new spiroplasma species.

It is remarkable that during the first decade of spiroplasma research, the discoveries of spiroplasmas occurred in almost inverse proportion to the ease with which they could be cultivated. For example, the first spiroplasma to be envisioned, manipulated in the laboratory and studied in detail (the sex ratio spiroplasma), has still not been culti-vated (Williamson and Poulson, 1979). The next spiroplasma to enter the laboratory, the suckling mouse cataract spiroplasma, also grows very slowly. The 277F agent grows more rapidly than SMCA, but not as fast as *S. citri*. The corn stunt agent had been studied in other ways for more than a decade, but difficulties were encountered in its cul-tivation. When the corn stunt agent was finally cultivated, and when soon thereafter the SMCA agent was cultivated, it appeared that, ten years after the report of Doi *et al.* (1967) had stimulated attempts at mycoplasma cultivation the world over, future mycoplasmas would turn out to be increasingly fastidious, and their cultivation would pose vexing problems for students of disease etiology. It therefore came as a surprise (even in an area where surprises had become commonplace) that a major habitat association literally packed with fast growing, readily cultivable spiroplasmas had not yet even been touched! This was the flower habitat.

The discovery began when Truman Clark of the Bioenvironmental Bee Laboratory in Beltsville discovered helical microorganisms in honey bees in his experimental hives (Clark, 1977). Clark recognised that the organisms were similar to spiroplasmas and began a collaborative study with R.E. Davis to elucidate their identity. Clark also recognised that the seasonality of the occurrence of the spiroplasmas indicated that they were probably transmitted from bee to bee in the sites where the bees foraged — in flowers. In the spring, the bees foraged to a major extent in the flowers of the tuliptree, *Liriodendron tulipifera*. Clark and Davis then set out, independently, to search for spiroplasmas in flowers. Their efforts were quickly rewarded (Clark, 1978; Davis, 1978), but in a surprising way. It turned out that spiroplasmas other than the bee spiroplasma commonly occurred in flowers. Also, various sterol-requiring and non-requiring mycoplasmas appeared to be present in the flowers. These nonhelical organisms have not as yet been typed, and their biology remains a complete mystery.

The spiroplasmas isolated from flowers have turned out to consist of three broad groups. The honey bee spiroplasma, upon character-isation and serological analysis, was found to be rather closely related to *S. citri*; species designation does not seem warranted by today's standards of microbial classification. However, two other groups (Clark's OBMG and Davis's 23-6A strain, and Davis's SR-3 strain) are considered candidate spiroplasma species. One of the candidate species appears to be very widespread and occurs in Connecticut (Davis, 1978), Maryland (Muniyappa and Davis, 1980), Florida (McCoy *et al.*, 1979), and the Mediterranean region (Vignault *et al.*, 1980; Tully *et al.*, 1980). Almost all the 'flower spiroplasmas' grow readily in simple media that do not support the growth of more fastidious spiroplasmas. Actually, these organisms are most likely to be associated with certain components of the arthropod assemblage that visits flowers.

In later years of spiroplasma study, attention has focused on arthropods as potential hosts for new spiroplasmas. Spiroplasmas discovered in the leafhopper *Oncometopia* (McCoy *et al.*, 1978) and in *Drosophila hydeii* (Ota *et al.*, 1979) were envisioned but not cultivated. On the other hand, three different spiroplasmas apparently occurred in the green leaf bug in Taiwan (Lei *et al.*, 1979). One closely resembles *S. citri* serologically, but another (LB-12) may represent a new spiro-plasma serovar or species; the third spiroplasma could not be cultivated (Lei *et al.*, 1979).

Further isolation attempts from ticks led to the discovery of yet another spiroplasma. The soft tick *Ixodes pacificus* is one of the ticks reputed to be aggressive towards humans. J.G. Tully recently initiated a collaborative study with C. Yunker at the Rocky Mountain Lab-oratory to search for spiroplasmas in this and other ticks of human medical importance. A spiroplasma, the Y-32 agent, emerged in at least six of the pools examined. In all, the potential for arthropods as reservoirs for spiroplasmas today seems, for all practical purposes, unlimited, and one wonders whether spiroplasmas, if all were catalogued, could turn out to be the dominant genus in the class Mollicutes.

7. Concluding Remarks

In conclusion, it is appropriate to acknowledge that grossly different coverage has been given various aspects of this chapter. We are aware of having emphasised our own perspectives and experiences and have given short shrift (or none at all) to other aspects. Hopefully, however, the details of these experiences will have imparted to the reader not only a sense of the work that has been done on plant and insect mycoplasmas but also, to some extent, what it was like to be working with these agents during the years before the discovery of their microbial identity. Perhaps workers who suffered through the difficult times when the etiological knots had yet to be unravelled or who even now are grappling with a mysterious disease, will find that their suffering was not a lonely one. We sincerely hope that there will be opportunities for other workers to present their own perspectives and experiences as we have done. Future historians will then have rich material to build an objective history of this fascinating scientific province.

Acknowledgements

We are indebted to E.C. Calavan for assistance on material relating to citrus stubborn disease, and to Ms Jane Wall of the National Technical Editing Staff of SEA-AR for many useful editorial comments.

References

Alstatt, G.E. (1945). A new corn disease in the Rio Grande Valley. *Plant Disease Reporter 29*, 533-4.
Ball, E.D. (1903). Food plants of some Bythoscopidae. *The Ohio Naturalist, 3*, 397-9.
Bascope, B. and Galindo, J. (1978). Mycoplasmic nature of the 'Mesa Central' corn stunt. *Abstracts of Third International Congress of Plant Pathology, Munich, W. Germany, 1978*, 78.
Bawden, F.C. (1950). *Plant Viruses and Virus Diseases*, 3rd ed. Waltham, Massachusetts: Chronica Botanica Co.
Beakbane, A.B., Slater, C.H.W. and Posnette, A.F. (1972). Mycoplasmas in the phloem of coconut, *Cocos nucifera* L., with lethal yellowing disease. *Journal*

of Horticultural Science (England) 47, 265.

Beijerinck, M.W. (1898). Ueber ein contagium vivum fluidum als Ursache der Fleckenkrankheit der Tabaksblätter. Verhandelingen der Koninklyke Akademie van Wettenschappen te Amsterdam 65, 3-21.

Black, L.M. (1941). Further evidence for multiplication of the aster-yellows virus in the aster leafhopper. Phytopathology 31, 120-35.

— (1943). Some properties of aster-yellows virus. Phytopathology 33, 2.

— (1950). A plant virus that multiplies in its insect vector. Nature 166, 852-3.

— (1959). Biological cycles of plant viruses in insect vectors. In The Viruses, Vol. 2, pp. 157-85, F.M. Burnet and W.M. Stanley (eds). New York: Academic press.

Black, L.M., Brakke, M.K. and Vatter, A.E. (1963). Purification and electron microscopy of tomato spotted-wilt virus. Virology 20, 120-30.

Bordet, J. (1910). La morphologie du microbe de la peripneumoniae des bovides. Annales de la Institut Pasteur (Paris) 24, 161-7.

Borrel, A., Dujardin-Beaumetz, Jeantet and Jouan. (1910). Le microbe de la péripneumoniae. Annales de la Institut Pasteur (Paris) 24, 168-79.

Bové, J.M. and Duplan, J.F. (1974). Les Mycoplasmes/Mycoplasmas. Les Colloques de l'Institut National de la Santé et de la Recherche Médicale 33, 450.

Bové, J.M. and Saillard, C. (1979). Cell biology of spiroplasmas. In The Mycoplasmas, Vol. 3, pp. 83-153, R.F. Whitcomb and J.G. Tully (eds). New York: Academic Press.

Bradfute, O.E., Nault, L.R., Robertson, D.C. and Toler, R.W. (1977). Maize bushy stunt – a disease associated with a nonhelical mycoplasma-like organism. Proceedings of the American Phytopathological Society 4, 171 (Abstract).

Brakke, M.K. (1953). Zonal separations by density-gradient centrifugation. Archives of Biochemistry and Biophysics 45, 275-90.

Brakke, M.K., Vatter, A.E. and Black, L.M. (1954). Size and shape of wound-tumor virus. Brookhaven National Laboratory, Upton, New York. Symposia in Biology 6, 137-56.

Brinton, L.P. and Burgdorfer, W. (1976). Cellular and subcellular organization of the 277F agent: a spiroplasma from the rabbit tick, Haemaphysalis leporis-palustris (Acari: Ixodidae). International Journal of Systematic Bacteriology 26, 554-60.

Calavan, E.C. and Christiansen, D.W. (1966). Effects of stubborn disease on various varieties of citrus trees. Israel Journal of Botany 15, 121-32.

Calavan, E.C. and Oldfield, G.N. (1979). Symptomatology of spiroplasmal plant diseases. In The Mycoplasmas, Vol. 3, pp. 37-64, R.F. Whitcomb and J.G. Tully (eds). New York: Academic Press.

Chanock, R.M., Hayflick, L. and Barile, M.F. (1962). Growth on artificial medium of an agent associated with atypical pneumonia and its identification as a PPLO. Proceedings of the National Academy of Science of the United States of America 48, 41-9.

Chapman, R. (1974). Control aspects of mycoplasma diseases: aster yellows disease. Les Mycoplasmes/Mycoplasmas. Les Colloques de l'Institut National de la Santé et de la Recherche Médicale 33, 251-3.

Chapot, H. (1959). First studies on the stubborn disease of citrus in some Mediterranean countries. In Citrus Virus Diseases, pp. 109-77, J.H. Wallace (ed). Berkeley: University of California, Division of Agricultural Science.

Chen, T.A. and Granados, R.R. (1970). Plant pathogenic mycoplasma-like organism: maintenance in vitro and transmission to Zea mays L. Science 167, 1633-6.

Chen, T.A. and Liao, C.H. (1975). Corn stunt spiroplasma: isolation, cultivation, and proof of pathogenicity. *Science 188*, 1015–17.

Childs, J.F.L., Nour-Eldin, F. and El-Hosseiny, N. (1956). Observations on Egyptian citrus diseases. *Citrus Industry 37 (10)*, 11–16.

Chiykowski, L. (1974). Yellows diseases and vectors. *Les Mycoplasmes/ Mycoplasmas. Les Colloques de l'Institut National de la Santé et de la Recherche Médicale 33*, 291–7.

— (1977). Cryopreservation of aster yellows agent in whole leafhoppers. *Canadian Journal of Microbiology 23*, 1038–40.

Cirillo, V.P. (1979). Transport systems, In *The Mycoplasmas*, Vol. 1, pp. 323–49, M.F. Barile and S. Razin (eds). New York: Academic Press.

Clark, H.F. (1964). Suckling mouse cataract agent. *Journal of Infectious Diseases 114*, 476–87.

Clark, H.F. and Rorke, L.B. (1979). Spiroplasmas of tick origin and their pathogenicity. In *The Mycoplasmas*, Vol. 3, pp. 155–74, R.F. Whitcomb and J.G. Tully (eds). New York: Academic Press.

Clark, T.B. (1977). *Spiroplasma* sp., a new pathogen in honey bees. *Journal of Invertebrate Pathology 29*, 112–13.

— (1978). Honey bee spiroplasmosis, a new problem for beekeepers. *American Bee Journal 118*, 18–19, 23.

Cole, R.M., Tully, J.G., Popkin, T.J. and Bové, J.M. (1973). Ultrastructure of the agent of citrus 'stubborn disease'. *Journal of Bacteriology 115*, 367–86.

Cole, R.M., Tully, J.G. and Popkin, T.J. (1974). Virus-like particles in *Spiroplasma citri. Les Mycoplasmes/Mycoplasmas. Les Colloques de l'Institut National de la Santé et de la Recherche Médicale 33*, 125–32.

Daniels, M.J. (1979). Mechanisms of spiroplasma pathogenicity. In *The Mycoplasmas*, Vol. 3, pp. 209–27, R.F. Whitcomb and J.G. Tully (eds). New York: Academic Press.

Davis, R.E. (1974). Spiroplasma in corn stunt-infected individuals of the vector leafhopper *Dalbulus maidis. Plant Disease Reporter 58*, 1109–12.

— (1978). Spiroplasma associated with flowers of the tulip tree (*Liriodendron tulipifera* L.) *Canadian Journal of Microbiology 24*, 954–9.

Davis, R.E., Dupont, G., Saglio, P., Roy, B., Vignault, J.C. and Bové, J.M. (1974). Spiroplasmas. Studies on the mircoorganism associated with corn stunt disease. *Les Mycoplasmes/Mycoplasmas. Les Colloques de l'Institut National de la Santé et de la Recherche Médicale 33*, 187–94.

Davis, R.E. and Worley, J.F. (1973). Spiroplasma: motile helical microorganisms associated with corn stunt disease. *Phytopathology 63*, 403–8.

Davis, R.E., Worley, J.F., Whitcomb, R.F., Ishijima, T. and Steere, R.L. (1972). Helical filaments produced by a mycoplasma-like organism associated with corn stunt disease. *Science 176*, 521–3.

de Bary, A. (1853). *Untersuchungen über die Brandpilze und die durch sie verursachten Krankheiten der Pflanzen mit Rücksicht auf das Getreide und andere Nutzpflanzen*. Müller, Berlin.

— (1861). *Die gegenwärtig herrschende Kartoffelkrankheit, ihre Ursache und ihre Verhütung*. Leipzig.

de Zoeten, G.A., Gaard, G. and Diez, F.B. (1972). Nuclear vesiculation associated with pea enation mosaic virus-infected plant tissue. *Virology 48*, 638–47.

Diener, T.O. and Raymer, W.B. (1967). Potato spindle tuber virus: a plant virus with properties of a free nucleic acid. *Science 158*, 378–81.

Dobroscky, I.D. (1929). Is the aster-yellows virus detectable in its insect vector? *Phytopathology 19*, 1009–15.

Doi, Y., Teranaka, M., Yora, K. and Asuyama, H. (1967). Mycoplasma or PLT group-like microorganisms found in the phloem elements of plants infected with mulberry dwarf, potato witches' broom, aster yellows, or Paulownia

witches' broom. *Annals of the Phytopathological Society of Japan 33*, 259–66.
Drake, D.C. and Chapman, R.K. (1965). Evidence for long distance migration of the six-spotted leafhopper into Wisconsin, *University of Wisconsin Research Bulletin 261*, Part 1, 3–20.
Dujardin-Beaumetz, E. (1900). *Le microbe de la péripneumonie et sa culture.* These de Paris, Paris, Octave Doin.
Eden-Green, S. (1979). Attempts to transmit lethal yellowing disease of coconut in Jamaica by leafhoppers (Homoptera: Cicadelloidae). *Tropical Agriculture, Trinidad 56*, 185–92.
Eden-Green, S. and Tully, J.G. (1980). Isolation of *Acholeplasma* spp. from coconut palms affected by lethal yellowing disease in Jamaica. *Current Microbiology 2*, 311–16.
Edward, D.G. ff. and Freundt, E.A. (1967). Proposal for *Mollicutes* as name of the class established for the order *Mycoplasmatales*. *International Journal of Systematic Bacteriology 17*, 267–8.
— (1970). Amended nomenclature for strains related to *Mycoplasma laidlawii*. *Journal of General Microbiology 62*, 1–2.
Elford, W.J. (1929). Ultrafiltration methods and their application in bacteriological and pathological studies. *British Journal of Experimental Pathology 10*, 126–44.
Elliott, K. and Birch, J. Jr. (eds). (1972). *Pathogenic Mycoplasmas. Ciba Foundation Symposium.* New York: Associated Scientific Poblishers.
Fawcett, H.S. (1946). Stubborn disease of citrus, a virosis. *Phytopathology 36*, 675–77.
Fawcett, H.S., Perry, J.C. and Johnston, J.C. (1944). The stubborn disease of citrus. *California Citrograph 29*, 146–7.
Fawcett, W. (1891). Report on the coconut disease at Montego Bay. *Bulletin of the Botanical Department of Jamaica 23*, 2.
Felt, E.P. (1906). Insects affecting park and woodland trees. *New York State Museum Memoirs 8*, 732.
Fox, G.E., Stackebrandt, E., Hespell, R.B., Gibson, J., Maniloff, J., Dyer, T., Wolfe, R.S., Balch, W., Tanner, R., Magrum, L., Zablen, L.B., Blakemore, R., Gupta, R., Bonen, L., Lewis, B.J., Chen, K.N. and Woese, C.R. (1980). The phylogeny of prokaryotes. *Science 209*, 457–63.
Frazier, N.W. (1945). A streak disease of corn in California. *Plant Disease Reporter 29*, 212–13.
Frazier, N.W. and Severin, H.H.P. (1945). Weed-host range of California aster yellows. *Hilgardia 16*, 621–50.
Freitag, J.H. (1964). Interaction and mutual suppression among three strains of aster-yellows virus. *Virology 24*, 401–13.
Freundt, E.A. (1974). Taxonomy and host relationships of mycoplasmas. *Les Mycoplasmes/Mycoplasmas. Les Colloques de l'Institut National Santé et de la Recherche Médicale 33*, 19–26.
Freundt, E.A. and Edward, D.G. ff. (1979). Classification and taxonomy. In *The Mycoplasmas*, Vol. 1, pp. 1–41, M.F. Barile and S. Razin (eds). New York: Academic Press.
Fudl-Allah, A.E.-S., Calavan, E.C. and Igwegbe, E.C.K. (1972). Culture of a mycoplasma-like organism associated with stubborn disease of citrus. *Phytopathology 62*, 729–31.
Giannotti, J. and Giannotti, D. (1978). Culture 'in vitro' d'un mycoplasme de plante agent de proliferation et de nanisme chez *Trifolium repens* L. *Annales de Phytopathologie 10*, 489–92.
Gierer, A. and Schramm, G. (1956). Infectivity of ribonucleic acid from tobacco mosaic virus. *Nature (London) 177*, 702–3.

Gilmer, R.M. and Blodgett, E.C. (1976). X-disease. In: *Virus Diseases and Non-infectious Disorders of Stone Fruits in North America*. United States Department of Agriculture Handbook *437*, 145–55.

Gogolak, F.M. and Weiss, E. (1950). The effect of antibiotics on agents of the psittacosis-lymphogranuloma group. II The effect of aureomycin. *Journal of Infectious Diseases 87*, 264–74.

Gourlay, R.N. (1970). Isolation of a virus infecting a strain of *Mycoplasma laidlawii*. *Nature (London) 225*, 1165.

Granados, R.R. (1969). Electron microscopy of plants and insect vectors infected with corn stunt disease agent. *Contributions from Boyce Thompson Institute 24*, 173–88.

Granados, R.R., Hirumi, H. and Maramorosch, K. (1967). Electron microscopic evidence for wound-tumor virus accumulation in various organs of an inefficient leafhopper vector, *Agalliopsis novella*. *Journal of Invertebrate Pathology 9*, 147–59.

Granados, R.R., Maramorosch, K., Everett, T. and Pirone, T.P. (1966). Leaf-hopper transmission of a corn stunt virus from Louisiana. *Phytopathology 56*, 584.

Granados, R.R., Maramorosch, K. and Shikata, E. (1968). *Mycoplasma*: Suspected etiologic agent of corn stunt. *Proceedings of the National Academy of Sciences of the United States of America 60*, 841–4.

Grylls, N.E. and Hunt, P. (1971). A review of the study of the aetiology of coconut lethal yellowing disease. *Oleagineux 26*, 311–15.

Hansen, H.P. (1952). On the so-called 'unknown disease' and related diseases on coconut palms in the West Indies. *Plant Disease Reporter 36*, 66–7.

Hartzell, A. (1935). A study of peach yellows and its insect vector. *Contributions from Boyce Thompson Institute 7*, 183-207.

Hayflick, L. (1969). Fundamental biology of the Class Mollicutes, Order Mycoplasmatales. In *The Mycoplasmatales and the L-phase of Bacteria*, pp. 15–47, L. Hayflick (ed). New York: Appleton-Century-Crofts.

Heinze, K.G., Petzold, H. and Marwitz, R. (1972). Beitrag zur Ätiologie der Tödlichen Vergilbung der Kokospalme. *Phytopathologische Zeitschrift 74*, 230–7.

Hershey, A.D. and Chase, M. (1952). Independent functions of viral protein and nucleic acid in growth of bacteriophage. *Journal of General Physiology 34*, 305–19.

Hibino, H. and Schneider, H. (1970). Mycoplasma-like bodies in sieve tubes of pear trees affected with pear decline. *Phytopathology 60*, 499–501.

Howard, F.W. and Thomas, D.L. (1980). Transmission of palm lethal decline to *Veitchia merilli* by the planthopper *Myndus crudus*. *Journal of Economic Entomology* (in press).

Igwegbe, E.C.K. and Calavan, E.C. (1970). Occurrence of mycoplasmalike bodies in phloem of stubborn-infected citrus seedlings. *Phytopathology 60*, 1525-6.

— (1973). Effect of tetracycline antibiotics on symptom development of stubborn disease and infectious variegation of citrus seedlings. *Phytopathology 63*, 1044-8.

Ishiie, T., Doi, Y., Yora, K. and Asuyama, H. (1967). Suppressive effects of antibiotics of tetracycline group on symptom development of mulberry dwarf disease. *Annals of the Phytopathological Society of Japan 33*, 267–75.

Ivanowski, D. (1892). Ueber die Mosaikkrankheit der Tabakspflanze. *St. Petersbourg Academi Imperiale des Sciences Bulletin 35* (nouvelle serie i.e. serie 4, v. 3), 67–70.

Jensen, D.D. (1959). A plant virus lethal to its vector. *Virology 8*, 164–75.

Jensen, D.D., Whitcomb, R.F. and Richardson, J. (1967). Lethality of injected peach western X-disease virus to its leafhopper vector. *Virology 31*, 532–8.

Jones, A.L., Whitcomb, R.F., Williamson, D.L. and Coan, M.E. (1977). Comparative growth and primary isolation of spiroplasmas in media based on insect tissue culture formulations. *Phytopathology 67*, 738–46.

Junca, P., Saillard, C., Tully, J., Garcia-Jurado, O., Degorge-Dumas, J.R., Mouches, C., Vignault, J.C., Vogel, R., McCoy, R., Whitcomb, R., Williamson, D., Latrille, J., and Bové, J.M. (1980). Caracterisation de spiroplasmes isolés d'insectes et de fleurs de France continentale, de Corse et du Maroc: Proposition pour une classification de spiroplasmes. *Comptes Rendus des Séances Hebdomadaires de l'Academie des Sciences, Paris, Série D 290*, 1209-12.

Kahane, I., Greenstein, S. and Razin, S. (1977). Carbohydrate content and enzymic activities in the membrane of *Spiroplasma citri*. *Journal of General Microbiology 101*, 173-6.

Klieneberger-Nobel, E. (1962). *Pleuropneumonia-like Organisms (PPLO): Mycoplasmataceae*. New York: Academic Press.

Koch, R. (1877). Untersuchungen über Bacterien. V. Die Aetiologie der Milzbrand-Krankheit, begründet auf die Entwicklungsgesichte des Bacillus Anthracis. *Beiträge zur Biologie der Pflanzen 2*, 277-310 (with 11 figures).

Kunkel, L.O. (1926). Studies on aster yellows. *American Journal of Botany 13*, 646–705.

— (1931). Studies on aster yellows in some new host plants. *Contributions from Boyce Thompson Institute 3*, 85-123.

— (1932). Celery yellows of California not identical with the aster yellows of New York. *Contributions from Boyce Thompson Institute 4*, 405-14.

— (1933). Insect transmission of peach yellows. *Contributions from Boyce Thompson Institute 5*, 19-28.

— (1937). Effect of heat on ability of *Cicadula sexnotata* (Fall.) to transmit aster yellows. *American Journal of Botany 24*, 316-27.

— (1938). Insects in relation to diseases of fruit trees and small fruits. *Journal of Economic Entomology 31*, 20.

— (1946). Leafhopper transmission of corn stunt. *Proceedings of the National Academy of Sciences of the United States of America 22*, 246-7.

— (1948). Studies on a new corn virus disease. *Archiv für die Gesamte Virusforschung 4*, 24-46.

— (1952). Transmission of alfalfa witches' broom to nonleguminous plants by dodder, and cure in periwinkle by heat. *Phytopathology 42*, 27-31.

— (1954). Maintenance of yellows-type viruses in plant and insect reservoirs. In *The Dynamics of Virus and Rickettsial Infections*, pp. 150-63, F.W. Hartman, F.L. Horsfall and J.G. Kidd (eds). New York: McGraw-Hill (Blakiston).

— (1955). Cross-protection between strains of yellows-type viruses. *Advances in Virus Research 3*, 251-73.

Kunkel, L.O., Blake, M.A. and Manns, T.F. (1951). Peach yellows. In *Virus Diseases and Other Disorders with Viruslike Symptoms of Stone Fruits in North America*, United States Department of Agriculture Handbook *10*, 1-3.

Lafleche, D. and Bové, J.M. (1970). Mycoplasmes dans les agrumes atteints de 'greening', de 'stubborn' ou de maladies similaires. *Fruits 25*, 455-65.

Leach, R. (1946). The unknown disease of the coconut palm in Jamaica. *Tropical Agriculture, Trinidad 23*, 50-60.

Lee, I.M., Cartia, G., Calavan, E.C. and Kaloostian, G.H. (1973). Citrus stubborn disease organism cultured from beet leafhopper. *California Agriculture 27 (11)*, 14-15.

Lei, J.D., Su, H.H. and Chen, T.A. (1979). Spiroplasmas isolated from green leafbug, *Trigonotylus ruficornis* Geoffroy. In *Proceedings of ROC* –

United States Cooperative Science Seminar on Mycoplasma Diseases in Plants. NSC Symposium Series I, 89-97. Taipei: National Science Council.

Liao, C.H. and Chen, T.A. (1975). A simple medium for the isolation and cultivation of corn stunt spiroplasma. *Proceedings of the American Phytopathological Society 2*, 100.

— (1977). Culture of corn stunt spiroplasma in a simple medium. *Phytopathology 67*, 802-7.

Loeffler and Frosch (1898). Berichte der Kommission zur Erforschung der Maulund Klauenseuch bei dem Institut für Infektionskrankheiten in Berlin. *Zentralblatt für Bakteriologie, Parasitenkunde und Infektionskrankheiten 23*, 371-91.

Lowe, S.K. and Raju, B.C. (1978). The morphology of spiroplasmas associated with aster yellows and pear decline diseases: A comparative study by negative staining *in vitro*. *Phytopathology News 12 (9)*, 216.

Malogolowkin, C. (1958). Maternally inherited 'sex-ratio' conditions in *Drosophila willistoni* and *Drosophila paulistorum*. *Genetics 43*, 274-86.

Malagolowkin, C. and Poulson, D.F. (1957). Infective transfer of maternally inherited abnormal sex-ratio in *Drosophila willistoni*. *Science 126*, 32.

Malogolowkin, C., Poulson, D.F. and Wright, E.Y. (1959). Experimental transfer of maternally inherited abnormal sex-ratio in *Drosophila willistoni*. *Genetics 43*, 274-86.

Manns, T.F. (1932). Dissemination of peach yellows and little peach – Is the periodical cicada responsible? *University of Delaware Agricultural Experiment Station Bulletin 179*, 46-7.

— (1934). The dissemination of yellows and little peach. *University of Delaware Agricultural Experiment Station Bulletin 188*, 36-8.

— (1942). Peach yellows and little peach. *University of Delaware Agriculture Experiment Station Bulletin 236*, 50.

Maramorosch, K. (1952). Direct evidence for the multiplication of aster-yellows virus in its insect vector. *Phytopathology 42*, 59-64.

— (1953). Incubation period of aster yellows virus. *American Journal of Botany 40*, 797-809.

— (1955). The occurrence of two distinct types of corn stunt in Mexico. *Plant Disease Reporter 39*, 896-8.

— (1958). Cross protection between two strains of corn stunt virus in an insect vector. *Virology 6*, 448-59.

— (1972). Letter to the editor: The enigma of mycoplasma in plants and insects. *Phytopathology 62*, 1230-1.

— (ed) (1973). Mycoplasma and mycoplasmalike agents of human, animal, and plant diseases. *Annals of the New York Academy of Sciences, 225*, 532.

Maramorosch, K., Granados, R.R. and Hirumi, H. (1970). Mycoplasma diseases of plants and insects. *Advances in Virus Research 16*, 135-93.

Maramorosch, K. and Kondo, F. (1978). Aster yellows spiroplasma: Infectivity and association with a rod-shaped virus. *Zentralblatt für Bakteriologie, Parasitenkunde, Infektionskrankheiten und Hygiene Erste Abteilung Originale, 241*, 196.

Markham, P.G., Townsend, R., Bar-Joseph, M., Daniels, M.J., Plaskitt, A. and Meddins, B.M. (1974). Spiroplasmas are the causal agents of citrus little-leaf disease. *Annals of Applied Biology 78*, 49-57.

Martyn, E.B. (1945a). Coconut diseases in Jamaica. 1. Bronze leaf wilt and other diseases affecting the bud of coconuts. *Tropical Agriculture, Trinidad 22*, 51-9.

— (1945b). Coconut diseases in Jamaica. 2. Diseases affecting the leaves, crown and stem of coconuts. *Tropical Agriculture, Trinidad 22*, 69-76.

Martyn, E.B. (1955). Diseases of coconuts. *Tropical Agriculture, Trinidad 32*, 162-9.

McCoy, R.E. (1979). Mycoplasmas and yellows diseases. In *The Mycoplasmas*, Vol. 3, pp. 229-64, R.F. Whitcomb and J.G. Tully (eds). New York: Academic Press.

McCoy, R.E., Tsai, J.H. and Thomas, D.L. (1978). Occurrence of a spiroplasma in natural populations of the sharpshooter *Oncometopia nigricans. Phytopathology News 12 (9)*, 217.

McCoy, R.E., Williams, D.S. and Thomas, D.L. (1979). Isolation of mycoplasmas from flowers. In *Proceedings of ROC – United States Cooperative Science Seminar: Mycoplasma Diseases of Plants.* NSC Symposium Series I, 75-81. Taipei: National Science Council.

McCubbin, W.A. (1928). Peach yellows report – 1927. *Pennsylvania Department of Agriculture General Bulletin 460*, 25pp. (Alternative notation: *Volume 11, Bulletin 6.*)

Merrett, C. (1666). *Pinax Rerum Naturalium Britannicarum*, London.

Moulder, J.W. (1966). The relation of the psittacosis group (Chlamydiae) to bacteria and viruses. *Annual Review of Microbiology 20*, 107-30.

Mudd, J.B., Ittig, M., Roy, B., Latrille, J. and Bové, J.M. (1977). Composition and enzyme activities of *Spiroplasma citri* membranes. *Journal of Bacteriology 129*, 1250-6.

Muniyappa, V. and Davis, R.E. (1980). Occurrence of spiroplasmas of two serogroups on flowers of the tulip tree (*Liriodendron tulipifera* L.) in Maryland. *Current Science 49*, 58-60.

Nasu, S., Jensen, D.D. and Richardson, J. (1970). Electron microscopy of mycoplasma-like bodies associated with insect and plant hosts of peach western X-disease. *Virology 41*, 583-95.

Nasu, S., Sugiura, M., Wakimoto, T. and Iida, T.T. (1967). On the pathogen of rice yellow dwarf virus. *Annals of the Phytopathological Society of Japan 33*, 343 (Abstract in Japanese).

Nault, L.R. (1980). Maize bushy stunt and corn stunt: A comparison of disease symptoms, host range and vectors. *Phytopathology 70*, 659-62.

Nault, L.R. and Bradfute, O.E. (1979). Corn stunt: Involvement of a complex of leafhopper-borne pathogens. In *Leafhopper Vectors and Plant Disease Agents*, pp. 561-86, K. Maramorosch and K. Harris (eds). New York: Academic Press.

Nault, L.R., Gordon, D.T., Gingery, R.E., Bradfute, O.E. and Loayza, J.C. (1979). Identification of maize viruses and mollicutes and their potential insect vectors in Peru. *Phytopathology 69*, 824-8.

Nocard, Roux, Borrel, Salimbeni and Dujardin-Beaumetz (1898). Le microbe de la peripneumonie. *Annales de la Institut Pasteur (Paris) 12*, 244-62.

Nour-Eldin, F. (1959). Citrus virus disease: research in Egypt. In *Citrus Virus Diseases*, pp. 219-27, J.M. Wallace (ed). Berkeley: University of California Division of Agricultural Sciences.

Oldfield, G.N., Kaloostian, G.H., Pierce, H.D., Calavan, E.C., Granett, A.L. and Blue, R.L. (1976). Beet leafhopper transmits citrus stubborn disease. *California Agriculture 30 (6)*, 15.

Oldfield, G.N., Kaloostian, G.H., Pierce, H.D., Calavan, E.C., Granett, A.L., Blue, R.L., Rana, G.L. and Gumpf, D.J. (1977). Transmission of *Spiroplasma citri* from citrus to citrus by *Scaphytopius nitridus. Phytopathology 67*, 763-5.

Orenski, S.W., Murray, J.R. and Maramorosch, K. (1965). Further studies on the feeding habits of aster-yellows virus-carrying corn leafhoppers. *Contributions from Boyce Thompson Institute 23*, 47-50.

Ota, T., Kawabe, M., Oishi, K. and Poulson, D.F. (1979). Non-male-killing spiroplasmas in *Drosophila hydei. Journal of Heredity 70*, 211-13.

Ozkal, I. (1958). Pleuropneumonia-like organism'ler (PPLO) uzerinde araspirmalar.
II. Kucuk kirmizi purp yapraklarindan izole edilen pleuropneumonia-like
organism'ler (PPLO). *Turk Veteriner Hekimleri Dernegi Dergisi 28*, 44-50
(with English summary).

Patt, J. (1964). Observations on the appearance of the 'little leaf' (stubborn)
disease of citrus. *Plant Disease Reporter 48*, 761-2.

Pereira, A.L.G. and Oliveira, B.S. (1971). Isolamento e trasmissao direta do agente
causal do enfezamento do milho (corn stunt) cultivado em meio artificial de
cultura. *Arquivos do Instituto Biologico, Sao Paulo 38*, 191-200.

Pickens, E.G., Gerloff, R.K. and Burgdorfer, W. (1968). Spirochete from the rabbit
tick *Haemaphysalis leporispaulustris* (Packard). *Journal of Bacteriology 95*,
291-9.

Plavsic-Banjac, B. and Maramorosch, K. (1972). Mycoplasma-like bodies associated
with lethal yellowing disease of coconut palms. *Phytopathology 62*, 298-9.

Poulson, D.F. and Sakaguchi, B. (1961). Nature of 'sex ratio' agent in *Drosophila.
Science 133*, 1489-90.

Rana, G.L., Kaloostian, G.H., Oldfield, G.N., Granett, A.L., Calavan, E.C., Pierce,
H.D., Lee, I.M. and Gumpf, D.J. (1975). Acquisition of *Spiroplasma citri*
through membranes by homopterous insects. *Phytopathology 65*, 1143-5.

Reichert, I. (1958). Citrus virus diseases in the Mediterranean and the New World.
FAO Plant Protection Bulletin 6, 180-3.

Reichert, I. and Perlberger, J. (1931). Little leaf disease of citrus trees and its
cause. *Hadar 4*, 193-4.

Romney, D.H. (1972). Past studies on and present status of lethal yellowing
disease of coconuts. *PANS: Pest Articles and News Summaries 18*, 386-95.

Saglio, P., L'Hospital, M., Laflèche, D., Dupont, G., Bové, J.M., Tully, J.G.
and Freundt, E.A. (1973). *Spiroplasma citri* gen. and sp. n. A mycoplasma-like
organism associated with 'stubborn' disease of citrus. *International Journal of
Systematic Bacteriology 23*, 191-204.

Saglio, P.H.M. and Whitcomb, R.F. (1979). Diversity of wall-less prokaryotes in
plant vascular tissue, fungi, and invertebrate animals. In *The Mycoplasmas*,
Vol. 3, pp. 1-36, R.F. Whitcomb and J.G. Tully (eds). New York: Academic
Press.

Severin, H.H.P. (1921). Minimum incubation periods of causative agent of curly-
leaf in beet leafhopper and sugar beet. *Phytopathology 11*, 424-9.

— (1929). Yellows disease of celery, lettuce, and other plants, transmitted by
Cicadula sexnotata (Fall.). *Hilgardia 3*, 543-83.

— (1945). Evidence of nonspecific transmission of California aster-yellows
virus by leafhoppers. *Hilgardia 17*, 21-59.

Shikata, E. and Maramorosch, K. (1965). Electron microscopic evidence for the
systemic invasion of an insect host by a plant pathogenic virus. *Virology 27*,
461-75.

Skripal, I.G. (1974). On improvement of taxonomy of the class Mollicutes and
establishment in the order Mycoplasmatales of the new family Spiroplasmataceae Fam. Nova. *Mikrobiologicheskii Zhurnal (Kiev) 36*, 462-7.

Smith, A.J. (1980). Maintenance *in vitro* of the aster yellows pathogen. MS
thesis, University of Florida, Gainesville, 51 pp.

Smith, E.F. (1888). Peach yellows: a preliminary report. *United States Department of Agriculture Botanical Division Bulletin 9*, 254 pp.

Smith, R.E. (1902). Growing china asters. *Hatch Experiment Station, Massachusetts Agricultural College, Bulletin 79*, 1-26.

Somerson, N.L., Kocka, J.P. and Del Giudice, R. (1980). Isolation of acholeplasmas from foods. *Proceedings of the 3rd Conference of the International Organization of Mycoplasmology, Custer, South Dakota, 1980, 44.*

Stalheim, O.H.V., Ritchie, A.E. and Whitcomb, R.F. (1978). Cultivation, serology, ultrastructure, and virus-like particles of spiroplasma 277F. *Current Microbiology 1*, 365-70.

Stanley, W.M. (1935). Isolation of a crystalline protein possessing the properties of the tobacco-mosaic virus. *Science 81*, 644-5.

Stearns, L.A. (1927). The Cicadellidae (Homoptera) of Virginia. *Virginia Agricultural Experiment Station Technical Bulletin 31*, 1-21.

Storey, H.H. (1925a). Streak disease of sugar cane. *Union of South Africa Scientific Bulletin 39*, 30 pp.

— (1925b). The transmission of streak disease of maize by the leafhopper *Balclutha mbila* Naude. *Annals of Applied Biology 12*, 422-39.

Subcommittee on the Taxonomy of Mycoplasmatales (1967). Recommendations on nomenclature of the Order Mycoplasmatales. *Science 155*, 1694-6.

— (1972). Proposal for minimal standards for descriptions of new species of the order *Mycoplasmatales. International Journal of Systematic Bacteriology 22*, 184-8.

— (1977). Minutes of interim meeting, 22 September 1976. *International Journal of Systematic Bacteriology 27*, 392-4.

Subcommittee on the Taxonomy of Mollicutes (1979). Proposal of minimal standards for description of new species of the class Mollicutes. *International Journal of Systematic Bacteriology 29*, 172-80.

Takami, N. (1901). Stunt disease of rice and *Nephotettix apicalis. Journal of the Agricultural Society of Japan 241*, 22-30.

Townsend, R., Archer, D.B. and Plaskitt, K.A. (1980). Purification and preliminary characterization of spiroplasma fibrils. *Journal of Bacteriology 142*, 694-700.

Tsai, J.H. (1979a). Vector transmission of mycoplasmal agents of plant diseases. In *The Mycoplasmas*, Vol. 3, pp. 265-307, R.F. Whitcomb and J.G. Tully (eds). New York: Academic Press.

— (1979b). Lethal yellowing of coconut palms; search for a vector. In *Leafhopper Vectors and Plant Disease Agents*, pp. 177-97, K. Maramorosch and K.F. Harris (eds). New York: Academic Press.

Tully, J.G. (1979). Special features of the acholeplasmas. In *The Mycoplasmas*, Vol. 1, pp. 431-49, M.F. Barile and S. Razin (eds). New York: Academic Press.

Tully, J.G., Rose, D.L., Vignault, J.C., Saillard, C., Bové, J.M., Garcia-Jurado, O., McCoy, R.E. and Williamson, D.L. (1980). Serological analysis of a new group of spiroplasmas. *Current Microbiology 3*, 369-72.

Tully, J.G., Whitcomb, R.F., Clark, H.F. and Williamson, D.L. (1977). Pathogenic mycoplasmas: Cultivation and vertebrate pathogenicity of a new spiroplasma. *Science 195*, 892-4.

Tully, J.G., Whitcomb, R.F., Williamson, D.L. and Clark, H.F. (1976). Suckling mouse cataract agent is a helical wall-free prokaryote (spiroplasma) pathogenic for vertebrates. *Nature 259*, 117-20.

Vignault, J.-C., Bové, J.M., Saillard, C., Vogel, R., Farro, A., Venegas, L., Stemmer, W., Aoki, S., McCoy, R., Albeldri, A.A., Larue, M., Tuzcu, O., Ozsam, M., Nhami, A., Abassi, M., Bonfils, J., Moutous, G., Fos, A., Poutiers, F. and Viennot-Bourgin, B. (1980). Mise en culture de spiroplasmes a partir de matériel végétal et d'insectes provenant de pays circum-méditerranéans et du Proche Orient. *Comptes Rendus des Séances Hebdomadaires de l'Academie des Sciences, Paris, Série D 290*, 1209-12.

Weikel, S. (1968). The effect of aureomycin on plant virus. Project Report:

Southern Appalachian Science Fair, Knoxville, Tennessee, 29 March 1968. 10 pp.

Weiss, E. (1950). The effect of antibiotics on agents of the psittacosis-lympho-granuloma group. I. The effect of penicillin. *Journal of Infectious Diseases* 87, 249-63.

— (1968). Comparative metabolism of rickettsiae and other host-dependent bacteria. *Zentralblatt für Bakteriologie, Parasitenkunde, Infektionskrankheiten und Hygiene. Erste Abteilung Originale, 206*, 292-8.

Whitcomb, R.F. (1981). The biology of spiroplasmas. *Annual Review of Entomology 15*, 405-64.

Whitcomb, R.F. and Davis, R.E. (1970). Mycoplasma and phytarboviruses as plant pathogens persistently transmitted by insects. *Annual Review of Entomology 15*, 405-64.

Whitcomb, R.F., Jensen, D.D. and Richardson, J. (1968a). The infection of leafhoppers by western X-disease virus. V. Properties of the infectious agent. *Journal of Invertebrate Pathology 12*, 192-201.

— (1968b). The infection of leafhoppers by western X-disease virus. VI. Cytopathological interrelationships. *Journal of Invertebrate Pathology 12*, 202-21.

Whitcomb, R.F. and Williamson, D.L. (1975). Helical wall-free prokaryotes in insects: Multiplication and pathogenicity. *Annals of the New York Academy of Sciences 266*, 260-75.

Williamson, D.L. (1974). Unusual fibrils from the spirochete-like sex ratio organism. *Journal of Bacteriology 117*, 904-6.

Williamson, D.L. and Poulson, D.F. (1979). Sex ratio organisms (spiroplasmas) of *Drosophila*. In *The Mycoplasmas*, Vol. 3, pp. 175-208, R.F. Whitcomb and J.G. Tully (eds). New York: Academic Press.

Williamson, D.L. and Whitcomb, R.F. (1974). Helical wall-free prokaryotes in *Drosphila*, leafhoppers and plants. *Les Mycoplasmes/Mycoplasmas. Les Colloques de l'Institut National de la Santé et de la Recherche Médicale 33*, 283-90.

— (1975). Plant mycoplasmas: A cultivable spiroplasma causes corn stunt disease. *Science 188*, 1018-20.

Windsor, I.M. and Black, L.M. (1973). Remission of symptoms of clover club leaf following treatment with penicillin. *Phytopathology 63*, 44-6.

Woese, C.R., Maniloff, J. and Zablen, L.B. (1980). Phylogenetic analysis of the mycoplasmas. *Proceedings of the National Academy of Sciences of the United States of America 77*, 494-8.

Wolanski, B.S. (1973). Negative staining of plant agents. *Annals of the New York Academy of Sciences 225*, 223-53.

Wolanski, B. and Maramorosch, K. (1970). Negatively stained mycoplasmas: Fact or artifact? *Virology 42*, 319-27.

Wolfe, H.R., Anthon, E.W., Kaloostian, G.H. and Jones, L.S. (1951). Leafhopper transmission of western X-disease. *Journal of Economic Entomology 44*, 616-19.

Wood, J.I. (1953). Three billion dollars a year. *United States Department of Agriculture Yearbook: Plant Diseases*, 1-9.

3 THE 'YELLOWS' PLANT DISEASES: PLANT HOSTS AND THEIR INTERACTION WITH THE PATHOGENS

P.G. Markham

1. Introduction

The 'yellows' are now a well-established group of plant diseases that occur in temperate and tropical regions. They infect over 300 genera of plants including monocotyledons and dicotyledons, trees and herbaceous plants. Most of the yellows diseases are associated with mycoplasma-like organisms (MLO) or with the spiroplasmas, but a few are associated with small bacteria or rickettsia-like organisms (RLO). The MLO, spiroplasmas and some of the RLO are found only in the phloem sieve cells, while other RLOs are found only in the xylem vessels of infected plants. Associating MLOs and RLOs with a disease syndrome has relied mainly on observing the symptoms and establishing the presence of organisms by electron microscopy (Chapter 4) or by implication following chemotherapy (Chapter 5).

2. Identification and Nomenclature

Until the late 1960s it was assumed that the yellows diseases were caused by viruses. Consequently the traditional nomenclature was used by plant pathologists, and the names were derived from the host plant, in which a disease was found, coupled with the most conspicuous disease symptom; for example clover phyllody, corn stunt.

Although about 100 of these MLO-associated diseases have now been reported it has not yet been possible to establish how many different species of organisms are implicated. At present the etiologic agent of only three of these diseases has been irrefutably established; corn stunt (Chen and Liao, 1975; Williamson and Whitcomb, 1975) and citrus stubborn (Markham *et al.*, 1974) are caused by spiroplasmas and Pierce's disease of grapes is caused by a bacterium or RLO (Davis *et al.*, 1978). The citrus stubborn spiroplasma is the only plant pathogenic mycoplasma which has been fully characterised and named, *Spiroplasma citri* (Saglio *et al.*, 1973). The relatedness of *S. citri* to other microorganisms is still under discussion (see Chapter 2).

This lack of information means that identification, at least at field level, relies on symptoms and host range studies, which can often be inconclusive. We now know that the agents may occur as different strains, which may give different symptoms in the same hosts, e.g. the celery and non celery infecting strains of aster yellows. It is also possible that different agents may cause the same symptoms in a single host species. Conversely the diseases clover phyllody and strawberry green petal are probably the same agent but in different hosts, while a Canadian isolate of clover phyllody infected 79 species in 22 families (Chiykowski, 1974). Similarly citrus stubborn and citrus little leaf are caused by the same spiroplasma which will also infect more than 30 species of plants in 13 families (Calavan and Oldfield, 1979).

It has also been shown that some field infections may be caused by a mixture of agents, e.g. MLO-virus complex (aster yellows and oat blue dwarf virus); MLO-MLO complex (as in some corn stunt-MLO infections) (Banttari and Zeyen, 1979; Nault and Bradfute, 1979). Double infections of *S. citri* and MLOs have also been found (Oldfield, 1980).

3. Symptomatology

A. Symptoms

It is evident from a study of a list of yellows diseases (Markham, 1978) that a number of descriptive symptoms occur repeatedly, e.g. virescence, phyllody, stunt, proliferation ('witches' broom'), etc. Many of the abnormalities in growth and development suggest that the cause may be due to an imbalance in levels of plant hormones such as gibberellins, auxins and cytokinins. How the MLO cause these hormonal imbalances is not yet understood. Other symptoms appear to be due to nutritional deficiencies which can be ameliorated by certain ions (Carr and Stoddart, 1963).

The yellowing of the foliage is a major characteristic of the group, but the leaves may develop with abnormal midveins and misshapen lamellae (Figure 3.1). The chlorosis may be anything from mild and localised to severe and affecting the entire plant. The first symptom is often vein clearing (Figures 3.1 and 3.4c). The extent of yellowing is often characteristic for a given disease-host combination, e.g. in *Vinca* infected with corn stunt the young leaves are chlorotic and the edges of the older leaves are yellowed and wavy (Figure 3.2c), while in maize the yellowing forms longitudinal stripes which may coalesce until the entire lamellae are yellowed (Figure 3.2b). The older leaves on many infected plants may abscise prematurely resulting in a 'bunchy' appearance of the branch tips (Figure 3.7).

Figure 3.1: Leaves of *Vinca* showing a Range of Typical Symptoms: Mild, Chlorosis, Yellowed Patches, Vein Clearing, Distortion of Mid-veins and Lamellae. Healthy leaves on left. Leaves taken from plants with different 'yellows' diseases.

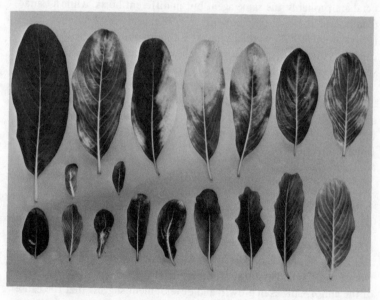

Figure 3.2: Corn Stunt Disease in (a, b) Maize and (c) Periwinkle

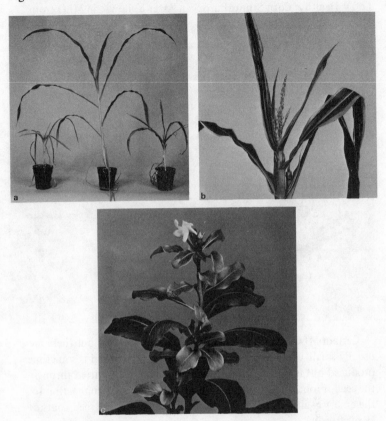

Growth is usually slower after infection resulting in shorter inter-nodes ('stunt') and small leaves ('little leaf') (Figures 3.2, 3.3, 3.4c and d), while in other diseases the shoots may be swollen (hypertrophy) or chlorotic or etiolated (Figure 3.4b). The proliferation of side shoots lead to 'bunchy' and 'witches' broom' symptoms (Figures 3.4c and d, 3.7).

Flowers may be reduced in size or initiation of flowers may cease. However a common symptom is a greening or virescence of flowers, which may later be replaced by a 'phyllody' (the growth of leaf-like structures instead of the normal floral parts (Figures 3.5 and 3.6)). This vegetative growth may produce other virescent and phyllody flowers which further accentuate the 'bushy' growths on the branches (Figure 3.7a).

Figure 3.3: Tips of Periwinkle Branches Infected with (Clockwise from Left): Healthy; Corn Stunt; European Aster Yellows; an MLO from Primula; an MLO from Cabbage

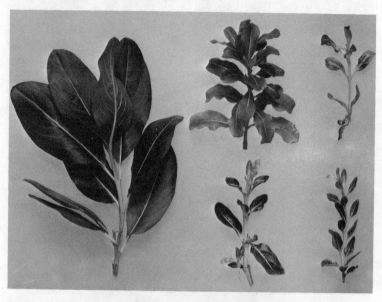

Certain MLO-infected plants may still produce fruit but these are usually small, often deformed and of poor quality. Seed is sometimes produced but is usually infertile. MLOs are not transmitted through the seed, probably because there is no direct vascular connection to the embryo, although *S. citri* may be isolated from the seed coats of citrus fruits.

B. Development of Symptoms

The symptoms are usually more extreme in herbaceous plants, although diseased plants may survive for many years. Large trees often decline slowly or infections may be localised for a number of years (Figure 3.8c). However a few diseases may kill the plants rapidly; in a few weeks, as for example in herbaceous plants infected with *S. citri*, or in a few months, as for example in the case of mature trees of elm infected with phloem necrosis and palms infected with lethal yellowing. This rapid decline in the vigour of these yellows-infected plants is not attributable to any physical plugging of the vascular tissue, despite the high numbers (10^9 per ml of phloem sap) that the MLOs are thought to reach, except in the case of xylem-restricted RLO. In the

Figure 3.4: (a) Early Symptoms of European Aster Yellows; (b) Early and (c) Late Symptoms of an MLO from Primula; (d) *Opuntia tuna* — Healthy (left) and 'Monstrose' Variant (right) Caused by MLO Infection

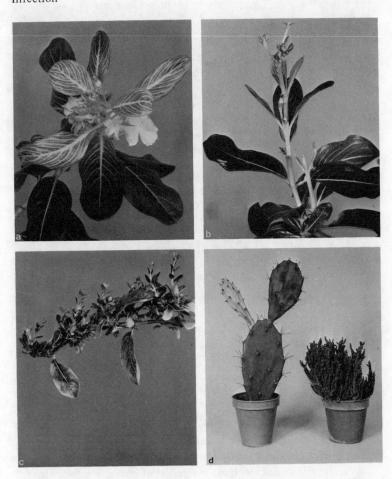

latter case the numbers of organisms and the production of poly-saccharide-like material may be the main cause of a wilting symptom. However of the MLO disorders *S. citri* is unusual since wilting follows the more typical yellows symptoms. In this case a toxin is produced (see Chapter 11) which seems to affect the roots and the uptake of water. Turgor can be re-established by placing the branches in water. Similarly a toxin may be involved in the rapid decline of elm necrosis

Figure 3.5: Clover Phyllody Symptoms in Flowers of Periwinkle. Normal flower (top left). Early symptoms are a greening (virescence) of the petals; the flowers then become increasingly leaf-like (phyllody).

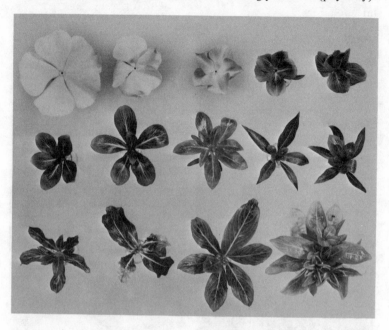

and lethal yellowing of palms (Figure 3.8a and b).

In general the younger the plant at the time of infection, the more severe are the symptoms. However, the MLO-associated lethal yellowing disease has not been observed in young palms less than two years old, and a similar situation is found with a disease of clove trees in Sumatra, which is probably caused by a xylem-restricted RLO (Dr P. Hunt, personal communication). Exceptions such as these may only reflect a lack of experimental data due to difficulty in transmitting the diseases or recognising plants with early symptoms.

With all yellows diseases there is a period of incubation following infection before the plant shows the first symptoms. In most cases where an experimental method of transmission is not available, the incubation period is unknown. The incubation is usually between two and six weeks, but periods of two months to a year have been recorded. The symptoms are usually seen first at the growing points nearest the site of inoculation. The MLO probably reach the highest concentration at the growing tips of roots and shoots just before the onset of severe

Figure 3.6: Clover Phyllody in Periwinkle. Early symptoms (a) and severe phyllody (c) with the leaves removed (b and d) to show the succession of flowers.

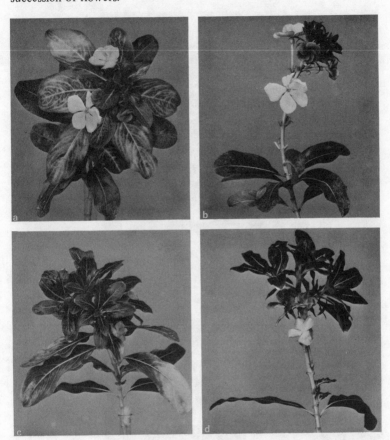

symptoms (Daniels *et al.*, 1981). They are also rapidly transported in the phloem sap and usually become systemic. There are two common features: (a) some branches may not show symptoms until a long time after the remainder of the plant becomes severely affected; (b) infected shoots often appear near the base of the plant, particularly in plants that have shown remission of symptoms.

By analogy to plant virology where infected but symptomless plants are known, there is the possibility that a similar effect may exist with MLO infections, although there are no reports to date. The 'monstrose' variants of *Opuntia* cactus appear 'healthy' despite the fact that the

Figure 3.7: Later Stages in Infection (a) Clover Phyllody, (b) an MLO from Primula. Loss of original foliage leaves gives 'bunchy' appearance to branches.

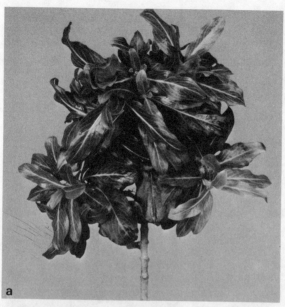

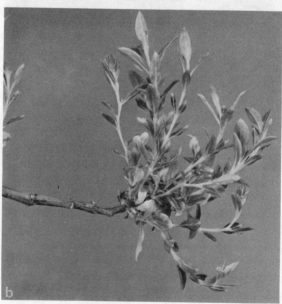

Figure 3.8: A Rapid Decline: Lethal Yellowing of Palms in (a) Jamaica and (b) Florida. Fronds turn yellow, the head rapidly disintegrates until only the trunk remains. A Slow Decline: (c) Sandle Spike Disease in India (photograph by permission of Dr R. Hull, John Innes Institute).

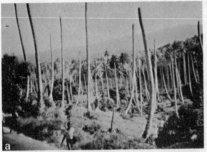
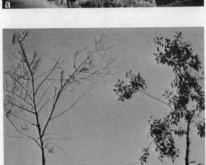
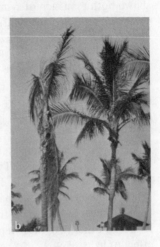

condition is induced by MLO infection, the main symptom being proliferation of axillary buds and dwarfing.

C. Symptoms and Environment

(1) Temperature. This is one of the most important factors in determining the length of the incubation period and the severity of symptoms. The optimal temperature may vary from disease to disease, e.g. the best symptoms are obtained at 30-32°C for *S. citri* and at 18-24°C for clover phyllody. Extremes of temperature may also affect the symptom expression. Very high air temperature (30-50°C) may cure plants of infection. Both hot air and hot water have been used for curing plant material (Nyland and Goheen, 1969). Both methods require careful control, especially the hot water treatment, since there is little difference between the effective inactivation point of the disease organisms and the temperature at which the plant tissues

are damaged. Although plants can stand high air temperatures for long periods, the hot water treatment must be rapid. Very low temperatures (several treatments of about seven hours at -12°C) have cured plant material of RLO infection (Purcell, 1977). MLO-infected plants have shown both remission of symptoms, and even recovery, following severe winters (Purcell, 1980). Where the effect was temporary the disease agent is thought to overwinter in the roots (McCoy, 1979). It has been noticed, with an RLO-associated disease of clover, that at temperatures below about 15°C the organisms could only be found in the stolon and roots, while at high temperatures the RLO were numerous in the leaves and petioles (Markham *et al.*, 1975).

(2) Light. It is possible that light (intensity, wavelength, and photoperiod) plays a part in the symptom expression of diseased plants. Mulberry dwarf symptoms vary in severity depending on the light intensity and photoperiod (Tahama, 1971, 1974). When aster yellows-infected plants were kept in darkness for long periods, the MLO showed abnormal development, probably due to the physiological and nutritional changes in these dark-treated plants (Chen and Hiruki, 1977). However, other than these reports very little is known about the effect of light.

(3) Plant Condition and Nutrition. Some of the most characteristic and obvious symptoms may only occur as a result of the initial challenge to infection, or as a consequence of favourable conditions and a flush of plant growth. Old plants or ones grown under poor conditions may show only mild symptoms, or symptoms may be masked by poor nutrition. For example, old plants which have been infected for months or years with clover phyllody may produce flowers which are smaller than normal, but which show no virescence. These plants, if repotted and placed in favourable conditions, will again produce virescence or phyllody flowers.

D. *'Symptoms' not Caused by MLO*

'Symptoms' alone are not sufficient proof of plant infection by MLO. Syndromes may be induced by factors such as mineral deficiency, insect damage (both mechanical and biochemical), herbicide damage (especially hormonal types), other agents (e.g. viruses), and genetic abnormalities. The distinctive phyllody condition may be of teratological origin in some field-collected material (Erith, 1924). Therefore it is always essential to establish the presence of MLO by some other criteria.

4. Transmission

A. Physical and Physiological Factors Affecting Transmission

When contemplating the transmission of a yellows disease both the organism and the vascular environment need consideration (Zimmerman, 1978; McCoy, 1978). The size, shape and structure of the pathogens are particularly important in relation to the pore size between the vascular cells. Most of the yellows-associated agents are MLOs which range in size from 300-800 nm and are both pleomorphic and pliable. The motile spiroplasmas are 3-6 μm long by 100 nm and although usually helical may be pleomorphic, especially when transmitted by the insect vector. Some MLO may be pleomorphic organisms with long branching filaments (Waters and Hunt, 1980). The RLO are small bacteria with a rigid cell wall and range in size from 200 to 400 nm in diameter by 1 to 3 μm long.

Most of the diseases are associated with agents which are found only in the phloem sieve cells. These cells are under considerable positive pressure, as high as 15 atmospheres or more (Milburn, 1975). There is usually a constant flow of concentrated (1M) sap from cell to cell via the sieve pores, which are on average about 2 μm in diameter, but may vary from less than 1 μm to several microns (Esau, 1965). If the sieve cell is damaged there is instantaneous coagulation of P-protein and a rapid deposition of callose in the sieve plates (Zimmerman, 1978). The P-protein and callose formation serve to plug the sieve pores and minimise further damage to the vascular system. The outflow of sieve cell contents may affect cells a considerable distance from the site of injury (McCoy, 1978). The phloem-restricted agents would normally be able to pass through sieve pores with ease (Figure 3.9); however once the cells are damaged and callose forms the organisms may block the pores, often causing considerable distortion of the organisms (Figure 3.10). Monocotyledons produce less callose than dicotyledons in response to damage (Baker, 1978). Thus special care is needed in the preparation of tissue for electron microscopy in order to avoid these artifacts (Chapter 4). MLO and RLO can therefore normally be transported rapidly throughout the plant in the cytoplasmic stream, and there is no evidence at the moment that the motility of spiroplasmas confers any added advantage. However it is not clear how the filamentous, branched organisms move from cell to cell unless there is some smaller form in the 'life cycle'.

The xylem is a system of interconnected vessels, which may vary in length from a few millimetres to a metre or more depending on the

Figure 3.9: Corn Stunt Organism in Maize Phloem Cells. Note the large sieve pore size in relation to the organism.

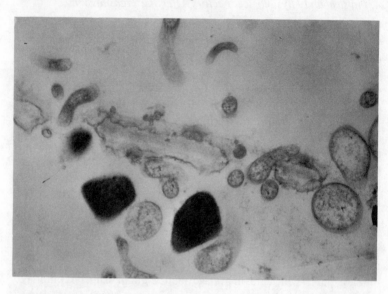

Figure 3.10: Clover Phyllody MLO in Clover. Note blockage of sieve pores with P-protein and MLO.

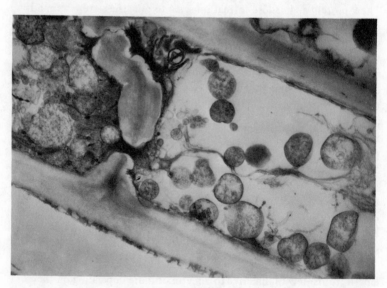

species of plant. The pores between the vessels are probably 20 nm or less, so that any damage to the vascular system would permit air to be drawn into only one or a few vessels. The air/water surface tension would prevent further movement through the pores. The osmotic potential of the xylem sap is very low, although water and nutrients may flow at high velocities. The yellows organisms which invade the xylem are small bacteria or RLO, 200-400 nm by 1-3 μm, with a cell wall to withstand the low osmotic pressure. The relatively large size of the organisms, compared to the pore size between vessels, would suggest that the bacteria would need to produce an enzyme to enlarge these pores. It also appears that these RLO move more easily to the vessels at either end than to those adjacent, suggesting the enzyme action is more effective at the end pores. Blocking of the vessels by these organisms and their metabolic products probably accounts for the wilting symptom commonly associated with these pathogens.

B. Transmission Methods

(1) Mechanical. The phloem-restricted agents have not as yet been re-liably transmitted mechanically, probably because of the rapid response of the phloem to injury. Introducing pathogens into the xylem has been achieved both by immersion of cut stems into cultures or by inoc-ulation with a needle, the problem of mechanical injury being less important in the xylem vessels. Conditions inducing rapid transpiration will assist penetration of the xylem vessels by the pathogen. Beneficial conditions for phloem infection have not yet been established but might include wilting a plant prior to infection, which would reduce the osmotic potential within the cell.

(2) Grafting. Commercial grafting of crops is often a means of dis-semination for the MLO diseases. It is also used experimentally for transmission. There are numerous techniques available (Garner, 1958). For example, stubborn is easily transmitted from citrus to citrus by inserting a small, young, infected leaf, under the bark of the recipient stock (J.M. Bové, personal communication). A simple method, par-ticularly suitable for *Vinca rosea*, is to insert a scion into the stem of the stock, either by making a cut in the side of the branch or a longi-tudinal cut down the stem after removing the growing tip. Stock and scion must be kept in close contact by binding, and the scion must be prevented from dessication for a few days (e.g. by covering with a polythene bag).

(3) Dodder. Infection of plants can sometimes be achieved using a parasitic plant called dodder. Species of the genus *Cuscuta* are usually

used. They are leafless climbing plants with no roots, which obtain
their nutrients from the vascular tissue of a host plant with the aid of
haustoria. These haustoria penetrate between the host cells and connect
with the cells of the vascular tissue via connections similar to plas-
modesmata (Dorr, 1968, 1969). It is still not understood how the
disease agents do pass from the infected plant to the dodder. However
once the dodder is infected it can also pass on the infection to another
susceptible plant.

(4) Insects. Insect transmission in dealt with in Chapter 10.

5. Growth and Treatment

The choice of host species may depend on the disease under study, the
feeding preference of a vector, and the ease with which a plant species
may be grown. The size, age and physiology of the plant may be dictated by experimental conditions. It is considered best to choose young
plants, since these are usually easier to infect and show the best
symptoms. It is essential that the plants are raised under pest-free
conditions as insect feeding damage can produce symptoms which may
be confused with the symptoms of MLO infection. For example, leaf-
hopper-feeding damage to a growing tip may result in deformed and
abnormal leaves similar to early symptoms. In the field, witches'
brooming may be caused by insect-feeding damage and not by MLO
infection. The pesticides used for control must be of short persistence
(e.g Mevinphos) as residual chemicals may affect vector transmission.
It is also reported that certain insecticides and fungicides may have a
direct effect on the MLOs in the phloem (Paddick *et al.*, 1971).

Since some yellows type symptoms are similar to certain mineral and
nutritional deficiencies particular attention must be given to the growth
of plants. Plants used for MLO transmission studies may have to be kept
for long periods, and it is therefore advisable to use either soil-based
composts or, if peat-based composts are used, then liquid fertiliser
should be applied regularly. Although most workers use plants which
are grown in composts under glasshouse conditions, hydroponic solutions have been successfully used both for propagating and maintaining healthy and MLO-diseased plants.

Whenever possible, and especially when direct comparisons of
symptoms are being carried out, the plants should be of cloned material.
The genotype may affect symptom expression, and therefore host
plants which may be vegetatively propagated are useful. Plants which

root easily from 'cuttings' are ideal but tissue culture methods are
available for many species (Murashige, 1974; Hussey, 1978).

Controlled conditions are also preferable. Plants should be protected
from sudden and large temperature changes, such as changes from stock
houses to experimental chambers or cages, and vice versa. Taking
plants from cages where the humidity and temperature may be high
and immediately removing them to a differing environment can cause
losses of young plants. Light intensity and particularly photoperiod are
factors in determining flowering, which may be important if floral
symptoms are required. The author has consistently noticed that transmission and symptom studies under glasshouse conditions are more
successful when carried out during winter than during summer in the
United Kingdom, probably due to difficulty in controlling temperatures
and lighting fluctuations during summer months.

6. *Vinca rosea (Catharanthus roseus)*

V. rosea, the Madagascar Periwinkle, is one of the most widely used
test plants for MLO work. It has large, dark green glossy leaves, the
flowers are large and it will flower continuously under long daylength
conditions. It will survive a wide range of temperatures. Plants are easy
to propagate from cuttings and to graft. For this reason it is one of the
most useful plants in which to maintain MLO diseases.

7. Plant Resistance

There are many cases where an MLO disease will fail, for unknown
reasons, to infect a particular plant species, but host range studies are
often limited by the techniques available for transmitting the disease,
e.g. vectors, dodder and grafting. For example, for many years corn
stunt was thought only to infect a limited number of monocotyledons,
but under experimental conditions it was shown to infect dicotyledons
(Markham *et al.*, 1977). Consequently there are limited data on plant
resistance and the mechanisms of resistance. On a field scale the most
successful example has been the resistance of the Malayan Dwarf
Coconut to lethal yellowing disease. In the Caribbean area the Malayan
Dwarf shows about 97 per cent resistance, but in West Africa reports
suggest that this variety is susceptible. Pear varieties (Westwood, 1976)
and maize hybrids (Nelson and Scott, 1973) have shown genetic

resistance to pear decline and corn stunt respectively, and in both cases it was an additive effect of many genes. In tests on a number of commercial crops for resistance to aster yellows only sunflowers have shown a qualitatively inherited trait (Schultz, 1973). However, there may be scope for breeding plants that discourage the vectors from feeding: by either producing a physical barrier, such as increasing the hairs on the surface, or by making the plant unpalatable to the vector, for example. There may also be mechanisms within the plant which could be developed to counter a challenge by the invading agent. Some resistance to ratoon-stunting disease (a xylem-RLO) has been found in sugar cane, and this possibly results from changes in the vascular anatomy which reduces movement of the organism (Teakle *et al.*, 1978). The 'tolerant' and 'resistant' varieties have reduced rates of water flow through the xylem. The lack of large continuous vascular bundles was the most important feature of the resistant varieties.

It has been shown that at least two vectors *Euscelis plebejus* (Markham *et al.*, 1974) and *Euscelidius variegatus* (Markham and Townsend, 1979) will transmit *S. citri* very inefficiently (usually less than 10 per cent) to plants despite the following factors: (1) all individuals are infected, (2) all salivary glands (tested) are infected, (3) insects are capable of transmitting organisms *in vitro* through parafilm membranes with efficiencies of up to 60 per cent. There are of course a number of possibilities for this discrepancy, only one of which may be some form of plant resistance.

Although breeding for resistance to MLO diseases is an attractive proposition it has met with little success so far.

References

Baker, D.A. (1978). *Transport Phenomena in Plants*. London: Chapman and Hall.

Banttari, E.E. and Zeyen, R.J. (1979). Interactions of mycoplasma-like organisms and viruses in dually infected leafhoppers, planthoppers and plants. In *Leafhopper Vectors and Plant Disease Agents*, pp. 327–44, K. Maramorosch and K.F. Harris (eds). New York: Academic Press.

Calavan, E.C. and Oldfield, G.N. (1979). Symptomatology of spiroplasmal plant diseases. In *The Mycoplasmas*, Vol. III, pp. 37–64, R.F. Whitcomb and J.G. Tully (eds). New York: Academic Press.

Carr, A.J.H. and Large, E.C. (1963). Surveys of phyllody in white clover seed crops, 1959–62. *Plant Pathology 12*, 121–7.

Carr, A.J.H. and Stoddart, J.L. (1963). The ameliorating effect of zinc on symptoms of phyllody virus (strawberry green-petal) in white clover. *Annals of Applied Biology 51*, 259–68.

Chen, M.H. and Hiruki, C. (1977). Effects of dark treatment on the ultrastructure of the aster yellows agent *in situ*. *Phytopathology 67*, 321–4.

Chen, T.A. and Liao, C.H. (1975). Corn stunt spiroplasma: isolation, cultivation and proof of pathogenicity. *Science 188*, 1015–17.

Chiykowski, L.N.(1974). Additional host plants of clover phyllody in Canada. *Canadian Journal Plant Science 54*, 755–63.

Daniels, M.J., Archer, D.B. and Stemmer, W.P.C. (1981). Interaction of wall-free prokaryotes with plants. In *Bacteria and Plants*, The Society for Applied Bacteriology, symposium series, (in press). London: Academic Press.

Davis, M.J., Purcell, A.H. and Thomson, S.V. (1978). Pierce's disease of grape-vines; isolation of the causal organism. *Science 199*, 75–7.

Dorr, I. (1968). Zur Lokalisierung von Zellkontakten zwischen *Cuscuta odorata* und verschiedenen höheren Wirtspflanzen. *Protoplasma 65*, 435–48.

— (1969). Feinstruktur int Razellular wachsender *Cusata-Protoplasma 67*, 123–37.

Erith, A.G. (1924). *White Clover (Trifolium repens L.) A Monograph*. London: Gerald Duckworth & Co.

Esau, K. (1965). *Anatomy of Seed Plants*. New York and London: John Wiley.

Garner, R.J. (1958). *The Grafter's Handbook*. London: Faber & Faber.

Hussey, G. (1978). The application of tissue culture to the vegetative propagation of plants. *Science Progress, Oxford 65*, 185–208.

Markham, P.G. (1978). Chemotherapy of plant diseases caused by mycoplasma-like and rickettsia-like organisms. *Proceedings 1977 British Crop Protection Conference 3*, 815–22.

Markham, P.G. and Townsend, R. (1979). Experimental vectors of spiroplasmas. In *Leafhopper Vectors and Plant Disease Agents*, pp. 413–45, K. Maramorosch and K.F. Harris (eds). New York: Academic Press.

Markham, P.G., Townsend, R., Bar-Joseph, M., Daniels, M.J. Plaskitt, A. and Meddins, B.M. (1974). Spiroplasmas are the causal agents of citrus little leaf disease. *Annals of Applied Biology 78*, 49–57.

Markham, P.G., Townsend, R. and Plaskitt, K.A. (1975). A rickettsia-like organism associated with diseased white clover. *Annals of Applied Biology 81*, 91–3.

Markham, P.G., Townsend, R., Plaskitt, K.A. and Saglio, P. (1977). Transmission of corn stunt to dicotyledonous plants. *Plant Disease Reporter 61*, 342–5.

McCoy, R.E. (1978). Passage of mycoplasma-like organisms through sieve pores? *Proceedings of ROC-United States Cooperative Science Seminar on Myco-plasma Diseases of Plants. NSC Symposium Series 1*, 15–18.

— (1979). Mycoplasmas and yellows diseases. In *The Mycoplasmas*, Vol. III, pp. 229–59, R.F. Whitcomb and J.G. Tully (eds). New York: Academic Press.

Milburn, J.A. (1975). Pressure flow. In *Transport in Plants*, Vol. I, *Phloem Transport*, pp. 3–38, M.H. Zimmerman and J.A. Milburn (eds). New York: Academic Press.

Murashige, T. (1974). Plant propagation through tissue cultures. *Annual Review of Plant Physiology 25*, 135–66.

Nault, L.R. and Bradfute, O.E. (1979). Corn stunt: Involvement of a complex of leafhopper-borne pathogens. In *Leafhopper Vectors and Plant Disease Agents*, pp. 561–86, K. Maramorosch and K.F. Harris (eds). New York: Academic Press.

Nelson, L.R. and Scott, G.E. (1973). Diallel analysis of resistance of corn (*Zea mays* L.) to corn stunt. *Crop Science 13*, 162–4.

Nyland, G. and Goheen, A.C. (1969). Heat therapy of virus diseases of perennial plants. *Annual Review of Phytopathology 7*, 331–54.

Oldfield, G.N. (1980). A virescence agent transmitted by *Circulifer tenellus* (Baker): Aspects of its plant host range and association with *Spiroplasma citri. Abstracts of 3rd Conference of The International Organisation for*

Mycoplasmology, Custer, South Dakota, 1980, 46.

Paddick, R.G., French, F.L. and Turner, P.L. (1971). Control of leafhopper-borne plant diseases possibly due to direct action of systemic biocides on mycoplasmas. *Plant Disease Reporter 55*, 291–3.

Purcell, A.H. (1977). Cold therapy of Pierce's disease of grapevine. *Plant Disease Reporter 61*, 514–18.

— (1980). Environmental therapy for Pierce's disease of grapevines. *Plant Disease 64*, 358–90.

Saglio, P., L'Hospital, D., Bonissol, C., Bové, J.M., Tully, J.G. and Freundt, E.A. (1973). *Spiroplasma citri* gen. and sp. n: a mycoplasma-like organism associated with 'stubborn' disease of citrus. *International Journal Systemic Bacteriology 23*, 191–204.

Schultz, G.A. (1973). Plant resistance to aster yellows. *Proceedings North Central Branch, Entomological Society of America 28*, 93–9.

Tahama, Y. (1971). Studies on the mulberry dwarf disease XIX. Effect of light intensity on manifestation of symptoms (Part 1). *Bulletin of Hiroshima Agricultural College 4*, 97–105.

— (1974). Studies on the mulberry dwarf disease XXII. Effect of light intensity on manifestation of symptoms (Part 2). *Bulletin of Hiroshima Agricultural College 5*, 23–33.

Teakle, D.S., Appleton, J.M. and Steindl, D.R.L. (1978). An anatomical basis for resistance of sugar cane to ratoon stunt disease. *Physiological Plant Pathology 12*, 83–91.

Waters, H. and Hunt, P. (1980). The *in vivo* three dimensional form of a plant mycoplasma-like organism by the analysis of serial ultrathin sections. *Journal of General Microbiology 116*, 111–31.

Westwood, M.N. (1976). Inheritance of pear decline resistance. *Fruit Varieties Journal 30*, 63–4.

Williamson, D.L. and Whitcomb, R.F. (1975). Plant mycoplasmas: A cultivable spiroplasma causes corn stunt disease. *Science 188*, 1018–20.

Zimmerman, M.H. (1978). Mycoplasma diseases and long distance transport in plants. *Proceedings of ROC-United States Cooperative Science Seminar on Mycoplasma Diseases of Plants. NSC Symposium Series 1*, 15–18.

4 LIGHT AND ELECTRON MICROSCOPY

Henry Waters

1. Introduction

Mycoplasma-like organisms (MLO) have been recognised as pathogens of plants and insects for only fourteen years (Chapter 2) and already the literature describing the application of light and electron microscopy to their study is considerable. The majority of contributions have relied only on straightforward transmission electron microscopy of ultrathin sections to confirm the association of MLO with plants exhibiting symptoms of disease (see Chapter 3). Perhaps because the study of MLO is still in its infancy few of the more specialised techniques have achieved the status of 'standard methods'. This chapter therefore contains references to some methods which have not been 'tried and tested' but nevertheless are worthy of consideration for development and wider use.

Apart from the competent application of methodology the successful microscopy of the MLO also requires an appreciation of the biology of their plant and insect hosts as well as the MLO themselves. Our knowledge of the biology, morphology and ultrastructure of MLO is derived largely by analogy from studies made over the last seventy years of species of *Mycoplasma* and *Acholeplasma*. Thus the microscopy of the MLO and mycoplasmas is inextricably linked. One difference between the two areas of study is that whilst most of the known mycoplasmas are amenable to culture the MLO are not (Chapter 7). The spiroplasmas neatly bridge this gap with the cultivable forms associated with, for example, corn stunt and citrus stubborn. Despite the disadvantages of this limitation it has encouraged the refinement of methods for the study of MLO in their natural environments rather than the unnatural environment of a culture medium.

This chapter attempts to draw together the relevant technical experience from the diverse fields of phloem anatomy and physiology, insect anatomy and physiology, mycoplasmal morphology and ultrastructure and the theoretical aspects of fixation of biological tissues so as to equip the microscopist with the necessary background to select rationally the most appropriate techniques.

Throughout the text the trivial definition 'mycoplasma' will be used to describe organisms belonging to the genera *Mycoplasma* and *Acholeplasma* of the class Mollicutes. The term 'mycoplasma-like organism', abbreviated to 'MLO', will be used to describe those structures present in plant phloem and insect tissues which have the ultrastructural characteristics of mycoplasmas although there is no evidence from cultured organisms to define their taxonomic status accurately. Finally, the term 'spiroplasma' will be confined to those organisms, whether taxonomically defined (i.e. *Spiroplasma citri*, Saglio *et al.*, 1973) or not, which have the ultrastructural characteristics of mycoplasmas and which, for at least part of their life cycle, exhibit helical filamentous morphology.

2. MLO and Spiroplasma Habitats

Before describing the microscopical techniques which have been or might be used for the study of MLO and spiroplasmas it is necessary to discuss those physical and biological properties of their plant and insect hosts which are relevant to the selection of appropriate methods. These factors are also significant to the proper interpretation of the results obtained.

A. *Plants*

In plants, MLO and spiroplasmas are restricted internally to the phloem (Maramorosch *et al.*, 1970; Whitcomb and Davis, 1970; Davis and Whitcomb, 1971; Whitcomb, 1973; Maramorosch, 1974, 1976; McCoy, 1979; Davis, 1979) and externally spiroplasmas have been found in the nectar of flowers (Davis, 1978) and *Acholeplasma* spp. on the surfaces of leaves of coconut palms (Eden-Green and Tully, 1979). The report of MLO in the mesophyll of pea leaves (Hampton *et al.*, 1969) was refuted after re-examination (Hampton *et al.*, 1976) in the light of evidence that the structures first identified as MLO were in fact membrane-bound vesicles associated with a viral disease.

Phloem is both anatomically and physiologically a complex tissue. It can be comprised of many different cell types (Esau, 1969) of which sieve tube elements, parenchyma and companion cells are of particular interest because it is in these cells that MLO have been reported to occur. McCoy (1979) recently critically assessed the validity of reports of MLO in phloem parenchyma and companion cells and concluded that much of the evidence supporting claims that MLO occur in these cells was often dubious and sometimes lacking because authors had either misidentified MLO or the cells in which MLO appeared.

Aside from this controversial point MLO are accepted to be inhabitants of the phloem sieve tube elements; one of the most fragile environments in a plant. This is because the individual sieve elements of angiosperm phloem are interconnected via sieve plates to form continuous conduits — the sieve tubes. In functional phloem sieve tubes are under positive hydrostatic pressures which range from 8 to 20 bars and may be as high as 30 bars (Weatherley, 1962; Hammel, 1968; Milburn, 1975). Any incision to remove phloem for microscopy will release this pressure 'explosively' (Srivastava, 1975) and affect cells distant to the cut. One effect of this pressure release is to disrupt the sieve tube contents and force them through sieve areas where some may lodge in the pores. It is important to recognise that pressure release affects MLO in the same way and will alter both their morphology and apparent distribution within individual sieve elements.

Sieve tube elements also respond physiologically to injury and disruption by plugging sieve plates with deposits of wound callose. Whilst this reaction may not directly affect MLO the presence of wound callose can be an indication of inadequate phloem fixation (Eschrich,

1975; Srivastava, 1975). Phloem anatomists agree that it is almost impossible to preserve undisturbed the integrity of sieve tube elements with any of the fixation methods presently available (Weatherley and Johnson, 1968; Srivastava, 1975).

B. Insects

MLO and spiroplasmas are transmitted from plant to plant by phloem-feeding insects and the majority of known vector species are leafhoppers (Homoptera; Cicadellidae) (Whitcomb and Davis, 1970; Hull, 1972; Williamson and Whitcomb, 1974). In these insects the piercing mouth-parts consist of paired maxillary stylets ensheathed by a pair of mandibular stylets to form a stylet bundle which at rest lies for most of its length in the rostral groove of the specialised labium (rostrum). During feeding the stylet bundle is exerted along the rostral groove by musculature within the head capsule. The mechanism of probing has been studied and reviewed by Pollard (1968, 1969, 1973) and most significantly it involves the formation of a salivary sheath around the stylets as they pass through the host plant's tissues. This salivary sheath does not always reach to the maximum extension of the maxillary stylets but the materials from which it is composed (Miles, 1972) originate within the salivary glands of the feeding insect and are forced down the salivary canal of the maxillary stylets by a salivary pump located within the head. It is thought that MLO from infectious insects are transferred to the phloem of susceptible host plants in the saliva although there is no evidence for MLO in salivary sheaths (Raine *et al.*, 1976). Whilst feeding, a leafhopper ingests sieve tube sap via the food canal which is formed by the interlocked maxillary stylets and it is at this time that insects acquire MLO or spiroplasmas from diseased plants. After acquisition insects remain non-infectious for an incubation period during which MLO and spiroplasmas are thought to pass from the alimentary canal through the gut wall into the hemolymph and from there to other organs including the salivary glands at which time the insect may become infectious (Maillet and Gouranton, 1971). Insects known to have transmitted disease have MLO or spiroplasmas in their salivary glands but not all insects with MLO or spiroplasmas in their salivary glands will transmit; this discrepancy remains unexplained (e.g. Townsend *et al.*, 1977).

Compared with the voluminous literature describing MLO and spiroplasmas in plants the relevant literature for insects is scanty. Table 4.1 summarises some of the published reports of MLO or spiroplasmas in leafhoppers to indicate the different organs in which

Table 4.1: The Different Leafhopper Organs in which MLO or Spiroplasmas Have Been Detected by Electron Microscopy

Nervous system	Gut	Salivary glands	Malpighian tubules	Fat body	Leafhopper sp.	Disease	Reference
+	+	+	-	-	Dalbulus elimatus	corn stunt	Granados et al. (1968)
-	+	+	+	-	Euscelis plebejus	clover phyllody	Giannotti et al. (1968a, c)
+	+	-	-	-	D. elimatus	corn stunt	Maramorosch et al. (1968a, b)
-	-	+	-	-	Macrosteles fascifrons	aster yellows	Hirumi & Maramorosch (1969a)
+	+	+	+	-	D. elimatus	corn stunt	Granados (1969)
+	+	+	+	-	D. maidis	corn stunt	Granados (1969)
-	-	-	-	+	D. maidis	corn stunt	Shikata & Maramorosch (1969)
-	-	-	-	+	M. fascifrons	aster yellows	Shikata & Maramorosch (1969)
-	+	+	-	-	M. fascifrons	clover phyllody	Sinha & Paliwal (1970)
-	-	+	-	-	E. plebejus	clover phyllody	Maillet (1970a)
+	-	+	-	+	Collodanus montanus	western X	Nasu et al. (1970)
-	+	-	-	-	E. lineolatus	clover phyllody	Maillet & Gouranton (1970)
-	-	+	-	-	E. lineolatus	clover phyllody	Maillet (1970b)
+	+	+	-	+	E. lineolatus	clover phyllody	Maillet & Gouranton (1971)
-	+	+	-	-	Orosius argentatus	legume little leaf	Bowyer & Atherton (1971)
-	-	+	-	-	M. fascifrons	aster yellows	Raine & Forbes (1971)
+	+	+	-	-	M. fascifrons	aster yellows	Sinha & Peterson (1972)
-	+	-	-	-	E. plebejus	clover phyllody etc.	Giannotti et al.(1973)
-	-	+	-	-	E. lineolatus	clover phyllody	Gourret et al. (1973)
+	-	-	-	-	C. montanus	western X	Nasu et al. (1974b)
-	+	-	-	-	C. montanus	western X	Nasu et al. (1974a)
-	+	+	-	-	M. orientalis	Cryptotaenia yellows	Okuda & Nishimura (1974)
+	-	+	-	-	D. elimatus	corn stunt	Granados & Meehan (1975)
-	-	+	-	-	M. fascifrons	aster yellows	Raine & Forbes (1976)
-	-	+	-	-	E. plebejus	Spiroplasma citri	Townsend et al. (1977)

these organisms have been located by electron microscopy.

C. Environmental Osmolarity

Microscopical studies of insects are not complicated by the pressure release problems attendant upon phloem fixation but in both the plant and insect environments the MLO are prey to changes in both morphology and ultrastructure induced by changes in osmolarity.

In plants MLO and spiroplasmas are bathed in sieve tube sap which is a complex medium containing inorganic anions and cations, organic acids, proteins, amino acids, lipids and carbohydrates in aqueous solution (Ziegler, 1975). In insects, for at least part of their life cycle, MLO reside in the hemolymph which like sieve tube sap is a complex aqueous solution of metabolites and assimilates (Saglio and Whitcomb, 1979). The constituents of sieve tube sap and hemolymph are osmotically active and exert osmolarities of 240 to 600 mOsmols kg^{-1} (Saglio and Whitcomb, 1979). Nothing is known of the effects that changes in osmolarity have upon the morphology or ultrastructure of MLO except by analogy with the mycoplasmas and spiroplasmas.

Different species of mycoplasmas vary in their sensitivity to osmotic shock (Razin, 1963) and this effect is temperature-dependent with cells showing greater resistance to lysis at $0°C$ than at $37°C$ when tranferred to hypotonic conditions (Razin, 1964). Cells of *Mycoplasma mycoides* remain filamentous when suspended in media hypertonic to the original (isotonic) culture medium, but in hypotonic solutions they become approximately spherical and increase in volume. Spherical cells from hypotonic media regain their characteristic filamentous form when returned to a hypertonic medium (Rodwell, 1965). Conversely *M. gallisepticum*, a coccoid to pear-shaped organism under isotonic conditions, becomes filamentous in hypotonic media whilst retaining viability for a limited period (Bernstein-Ziv, 1971).

The stability of the helices of spiroplasmas in early log phase cultures is a sensitive indicator of hypotonic conditions. *S. citri* will despiral and appear filamentous when transferred from SMC culture medium to hypotonic solutions (Table 4.5, Cole *et al.*, 1973). The corn stunt spiroplasma behaves similarly when removed from plant sap to hypotonic negative staining solutions (see Section 8).

3. MLO and Spiroplasmal Ultrastructure and its Interpretation

It was against the background of studies of mycoplasmas that MLO were discovered (Doi *et al.*, 1967) to be associated with plant disease almost by serendipity (Maramorosch, 1976). Like mycoplasmas, MLO and spiroplasmas present in ultrathin sections a range of smoothly outlined profiles which may be circular, elliptical, sausage-shaped, filamentous, dumbbell-shaped or multiply-lobed. All profiles are devoid of a cell wall, the organisms being separated from their surroundings by only a single membrane. Within this membrane the cytoplasm contains ribosomes and DNA, the appearance of which can be influenced by the conditions of fixation. In well-preserved specimens the DNA appears as fine filaments forming a reticulate network. These ultrastructural features are characteristic of organisms belonging to the class Mollicutes (Maniloff and Morowitz, 1972; Razin, 1978; Tully, 1978; Freundt and Edward, 1979; Figure 4.1).

Some species of *Mycoplasma* exhibit specialised modifications to this generalised ultrastructure, e.g. the striated axial fibre in the Rho form of *M. mycoides* var. *mycoides* (Rodwell *et al.*, 1973); the structured tip of *M. pneumoniae* (Wilson and Collier, 1976) and the terminal bleb of *M. gallisepticum* (Maniloff *et al.*, 1965; Allen *et al.*, 1970).

The regular occurrence of specialised intracytoplasmic structures in MLO or spiroplasmas has not been reported. Many references have been made to the presence of membrane-bound vacuoles inside MLO but on close examination the evidence for such structures is wanting. Similar structures can also be present in mycoplasmas and significantly they appear most frequently in cells from colonies in the decline phase or organisms fixed in strongly hypertonic media (Lemcke, 1972). There is no evidence to correlate the presence of membrane-bound inclusions in MLO with the conditions of fixation. Razin (1969) was sceptical about reports describing intracytoplasmic vacuoles and in later reviews of mycoplasmal ultrastructure their presence is ignored (e.g. Boatman, 1979).

Hirumi and Maramorosch (1969a) first observed membrane-bound 'inclusion bodies' in some aster yellows MLO in the salivary glands of leafhoppers. Subsequently they reported that similar structures could be observed in the same MLO in phloem parenchyma cells (now thought to be sieve elements (McCoy, 1979) and hypothesised that they were associated with intracytoplasmic reproduction (Hirumi and Maramorosch, 1973a). This form of reproduction was considered possible for myco-plasmas but it is no longer accepted (Freundt, 1969; Anderson, 1969). Similar inclusions were also reported for normal (Hirumi and Mara-morosch, 1973b; Esau *et al.*, 1976) and senescent aster yellows MLO (Hirumi and Maramorosch, 1972) as well as the MLO associated with Salix yellows (Holmes *et al.*, 1972) and lethal decline of palms (Thomas, 1979). Sinha (1976) found membrane-bound inclusions in purified extracts of the clover phyllody MLO but they were absent from the same MLO *in vivo* (Sinha and Paliwal, 1969).

Esau *et al.* (1976) pointed out that the inclusions described within MLO profiles were either sinuously rod-shaped (Figure 4.3) or approximately circular (Figures 4.2 and 4.4). Several of the rod-shaped forms described (Holmes *et al.*, 1972 Figure 8; Hirumi and Mara-morosch, 1973b Figures 12, 13, 17 and 19) do not have well-defined membranes and are like the clumped DNA artefact sometimes induced by osmium tetroxide fixatives (see Section 7.C). Other rod-shaped forms (Hirumi and Maramorosch, 1973b Figures 14, 15 and 16) do have clear membranes and probably are very steeply invaginated regions of the MLO membrane (Figure 4.5).

Circular membrane-bound inclusions exist in two forms (Figures 4.2 and 4.4); in the first the lumen has amorphous contents and in the

Figures 4.1 to 4.4: MLO Profiles from Sieve Elements of *Vinca rosea* Naturally Infected with a Phyllody Disease in Jamaica. Figure 4.1: Normal Approximately Circular Profiles Showing the Characteristic Membrane, Ribosomes and Finely Stranded DNA. Figure 4.2: Doughnut-shaped MLO Profile with an Apparently Intracellular 'Vacuole'. Figure 4.3: Sinuously Rod-shaped Membranous Structures (Arrowed) inside MLO Profiles. Figure 4.4: MLO Apparently within MLO (Arrowed). (Scale Bar 100 nm.)

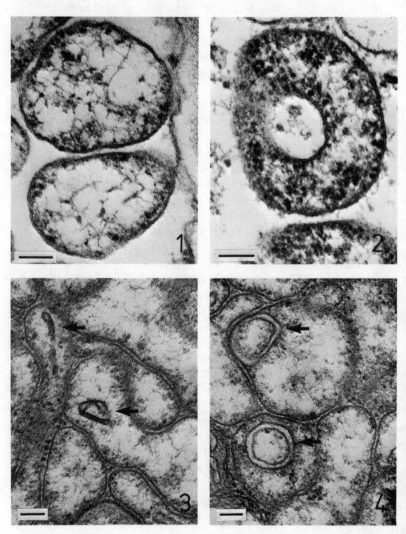

Figure 4.5: Diagrams of MLO Profiles (Below) to Illustrate the Probable Origin of Apparently Intracellular Rod-shaped Structures (A) and Vacuoles (B) in Relation to the Planes of Sectioning, Indicated by the Hatched Area in the Upper Drawings (Not to Scale)

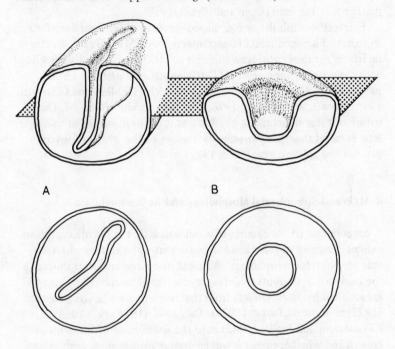

A B

second the lumen contains a complete MLO profile. The first type has been investigated by freeze-etching and serial sectioning (Braun, 1977). The use of freeze-etching was unable to resolve whether the inclusions were truly intracytoplasmic. The four adjacent 70 to 80 nm thick serial ultrathin sections figured by Braun (1977) do not provide convincing evidence for an entirely intracytoplasmic membrane-bound vesicle but rather a ring-shaped structure. At a section thickness of 70 to 80 nm a vesicle about 120 nm in diameter such as described by Braun (1977, Figure 9) would have to be represented in at least two or possibly three serial sections; the structure described appears in one. Braun's (1977) serial sectioning study appears to be the only one made of apparently intracytoplasmic vesicles and until further substantiated their existence remains equivocal. In the absence of serial sections, the circular membrane-bound inclusions in MLO profiles are best interpreted as invaginations included within the plane of sectioning (Figure 4.5).

There is no doubt from the analysis of serial ultrathin sections that the appearance of an MLO within an MLO (Figure 4.4) is a function of the plane of sectioning in relation to the orientation of two closely juxtaposed organisms (Chen and Hiruki, 1977).

Extracellular tubular or rod-shaped structures have been described from both plant and insect tissues infected with MLO. These structures lie free in the host cytoplasm adjacent to MLO or are directly associated with the outer membrane of MLO (Giannotti *et al.*, 1969a, 1973; Ploaie, 1971; Allen, 1972; Gourett *et al.*, 1973; Cadilhac and Giannotti, 1975; Marwitz and Petzold, 1976; Chen and Hiruki, 1978a, b). The nature of these structures is obscure and it has been suggested that at least some of them are virus-like by analogy to the viruses of mycoplasmas and spiroplasmas (Cole, 1979).

4. MLO and Spiroplasmal Morphology and its Interpretation

A concomitant of the absence of a cell wall is that mollicute organisms exhibit plasticity of form and this in turn gives rise to their characteristic pleomorphic morphology. A thread of controversy runs through the many early attempts to define mycoplasmal morphology (here exemplified by *M. mycoides*) from the pioneering studies of Ørskov (1927) to those of Turner (1935), Tang *et al.* (1935, 1936) and Klieneberger and Smiles (1942) as to the significance of filamentous growth and whether or not it was an artefact of specimen preparation. Hand in hand with this controversy, arguments also prevailed over the mode of mycoplasmal reproduction. The realisation (Freundt, 1952) that the nature of the culture medium and the age of sampled cultures could affect profoundly the morphology of intact cells as perceived by light or electron microscopy, as much as the microscopical methodology, cut through the controversy and led to the conclusion that filamentous growth was a normal part of mycoplasmal growth (Freundt, 1960). Confirmation of filamentous growth in eleven species of *Mycoplasma* and *Acholeplasma laidlawii* was provided by Razin and Cosenza (1966) and Razin *et al.* (1967). All the species examined produced, during early logarithmic growth, filaments 0.3 to 0.4 μm wide the length of which was species-dependent. As the cultures aged the filaments broke up into chains of coccoid bodies which in turn fragmented to produce shorter chains and coccoid bodies which were 0.6 to 0.8 μm in diameter. The decline phase of cultures was marked by the appearance of large non-viable cells up to 20 μm in diameter. These observations were confirmed by Bredt (1970) who, in a time-course study of individual organisms using phase contrast light microscopy, also provided the crucial evidence that multiplication during the early stages was by binary fission of approximately coccoid bodies and later by fragmentation of filaments or rings. Daughter-cell separation followed a constriction process which Metz and Bredt (1971) later showed did not involve the formation of a septum. Bredt *et al.* (1973) went on to demonstrate, using microcinematography, that cells of *M. hominis* underwent dynamic changes of form and that sometimes these changes were reversible even within periods as short as seven seconds.

This pattern of changes in morphology with increasing age and transitory morphological changes can be expected in the MLO and this complicates the interpretation of MLO morphology. By comparison with the mycoplasmas and spiroplasmas the morphology of the MLO is only poorly understood. In large part this is because the MLO have so far resisted cultivation and also because it is not yet possible to extract organisms from a living host and observe them by light microscopy or electron microscopy of negatively-stained preparations. It has therefore been necessary either to infer MLO morphology *in vivo* from ultrathin sections or to observe fractured sieve elements by scanning electron microscopy (see Section 9). The two-dimensional MLO profiles presented by numerous authors have almost always been interpreted in terms of the simplest plausible three-dimensional form despite the evidence that mycoplasmas can be morphologically complex.

Clearly it is important to understand how profile shape relates to the intact form of MLO and spiroplasmas. In ultrathin sections of their plant hosts or centrifuged pellets from cultures the helical form of spiroplasmas can be recognised by the regular spacing of profiles associated with a sectioned helix (e.g. Davis and Worley, 1973; Cole *et al.*, 1973; Markham *et al.*, 1974). The helical form is particularly obvious in sections 300 to 600 nm thick observed by transmission electron microscopy (Figure 4.6) and such sections are routinely used to diagnose spiroplasmal helices (e.g. Markham *et al.*, 1977).

By contrast MLO (references in Tables 4.2 and 4.3) and spiroplasmas when nonhelical (e.g. Granados, 1969; Wolanski, 1973; Igwegbe and Calavan, 1970) present a bewildering range of profile shapes like those of sectioned mycoplasmas.

The most commonly encountered MLO profile in both plant and insect tissues is circular, and diameters from 80 nm to several

Figure 4.6: The Spiroplasma Associated with Corn Stunt in Jamaica in a Thick (c. 400 nm) Electron Microscope Section (Scale Bar 250 nm)

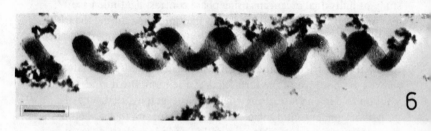

micrometres have been reported. Profiles at the smaller end of this range have often been interpreted as representing sections through 'elementary bodies'. The presence of elementary bodies was once considered to be significant because it was thought that they were the minimal reproductive unit for the mycoplasmas. This notion has now been discredited (Morowitz and Wallace, 1973). Spherical bodies of the dimensions of elementary bodies (i.e. 0.1 to 0.2 μm in diameter) are inviable and are associated with the decline phase of colonies (Robertson *et al.*, 1975a). The larger circular profiles have most frequently been described as being sections through spherical organisms although some authors have suggested that such profiles might also be sections through filaments. In support of this suggestion long filamentous profiles may sometimes be seen in ultrathin sections of sieve elements where organisms have fortuitously been orientated within the plane of sectioning (e.g. Granett and Gilmer, 1971; MacBeath *et al.*, 1972; Jones *et al.*, 1974; Hearon *et al.*, 1976; Thomas, 1979). There is also evidence that filaments may be branched (e.g. Hirumi and Maramorosch, 1973b; Sinha and Paliwal, 1969; Lombardo *et al.*, 1970; Cousin *et al.*, 1971b; Dabek, 1977; Thomas, 1979) or beaded (e.g. Ploaie and Maramorosch, 1969; Zelcer *et al.*, 1971; Hooper *et al.*, 1971; Hirumi and Maramorosch, 1973b; Hearon *et al.*, 1976; Thomas, 1979). Filamentous MLO profiles are not found in insect tissues and there is no evidence to suggest that spiroplasmas retain their helical or even filamentous form in insect tissues other than the hemolymph (Whitcomb and Williamson, 1975; Granados and Meehan, 1975; Townsend *et al.*, 1977; Davis, 1979) except for the report by Chen *et al.* (1973) of filaments in the salivary glands of the psyllid (*Diaphorina citri* Kuw.) vector of citrus likubin disease.

   Other MLO profile shapes are encountered in sectioned sieve elements. Dumbbell-shaped and multiply-lobed profiles have been frequently reported and usually interpreted as representing organisms undergoing binary fission (e.g. Hirumi and Maramorosch, 1973b; Worley, 1970; Ushiyama *et al.*, 1969; Parthasarathy, 1974; Seliskar *et al.*, 1974; Esau *et al.*, 1976). Curious 'octopus-like' structures (Hearon *et al.*, 1976) or rings (Begtrup and Lange, 1977), both composed of beaded profiles, were analysed by serial sectioning and they most closely resemble the ring forms of *M. hominis* associated with multiplication by fragmentation (Bredt, 1970).

The observation of electron micrographs from 300–600 nm thick sections viewed either by stereoscopy (Graf *et al.*, 1978) or directly (Braun, 1977; Thomas, 1979) indicates that the morphology of MLO is usually more complex than a traditional interpretation of profiles in ultrathin sections might have suggested. This impression is confirmed by the stereoscopic analysis of serial electron micrographs described by Florance and Cameron (1978).

The analysis of long ribbons of serial ultrathin sections (Waters and Hunt, 1978; 1980) allowed the relationship between profile shape and morphology to be explained by reference to reconstructional drawings of the coconut lethal yellowing MLO (Figure 4.7). These authors also suggested that the MLO could be classified on the basis of their morphology (Figure 4.7) and that often certain profile shapes were associated with particular morphotypes. The morphotypes recognised were analogous to those now recognised as usual for many species of *Mycoplasma* and *Acholeplasma* during the later stages of development. In the serially-sectioned sieve elements small, approximately spherical, organisms were uncommon and most usually MLO were filamentous, branched and ramified through the cell lumen, some organisms being up to 16 μm long. On the basis of this study and those of Braun (1977), Florance and Cameron (1978), Graf *et al.*, (1978), Haggis and Sinha (1978) and Thomas (1979) it seems likely that many of the previous interpretations of MLO morphology based only on single ultrathin sections have been too simple.

5. Aberrant MLO Ultrastructure

Apart from fixation artefacts, MLO are altered by changes in their environment. In many plants affected by MLO diseases the phloem undergoes necrosis and in response to this the MLO show membrane disruption and either increased electron density of the cytoplasm or complete loss of cytoplasmic ultrastructure (Hirumi and Maramorosch,

Figure 4.7: Reconstructional Drawings of Mycoplasma-like Organisms Prepared from Ultrathin Serial Sections of Sieve Elements from Coconut Palms Affected by Lethal Yellowing Disease. The six organisms are classified (Waters and Hunt, 1980) as saccate (A), filiform (B), erythrocyte-like (C), moniliform (D & F) and cylindrical (E) and show how individual profiles contribute to form. Highlighted are profiles which are filamentous (G), dumbbell-shaped (H), sausage-shaped (I), small circular (J) or three-lobed (K). In the drawings each step represents the shape and thickness of a single MLO profile. Unlabelled arrows indicate that an organism continued out of the set of serial sections at either one or both ends. The set of serial sections themselves represent approximately 3.5 μm.

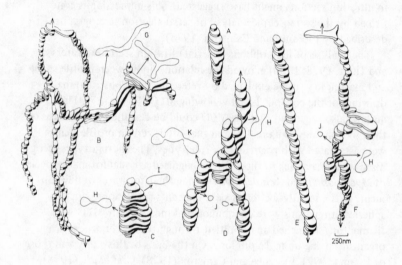

1972; Hiruki and Dijkastra, 1973b; Chen and Hiruki, 1977). MLO profiles may also be strongly dumbbell-shaped, perhaps indicating cellular collapse (Chen and Hiruki, 1977). Dumbbell-shaped profiles are also associated with MLO in plants after dark treatments (Chen and Hiruki, 1977). In insect vectors and plants treated with tetracylines the MLO also show membrane disruption and loss of cytoplasmic ultrastructure (Sinha and Peterson, 1972). The maintenance of MLO-infected periwinkle at 40°C initially induces the organisms to produce numerous buds and thereafter the loss of cytoplasmic contents and the formation of membranous inclusions (Zelcer *et al.*, 1972).

Strongly dumbbell-shaped and bizarrely stretched MLO profiles are often encountered in sections through sieve plates and it is frequently claimed that this is evidence for the translocation of MLO through sieve pores (e.g. Jacoli, 1974). Clearly MLO must pass through sieve pores to initiate systemic infection but, as McCoy (1979) points out, the ultrastructural evidence for the passage of MLO through sieve pores is really only evidence for the release of the phloem hydrostatic pressure during sampling.

6. Light Microscopy

A. *Direct Observation of Organisms*

Although MLO, spiroplasmas and mycoplasmas are so small as to be near the limit of resolution by light microscopy, valuable studies can be made of their gross morphology and the effects on this of various physical, chemical and biological factors. The opportunities for the study of MLO are restricted by the present inability to cultivate the organisms and the inadequacy of methods to distinguish these highly pleomorphic structures from a background of host cell debris in extracts from either plants or insects. So far the reported studies are restricted to the spiroplasmas and the mycoplasmas.

The earliest descriptions of mycoplasmal morphology were derived from observations made using either dark-field microscopy of broth cultures or bright-field microscopy of superstained smear preparations (see reviews: Turner, 1935; Freundt, 1969). Subsequently dark-field and phase-contrast microscopy have played an important role in the description of mycoplasmal morphology and reproduction. The optimum conditions for the observation of mycoplasmas and spiroplasmas from liquid culture are achieved using freely floating organisms (Anderson, 1969; Cole *et al.*, 1973). For organisms in colonies on solid media the method suggested by Ørskov (1927) is probably best. Blocks of agar carrying colonies are placed in liquid medium and separated from the colony surface by wisps of nonabsorbent cotton wool. Preparations of living organisms made by these methods are prey to artefacts which may be caused by capillarity forces, contact with either the cover glass or slide, centrifugation of organisms prior to examination, movements of the cover glass or chemical fixation (Anderson, 1969; Cole *et al.*, 1973).

It was in 1970 using phase-contrast microscopy of sap extracted from corn plants affected by corn stunt that Davis *et al.* (1972) discovered the helical morphology now associated with the spiroplasmas.

Poulson and Sakaguchi (1961) described from light microscope observations a 'spirochete' related to the maternally transmitted sex
ratio condition of *Drosophila* spp. which was later identified as a
spiroplasma (Williamson and Whitcomb, 1974). Apart from their
intrinsic interest the observations by Poulson and Sakaguchi (1961)
showed that, following formaldehyde vapour fixation of drops or
smears of *Drosophila* hemolymph, conventional bacteriological
staining methods (Lillie, 1954) could be successfully used to make
permanent preparations of the sex ratio spiroplasma. These applications of light microscopy to the detection of mollicutes in cultures
and extracts from plants or insects have not been extended to any of
the MLO diseases.

Colonies. Colonies of mycoplasmas and spiroplasmas on solid media
exhibit a characteristic 'fried egg' or 'umbonate' form. This may be
demonstrated with a binocular dissecting microscope using oblique
illumination to improve the view in relief (Edward, 1954). A compound microscope can also provide a similar effect if used in an
unconventional way (Muelas and Ales, 1973). In this method the
condenser is lowered and an objective of an appropriate magnification
on a revolving nosepiece is set slightly off centre to provide a form of
oblique illumination which shows colonies in relief and emphasises
the characteristic umbo.

B. Demonstration of MLO in Tissues

The attempts so far made to detect MLO in either plant or insect
tissues have relied upon histochemical methods for the detection of
DNA or RNA. Giannotti *et al.* (1968a) experimented with the clover
phyllody MLO both in the plant (*Trifolium repens* L.) and an insect
vector (*Euscelis plebejus* Fall.). They used the Feulgen reaction and
methyl green to detect DNA and pyronin Y to detect RNA as well
as complementary DNAase and RNAase treatments to confirm the
staining reactions observed. This kind of enzymatic treatment is an
essential adjunct to the histochemical demonstration of nucleic
acids using these stains (Pearse, 1968). Feulgen positive reactions
were obtained in the cells of the gut and salivary glands of insects as
well as the phloem of diseased plants. Confirmation that MLO were
present in similar tissues, but not contiguous samples, was obtained by
electron microscopy. Subsequently the Feulgen reaction has been
convincingly used to detect plant and insect cells containing MLO
(Giannotti, 1969; Cousin *et al.*, 1969b, 1972; Maillet and Gouranton,
1971; Cousins and Kartha, 1975; Purohit *et al.*, 1978).

The light microscopic detection of MLO in plants has also been claimed following haematoxylin staining of cryostat sections (Borges and David-Ferreira, 1968) or fixed (Navashin's fluid) wax embedded sections (Cousin, 1975). The worth of this stain for the detection of MLO will remain doubtful until more critically appraised because the staining reaction probably only reflects phloem damage associated with disease.

In many electron microscope laboratories it is routine practice to collect sections 1 to 2 μm thick from epoxy embedded tissues and stain them with toluidine blue O (TBO) in borax (Lewis and Knight, 1977) to locate areas by light microscopy for subsequent ultrathin sectioning. Obviously those studying the ultrastructure of MLO have searched sections so stained in an effort to detect MLO-containing cells. Very few reports (Cousin *et al.*, 1970, 1971a; Hooper *et al.*, 1971) exist in the extensive literature describing the electron micros-copic detection of MLO to suggest that MLO can be detected by TBO staining. The method applied to tissues from coconut palms affected by lethal yellowing has never given any indication of MLO positive sieve elements (Waters, unpublished observations). This probably reflects the very low concentration of MLO in the sieve elements of lethal yellowing affected palms. Hooper *et al.* (1971) emphasised that the light microscopic detection of MLO in 1 to 2 μm sections could only be demonstrated in cells containing high concentrations of MLO as confirmed by electron microscopy of contiguous ultrathin sections.

These indications that TBO staining might be used for the light microscopic detection of MLO are really only asides gleaned from electron microscope studies. The optimum conditions for the use of TBO as a metachromatic stain for nucleic acids follow acrolein fix-ation (glutaraldehyde is only suitable for some tissues) and either ester wax or methacrylate embedding (Feder and Wolf, 1965; Feder and O'Brien, 1968). No one appears to have explored the application of such methods; perhaps the time is ripe for such investigations. In this context Feder and O'Brien (1968) also describe other histochemical reactions for the localisation of DNA and RNA which might reward study.

Russell *et al.* (1975) showed that DAPI (4′-6-diamidino-2-phenylin-dole), a DNA binding fluorochrome, could be used to detect mycoplas-mal contamination of tissue cultures. Seemüller (1976) was quick to recognise that DAPI and a benzimidole derivative 33258 Hoechst could be used as fluorochromes to detect MLO in plant phloem. He used the phloem from trees affected by pear decline, a disease known to be associated with MLO in America (Hibino and Schneider, 1970), as well as healthy control trees. Tissue samples fixed in 5% glutaraldehyde (formaldehyde gave equally good results) in 0.1M phosphate buffer at 4°C were sectioned at 20 to 30 μm with a freezing microtome and incubated in DAPI or 33258 Hoechst (1 μg ml^{-1}) at room temperature for 20 to 30 min. Positive DNA/DAPI fluorescence was recorded in 14 of 16 samples from diseased trees and none from 18 healthy trees. That the positive reaction was associated with MLO could not be confirmed by electron microscopy. This study by Seemüller (1976) appears to be the only one using similar methods. The affinity of 33258 Hoechst for DNA is emphasised by Lemcke *et al.* (1978) in their studies of fungal nuclei. These authors also provide additional experimental methods which might be useful in studies of MLO *in vivo* or extracts.

C. Indirect Methods for the Detection of MLO Diseases

Cousin and Grison (1966) and Cousin (1975) reported high levels of autofluorescence in the lateral walls of sieve elements from the hyperplasic phloem of solanaceous plants with MLO diseases. This effect was not observed in healthy plants. Carle (1965) also showed that abnormally high levels of fluorescence could be detected in the phloem of vines affected by Flavescence dorée when treated with the fluorochromes thioflavin T or acridine orange. The cause of the fluorescence reported in these three studies remains unexplained and until it is there is little to recommend such non-specific techniques.

Phloem cells respond to injury with the production of wound callose and various authors have suggested that the detection of abnormally high levels of callose in sieve elements might be used as an indirect method for the diagnosis of MLO infected plants.

Two light microscopic methods for the detection of callose have achieved wide acceptance among phloem anatomists. The first for conventional bright-field microscopy relies on staining callose with alkaline solutions of lacmoid (resorcin blue) (Cheadle *et al.*, 1953) and the second on the use of analine blue as a callose-specific fluorochrome (Eschrich and Currier, 1964). Using the first method Braun and Sinclair (1976) showed that callose deposition preceded the necrosis of sieve elements of elm trees with phloem necrosis disease.

Hiruki and Shukla (1973) showed that aniline blue staining could be used to differentiate between phloem from diseased and healthy bleeding heart (*Dicentra spectabilis*) by inducing more fluorescence in the diseased sieve elements than the healthy. The same method applied

to *Vinca* plants infected with the sandal spike MLO showed a similar
response (Hiruki and Dijkstra, 1973a) which is illustrated by colour
plates by Hiruki *et al.* (1974). Whilst recognising that the fluorescence
they saw in diseased sieve elements was derived from callose Hiruki
and Dijkstra (1973a) suggested that the MLO assumed to be present
were also contributing to the observed fluorescence. This suggestion
was discounted following studies of aniline blue staining of cultured
mycoplasmas when no fluorescence was seen (Hiruki *et al.*, 1974).
Using plants affected by different diseases Goszdiewski and Petzold
(1975) and Seemüller (1976) confirmed the observations made by
Hiruki and his collaborators. The aniline blue fluorescence method
was thus established for detecting differences between the phloem of
healthy and MLO affected plants though of course it cannot be used
in isolation because it does not detect MLO. Dijkstra and Hiruki (1974)
discussed the usefulness of the method for the early detection of sandal
spike disease and emphasised that samples should be taken from young
wood to avoid confusion with definitive callose (Esau, 1969) in nonfunctional sieve elements and that sampling and staining methods
should be standardised to avoid discrepancies related to the unpre-
dictable formation of wound callose.

Serological Methods. Several serological methods for the characterisation of MLO and spiroplasmas rely on light microscopy and these are
described in Chapter 8.

7. Electron Microscopy: Specimen Preparation for Ultrathin Sectioning

Simply stated the preparation of tissues for ultrathin sectioning requires
that samples be collected, fixed, dehydrated, and finally impregnated
and embedded in epoxy resin. Sampling and fixation are the two most
crucial steps in this sequence and the ones where most control is
required but perversely where control is most difficult to achieve. For
these reasons and because of the constraints of space this section is
largely confined to a description of sampling and fixation methods
and the reader is referred to textbooks of electron microscopical
technique for details of the remaining stages.

A. Sampling

Plants. During sampling phloem sieve tubes undergo disruptive pressure
release. Very few attempts (Parthsarathy, 1974; Braun and Sinclair,
1976; Thomas, 1979; Waters and Hunt, 1980) have been made by those

studying MLO in plants to minimise the deleterious effects of pressure release. Most authors have followed the methods described in textbooks which suggest that samples should be 'minced' in fixative and that tissue blocks should be approximately 1 mm^3. Such methods might be correctly applicable to animal tissues but they are unnecessary and disastrous when applied to plants. Phloem anatomists have gone to extraordinary lengths to reduce pressure release, for example by flash-freezing intact plants with liquid nitrogen, injecting fixatives into hollow stems, or immersing stems and twigs in vats of fixatives prior to cutting the phloem. Clearly these precautions are not always applicable to plants with MLO diseases; imagine for example trying to flash-freeze a coconut palm with lethal yellowing!

Obviously the precise way in which sampling is carried out will be dictated by the form of the plant to be studied and the method which follows is meant to illustrate the principles that must be adhered to. Stem pieces 10 to 15 cm long (or as long as practicable) should be removed from the parent plant and immediately placed in fixative. One to 2 cm lengths of tissue cut from the middle of these lengths should be split longitudinally into slivers of sides approximately 2 to 3 mm and transferred to vials of fixative. Leaves or flowers should be removed with some attached stem and then sampled under fixative like stems. Although this method does not prevent pressure release it minimises its effects and it has the additional advantage of minimising the formation of wound callose but only if fixation is begun immediately and fast-penetrating fixatives are used. It is unlikely that wound callose formation can be prevented since it may appear within 30 s of injury (Eschrich, 1975).

Insects. Insects to be sampled should be first anaesthetised with carbon dioxide. Two approaches to the sampling of insects have been used. In the first insects are dissected (e.g. Sinha and Black, 1963) under fixative and the organs removed for further processing. This method is very disruptive and it is better to use intact insects but, since fixatives do not readily penetrate the cuticle, incisions must be made in the cuticle under fixative at sites away from the organs to be studied (e.g. Bowyer and Atherton, 1971).

Cultures. Liquid cultures may be sampled either as centrifuged pellets or on the surfaces of membrane filters (Lemcke, 1971). The latter method is the easier to use but note that cellulose acetate filters dissolve in acetone so ethanol dehydration must be used after fixation. Cultures on solid media should be fixed initially *in situ* by flooding with fixative after which blocks of medium carrying the colonies can be excised for the completion of fixation.

B. Fixation

Quality of Fixation. The assessment of the quality of fixation is usually subjective and therefore difficult to define. It is generally accepted that 'a good fixation' should not disturb cells or their contents and that all the cells in a sample should be uniformly well fixed. Membranes should be regular in width and continuous, nuclear membranes should be sharply defined and without discontinuities in the perinuclear space, mitochondria should show no signs of swelling or disruption, the cytoplasm should be uniform and without empty spaces and the tissues should not be markedly shrunken. In plant cells the tonoplast and fine transcellular strands should be intact. MLO and spiroplasmas should have sharply defined membranes, their cytoplasm should not be strongly electron dense and the DNA should appear finely stranded.

For the microscopist studying MLO or spiroplasmas *in vivo* this ideal state of affairs is often difficult if not impossible to achieve. Sieve elements undergo unavoidable pressure release and the uniform fixation of the various phloem cells is made complicated because of the very different osmolar environments in the sieve elements and companion cells compared with the phloem parenchyma cells (McCoy, 1979). Insect and plant tissues often respond adversely to infections with MLO or spiroplasmas and show histopathological changes that can be detected at the light and electron microscope levels (e.g. Littau and Maramorosch, 1956, 1960; Whitcomb *et al.*, 1967, 1968a, b; Schneider, 1973; Braun and Sinclair, 1976; Esau *et al.*, 1976; Esau, 1977). These cytopathological events cause changes to the normal appearance of cells and their organelles and thereby cloud the definition of a 'good fixation'. These effects should be borne in mind when interpreting micrographs prepared from such tissues. Against this background of naturally-induced artefacts the microscopist is faced with the task of overcoming the possibility of introducing further artefacts during fixation.

Double Fixation. This method of fixation introduced by Sabatini *et al.* (1963) is now the most widely used technique for the preservation of biological tissues for electron microscopy. As originally proposed primary fixation was for 0.5 to 4 hr in 4 to 6.5% glutaraldehyde buffered to pH 7.2 with either 0.1M phosphate or 0.1M sodium cacodylate and post-fixation after rinsing in buffer was for 2 to 4 hr in 2% (w/v) osmium tetroxide again buffered to pH 7.2 with either 0.1M phosphate or sodium cacodylate plus 0.2M sucrose. Clearly numerous permutations on this basic regime are possible involving changes to the concentration of glutaraldehyde, the nature and concentrations of the buffers, the temperature and times of fixation and the concentration of osmium tetroxide. Table 4.2 lists some of the many reports describing the application of double fixation to the preservation of MLO in plant tissues and gives some indication of the permutations that are possible. Other authors have used modified primary fixatives which have consisted of mixtures of glutaraldehyde with either acrolein or formaldehyde (Table 4.3). Both these tables are far from exhaustive in listing the papers describing MLO in plants; others might have been included had the authors given sufficiently accurate descriptions of the methods used. When reporting studies of organisms as pleomorphic and osmotically labile as MLO and spiroplasmas the accurate and complete description of the fixation method used is essential. In the past these details have been absent more often than they have been given. The bewildering array of methods (Tables 4.2 and 4.3) is confusing because there is very little pattern to correlate the quality of fixation with the conditions of fixation. Rather than get bogged down in a discussion of the results obtained by the authors listed in Tables 4.2 and 4.3 in an attempt to identify methods which might be recommended for wider application I have chosen to examine the theoretical aspects of tissue fixation and from this suggest methods which in the light of previous experience are likely to give satisfactory results and minimise artefacts.

Glutaraldehyde as a Fixative. Hopwood (1972) and Glauert (1974) have discussed the theoretical and practical aspects of animal and plant tissue fixation with glutaraldehyde and their conclusions are summarised here.

(1) Glutaraldehyde penetrates tissues relatively slowly but reacts rapidly with proteins and stabilises structures by cross-linking.

(2) The time required for fixation is reduced in the presence of monovalent or divalent ions or sucrose.

(3) Glutaraldehyde does not preserve lipids and it solubilises phospholipids which can reappear on subsequent osmium tetroxide postfixation as myelin figure artefacts which can be prevented by the addition of calcium chloride (1 to 3mM) to the fixative solution. The addition of calcium chloride also improves the preservation of lipids and mitochondria.

(4) Glutaraldehyde does not destroy the osmotic properties of plant and animal cells or their organelles. Mycoplasmas behave differently. According to Lemcke (1972) initial fixation of mycoplasma in isotonic

Table 4.2: Examples of Double Fixation Schedules That Have Been Used for the Preservation of MLO in their Plant Hosts

	Primary (1°) Fixation				Buffer rinse	OsO_4 Conc. %	Duration of fixation h	Post Fixation			Disease	Reference
GA Conc. %	Duration of fixation h	Buffer	pH	°C				Buffer	pH	°C		
2.5	3	0.1M sodium cacodylate	6.8	A	+	2	2	ditto 1° fix.	6.8	4	F aster yellows in spinach	Esau (1977)
2.5	2	0.1M sodium phosphate	-	-	+	+	4	-	-	A	- peach rosette	Kirkpatrick et al. (1975)
2.5	1.5	0.1M sodium cacodylate	7.2	-	+	1	1	ditto 1° fix.	7.2	-	- clover phyllody	Gourret et al. (1973)
2.5	24	0.1M sodium cacodylate	7	-	+	1	2	ditto 1° fix.	7	-	F citrus stubborn	Smets et al. (1977)
2.5	3	0.15M phosphate	7.4	4	+	1	1	ditto 1° fix.	7.4	4	- citrus stubborn	Igwegbe & Calavan (1970)
3	-	0.15M phosphate	7	-	+	2	3	ditto 1° fix.	7	-	- aster yellows	Worley (1970)
3	-	0.1M phosphate	6.9	-	+	1	2	ditto 1° fix.	-	-	S clover dwarf	Lombardo et al. (1970)
3	1	0.025M phosphate	7.4	-	+	1	1	-	-	F	F sandal spike in Vinca	Hiruki & Dijkstra (1973a, b)
3	2	0.2M phosphate + 3% sucrose	7.3	-	+	2	4	-	-	-	- hydrangea virescence	Weivaert et al. (1975)
3	12	- phosphate	6.8	-	+	2	2	-	-	-	- elm phloem necrosis	Wilson et al. (1972)
3	5	0.08M phosphate	7	A & 4	+	2	12 - 18	ditto 1° fix.	7	4	- elm phloem necrosis in Vinca	Braun (1977)
3	1	0.1M sodium cacodylate	7.3	4	+	2	2	0.2M phosphate[b]	7.3	4	- aster yellows in Nicotiana	Hirumi & Maramorosch (1972)
3	24+	0.05M sodium cacodylate	7	A	+	2	1	-	-	S	- lethal yellowing of coconuts	Niemhaus & Steiner (1976)
3	2	0.1M phosphate	ca 7	A	+	2	2	ditto 1° fix.	7.2	A	- pecan bunch	Seliskar (1974)
3	2	0.1M sodium cacodylate	6.9	4	+	1	0.75	ditto 1° fix.	6.9	-	- Vinca phyllody	Lombardo & Pignonetelli (1970)
3	12 - 18	0.1M phosphate	6.8	4	+	2	2	-	-	A	- black locust witches'-broom	Seliskar et al. (1973)
3.5	3	0.1M phosphate	7.3	4	+	4	2	aqueous	-	-	- ash witches'-broom in dodder	Hibben & Wolanski (1971)
4	22	0.1M sodium cacodylate	7.2	A - 4	+	2	2	ditto 1° fix.	7.2	-	- lethal yellowing of coconuts	Dollet et al. (1976)
4	over night	0.1M sodium cacodylate	6.8	5	+	2	3	phosphate	6.8	5	- elm phloem necrosis	Braun & Sinclair (1976)
4	4	0.1M phosphate	-	-	+	-	3	phosphate	-	-	- pear decline	Hibino & Schneider (1970)
4	2	0.1M phosphate	7.2	4	+	2	2	ditto 1° fix.	7.2	4	- apple witches'-broom	Marwitz et al. (1973)
4	-	0.07M phosphate +0.25M sucrose	7.4	5	+	1	1	-	-	-	- citrus stubborn & greening	LaFleche & Bové (1970)
4.1	20	0.1M sodium cacodylate	7.4	4	+	1	1	0.05M phosphate	7.4	-	- lethal yellowing of coconuts	Heinze et al. (1972)
5	12	0.125M sodium phosphate	7	A	+	1	20	ditto 1° fix.	7.2	-	- legume little leaf disease	Bowyer & Atherton (1970)
5	2	0.1M phosphate	7	4	+	4[a]	6 - 8	+[a]	-	4	- albino disease of Prunus avium	Florence & Cameron (1978)
5	2	0.1M phosphate	7	4	+	2	1,2	ditto 1° fix.	7	4	- citrus little leaf	Rishi et al. (1973)
5	1.5	0.1M phosphate	7	4	+	2	2	aqueous	-	4	- citrus little leaf	Zeicer et al. (1969)
6	1	- sodium cacodylate	7.2	-	+	1	1	veronal acetate	7.2	-	F white leaf of sugar cane	Jacoli (1976)
6	1.5	- sodium cacodylate	7.2	-	+	1	over night	-	-	-	- aster yellows in callus tissue	Cousin et al. (1971b)
6	6 - 8	0.1M phosphate	7	5	+	2	4	ditto 1° fix.	7	5	- dépérissement jaune of lavender	Sinha & Paliwal (1969)
6	2	- sodium cacodylate	7	-	+	2	2	phosphate	7	-	- clover phyllody	Chen (1971)
6	2	0.1M sodium cacodylate	7.4	A	+	2	2	phosphate	7.4	4	- blueberry & cranberry diseases	Giannotti et al. (1969b)
6	2	0.1M phosphate	7.2	A	+	2	2	ditto 1° fix.	7.2	A	- apple proliferation	Granados (1969)
6	1	Millong's phosphate	7.4	A	+	2	1	Millong 50%	7.4	A	- corn stunt	Ushiyama et al. (1969)
6	24+	0.1M phosphate	7	4	+	2	2	-	-	-	S Phormium yellows	Phatak et al. (1975)
6	6	0.125M phosphate	7	-	+	2	2	0.1M phosphate	-	-	S aster yellows	Allen (1972)
6	2 - 3	0.2M phosphate	7.2	-	+	1	1	-	-	-	- line pattern of hazel	Ragozzino et al. (1971)
6.25	1	- phosphate	7.3	4	+	1	0.5	ditto 1° fix.	-	A	S potato witches'-broom	Brčák et al. (1969)

Notes: a. Chrome osmium fixative (Dalton 1955). b. Plus 5% sucrose. Abbreviations: F, uranyl acetate fixed; S, uranyl acetate block stained; A, ambient temperature; GA, glutaraldehyde.

Table 4.3: Examples of the Glutaraldehyde Containing Fixative Mixtures That Have Been Used to Preserve MLO and Spiroplasmas in Plant Tissues

Primary (1°) Fixation							Post Fixation							Disease	Reference
Fixative & conc. %			Duration of				OsO_4	Duration of							
AC	FA	GA	fixation h	Buffer	pH	°C	Conc. %	fixation h	Buffer	pH	°C				
0	3	3	over night	0.1M sodium cacodylate	6.8	5	2	3	ditto 1° fix.	6.8	5	F	elm phloem necrosis	Braun & Sinclair (1977)
1.5	0	3	3	Millonig's phosphate	7.4	-	2	4	ditto 1° fix.b	-	-		aster yellows	Chen & Hiruki (1977)
0	2	2	2	- phosphate	7.2	4	1	2	ditto 1° fix.	-	-		Hydrangea virescence	Hearon et al. (1976)
0	4	5	4	0.08M sodium cacodylate	7.2	4	2	17	-	4	4		Cirsium, Stellaria & Epilobium yellows	Begtrup & Thoasen (1975)
3	0	3	-	0.02M phosphate	7.3	-	2	-	ditto 1° fix.	-	-		Opuntia tuna monstrosa	Leseman & Casper (1970)
0	3	3	3	0.05M sodium cacodylate[a]	7.2	30	2	2	ditto 1° fix.	7.2	21	F	lethal yellowing of coconuts	Waters & Hunt (1980)
0	2	2	18	0.1M collidine	7.4	4	2	6	ditto 1° fix.	7.4	4	S	lethal yellowing of coconuts	Thomas (1979)
0	4	5	4	0.08M sodium cacodylate	7.2	4	1	17	0.2M sucrose	-	-		MLO in Silene & Agrostema	Begtrup & Lange (1977)

Notes: a. Buffer also contained 0.15M sucrose and 2mM calcium chloride.
b. Buffer also contained 1% sucrose.
Abbreviations: AC, acrolein; FA, formaldehyde; GA, glutaraldehyde; F, uranyl acetate fixed; S, uranyl acetate block stained.

solutions protects them from alterations in ultrastructure or profile shape if later they are transferred to hypotonic or hypertonic conditions.

(5) Glutaraldehyde does not contribute to the effective osmolarity of the fixation medium. Osmolarity must therefore be controlled by the buffering medium (Bone and Denton, 1971; Rasmussen, 1974).

(6) Sabatini *et al.* (1963) recommended glutaraldehyde concentrations of between 4 and 6.5%. There has been more recently a tendency to reduce the concentration of glutaraldehyde for primary fixation (Table 4.2). The results referred to in Table 4.2 have been obtained using concentrations of glutaraldehyde ranging from 2 to 6.5% and there is no evidence to suggest that any one concentration is to be preferred.

Glutaraldehyde Containing Fixative Mixtures. Karnovsky (1965) introduced a primary fixative which was a mixture of formaldehyde (4%) and glutaraldehyde (5%) buffered to pH 7.2 in 0.08M sodium cacodylate to which calcium chloride was added (5mM). The use of other mixtures of aldehydes containing acrolein, formaldehyde and glutaraldehyde has also been advocated (e.g. Mollenhauer and Totten, 1971). The rationale for the use of either acrolein and/or formaldehyde is that while they are not suitable as fixatives by themselves, they penetrate tissues more rapidly than glutaraldehyde. In this way structure is stabilised prior to complete fixation by the more slowly penetrating glutaraldehyde. Note that commercial solutions of formaldehyde contain about 11% of methanol as a stabiliser and they cannot be used for the preparation of fixative solutions. Only formaldehyde prepared from freshly depolymerised paraformaldehyde should be used.

Osmium Tetroxide Post-fixation. To complete the satisfactory preservation of tissues fixed in glutaraldehyde or aldehyde mixtures, post-fixation in a solution of osmium tetroxide is essential (Sabatini *et al.*, 1963; Karnovsky, 1965). Fixation with osmium tetroxide destroys the osmotic properties of membranes but, empirically, control of the osmolar environment during post-fixation is to be preferred. The preservation of membranes, microtubules and nervous tissue is improved by the addition of calcium chloride (1-3mM) and sucrose may be added to control osmolarity.

Uranyl Acetate Fixation. Ryter *et al.* (1958) found that the nuclear material of bacteria was stabilised after osmium tetroxide fixation by rinsing cells in 0.25 to 2% aqueous uranyl acetate. More recently uranyl acetate has been used as a third fixative for a wide variety of tissues and been found to improve the preservation of membranes as well as prokaryotic DNA. Precipitation occurs in cacodylate and phosphate buffers on the addition of uranyl acetate. For this reason tissues post-fixed in either of these buffers should be well rinsed with distilled water before uranyl acetate fixation. Some authors use uranyl acetate in either the ethanol or acetone solutions used for dehydration (so called block staining). It is unlikely, because of the extractive nature of these organic solvents, that the same beneficial effects of aqueous uranyl acetate fixation will accrue.

Buffers. With the exception of uranyl acetate all the fixatives for electron microscopy are prepared as buffered solutions. It is important to recognise that the medium, together with any additives, which is used to buffer the primary fixative can have profound effects upon the quality of fixation.

Equally good fixation of animal tissues (Sabatini *et al.*, 1963) and mycoplasmas (Lemcke, 1972) is obtained using either phosphate buffer prepared according to Sorensen (Glauert, 1974) or sodium cacodylate. A comparison of the better results from the references in Tables 4.2 and 4.3 confirms that there is no difference in the quality of fixation which can be associated with the type of buffer used.

Similarly the pH of the buffer, providing it is near neutrality, does not appear to affect the fixation of host tissues and this is probably because of the natural buffering activity of the cell contents. Mycoplasmas are not adversely affected by fixation at pH values from 5.4 to 7 (Lemcke, 1972).

The proper control of buffer osmolarity is very important, especially now it is recognised that during the fixation of plant and animal tissues glutaraldehyde and the other aldehydes do not contribute to the effective osmolarity of the solutions used. Evidence from studies of spiroplasmas and mycoplasmas shows that the same conditions apply to these organisms. Cole *et al.* (1973) found that *S. citri* inexplicably lost its helical form when exposed to different concentrations of glutaraldehyde in 0.02M sodium cacodylate buffer even when the osmolarity was apparently approximately isotonic to the culture medium (see Table 4.5). An examination of their results reveals that the effective osmolarity of their fixation medium was only about 40 mOsmols kg^{-1} (i.e. the osmolarity of 0.02M sodium cacodylate) and therefore apart from distilled water was the lowest osmolarity used in their experiments (Table 4.5). Lemcke (1972) observed that the quality of fixation of *A. laidlawii* was nearly as good in 2.5% glutaraldehyde as in 0.25% glutaraldehyde although the osmolarities of the solutions were 460 and 231 mOsmols kg^{-1} respectively. In fact the effective osmolarity of the two solutions was the same and the organisms were fixed in nearly isotonic conditions.

The osmolarity of buffers can be adjusted by the addition of sucrose. Figure 4.8 shows graphically the osmolarities of solutions of Sorensen's phosphate buffer, sodium cacodylate and sucrose and it

Figure 4.8: The Osmolarities of Sucrose ($\triangle$), Sodium Cacodylate ($\square$), and Sorensen's Phosphate Buffer ($\bigcirc$) at Different Molarities. The data for Sorensen's buffer are from Glauert (1974).

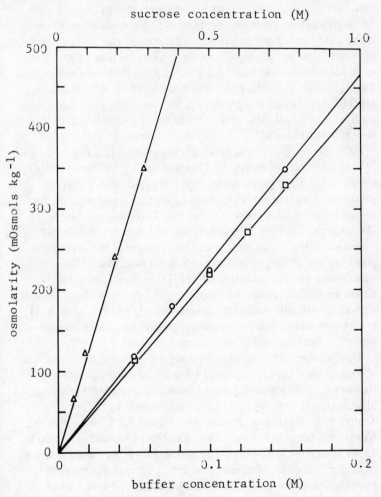

can be used to estimate the effective osmolarity of buffered fixation media because the osmolarities of mixtures are cumulative. The addition of 2mM calcium chloride increases osmolarity by 11 mOsmols kg^{-1} (Waters, unpublished) and 2% (w/v) osmium tetroxide adds approximately 70 mOsmols kg^{-1} to the buffer osmolarity (Rasmussen, 1974).

No experimental evidence is available to indicate the optimum effective osmolarity of fixatives for the preservation of MLO *in vivo*. Inspection of Tables 4.2 and 4.3 in conjunction with Figure 4.8 indicates that most often the effective osmolarities of the buffers so far used for the preservation of plants have been between 210 and 290 mOsmols kg^{-1}. Insect tissues have also been fixed under similar osmolar conditions. These values are near the lower end of the range for both sieve tube sap and insect hemolymph (see Section 2.C).

At very low osmolarities e.g. 55 mOsmols kg^{-1} (Hiruki and Dijkstra, 1973a, b) there is evidence of membrane disruption in most of the MLO figured. The same organism was well preserved when fixed in a medium with an effective osmolarity of about 230 mOsmols kg^{-1} (Dijkstra and Lee, 1972).

At higher osmolarities in Millonig's phosphate buffer (440 mOsmols kg^{-1}, Glauert, 1974) as used by Chen and Hiruki (1977) some MLO show increased cytoplasm density and strongly dumbbell-shaped profiles such as Lemcke (1972) found after fixation of mycoplasmas at high osmolarities. Chen and Hiruki (1977) considered that the abnormal profiles were either associated with dark-treated plants or senescent MLO. Ushiyama *et al.* (1969) also used Millonig's phosphate buffer and their results would indicate that, whilst high osmolarities may not adversely affect MLO in plant tissues, insect tissues are not well preserved. Welvaert *et al.* (1975) also used a buffer with a high effective osmolarity (approximately 885 mOsmols kg^{-1}) but unfortunately their figures are not at sufficiently high magnification to assess the quality of fixation.

On the basis of the evidence presently available and in the absence of experimental confirmation, the effective osmolarity of primary fixatives for both insect and plant tissues containing MLO or spiroplasmas should be between 250 and 300 mOsmols kg^{-1}.

Temperature of Fixation. From Tables 4.2 and 4.3 it can be seen that fixation has been carried out either at ambient temperatures (c. 20 to 25°C) or at about 4°C. There is no evidence from the results described to suggest that either temperature is to be preferred. From experiments with coconut palm tissues fixation at ambient temperature

(c. 20 to 30°C) produces better results than fixation at 4°C (Waters, unpublished results).

Fixation at Reduced Pressures. Several authors have fixed specimens at reduced pressures in an attempt to improve the penetration of fixatives by removing included air (Brčak *et al.*, 1969; Allen, 1972; Braun, 1977; Florance and Cameron, 1978). Whether such procedures actually improve fixation has not been investigated but there is no evidence from the results obtained to suggest improved fixation when compared with fixations at normal atmospheric pressure.

Fixation Schedule for Plant and Insect Tissues. On the basis of the previous studies of MLO in plants and insects and the theoretical aspects of tissue preservation the following schedule for the fixation of tissues is suggested. It is hoped that the wider use of a standard method will allow a more ready comparison of results than is presently possible.

(1) Sampling. This should be carried out under fixative taking the precautions described in Section 7.A.

(2) Primary fixation. For 3 to 4 hr at room temperature and at normal atmospheric pressure in 3% formaldehyde plus 3% glutaraldehyde in a buffer pH 7 to 7.2 containing 2mM calcium chloride. Either Sorensen's phosphate or sodium cacodylate may be used as the buffer and the concentration is a matter of personal choice but care must be taken to adjust the osmolarity to between 250 and 300 mOsmols kg^{-1} using sucrose if necessary.

(3) Buffer rinse. Three changes over 2 hr at room temperature in the same medium, minus the fixatives, used at stage (2) is sufficient. Plant samples should be trimmed at this stage (see Section 7.A). Protracted rinsing in buffer is to be discouraged because extraction can occur, but if it is necessary to store specimens temporarily it can be done at this stage at 4°C overnight.

(4) Post-fixation. For 1 to 2 hr at room temperature in the same medium used at stage 3 in 1% osmium tetroxide.

(5) Rinse. Three changes over 2 hr in distilled water at room temperature.

(6) Uranyl acetate fixation. For 3 hr at room temperature in 1% (w/v) aqueous uranyl acetate.

(7) Dehydration. Through an ascending acetone series.

(8) Impregnation and embedding. Since relatively large tissue pieces will have been used in the preceding stages Spurr's (Spurr, 1969) low viscosity resin is recommended.

Fixation Schedule for Cultured Organisms. For cultures in liquid media the following schedule is suggested.

(1)   Fixation. For 0.5 to 1 hr at room temperature in the culture medium itself by the simple expedient of adding concentrated glutaraldehyde to achieve a final concentration of 2 to 3% glutaraldehyde in slightly diluted buffer (e.g. Lemcke, 1972; Cole *et al.*, 1973).

(2)   Sampling. Either by filtration or centrifugation. Centrifuged pellets are usually quite fragile and therefore the cells must be supported in agar made up in culture medium (Glauert, 1974) which should be diced into blocks about 1 mm^3.

(3)   Buffer rinse. Three changes over 1 hr at room temperature in either Sorensen's phosphate or sodium cacodylate buffer at a pH and osmolarity approximately the same as the culture medium.

(4 to 8) The remaining stages are the same as those described for plant and insect tissues except that the times for post-fixation and uranyl acetate fixation can be halved.

For cultures on solid media the following schedule is suggested.

(1)   Sampling. As described in Section 7.A.

(2)   Fixation. Initially *in situ* for 0.5 hr at room temperature in 2 to 3% glutaraldehyde in the culture medium, minus the agar of course! After initial fixation excised blocks carrying colonies are fixed for a further 0.5 hr at room temperature in 2 to 3% glutaraldehyde solution prepared as above.

(3 to 8) The remaining stages are the same as those suggested for liquid cultures.

Fixation Schedule for Shipping Specimens. Workers in developing countries often require electron microscopic diagnosis of MLO infections in plants and this necessitates the shipping of specimens to electron microscope laboratories. It cannot be over-emphasised that the most detailed possible instructions be given to the collectors and as far as possible all the materials that they are likely to require should be sent to them. One cannot hope to obtain perfect results using material shipped halfway round the world but adequate results can be obtained (e.g. Dollet *et al.*, 1976; Nienhaus and Steiner, 1976; Table 4.2). The following schedule is suggested and is based on one used by Waters (1978).

(1)   Sampling. As far as possible the methods described in section 7.A should be used.

(2)   Fixation. For 3 to 4 hr at ambient temperatures in 3% glutaral-

dehyde plus 3% formaldehyde in a buffer mixture (pH 7.2)
containing 0.05M sodium cacodylate 0.15M sucrose and 2mM
calcium chloride. Sodium cacodylate is recommended because it
contains arsenic and therefore inhibits bacterial or fungal contamination of specimens in transit. Collectors of specimens should
be warned that both the fixative medium and the buffer are
poisonous.

(3)   Buffer rinse. Specimens should be rinsed in the buffer used in
stage (2) at ambient temperatures using two changes each of
1 hr. The samples should then be placed in fresh buffer and
shipped by the quickest means possible.

(4 to 8) The remaining stages are the same as those suggested for plant
and insect tissues except that on receipt the specimens should
be rinsed in fresh buffer for 30 min.

C. Osmium Tetroxide Fixatives

Variously buffered solutions of osmium tetroxide were widely used as
fixatives of biological tissues early in the history of electron microscopy
but today its use as a primary fixative has been superseded by the
aldehydes. Reports however exist describing MLO in plant and insect
tissues after fixation with osmium tetroxide. The quality of preservation achieved by Cousin *et al.* (1969a) and Dijkstra and Ie (1969)
was poor with evidence of both phloem disruption and damage to the
MLO membranes. In the latter example part of the damage was probably
caused because the tissues were embedded in methacrylate, a medium
known to cause tissue swelling and distortion (Pease, 1964). On the
other hand fixation of MLO with osmium tetroxide can preserve the
typical mycoplasmal ultrastructure (Ploaie, 1969; Smith *et al.*, 1976).

Frequently (Table 4.4) the typically delicate DNA ultrastructure
is absent from the profiles of osmium tetroxide-fixed MLO and is
replaced by approximately central irregularly shaped electron dense
bodies which are presumed to be clumped DNA. In other prokaryotes
such as mycoplasmas (e.g. Hummeler *et al.*, 1965) and bacteria (Ryter
et al., 1956) the DNA also shows similar clumping after osmium tetroxide fixation. In both instances it is regarded as an artefact of
fixation (Ryter *et al.*, 1958; Gourret, 1974; Esau, 1977).

It is apparent from Table 4.4 that there is very little pattern to
associate DNA clumping with either a particular concentration of
osmium tetroxide or any one buffer. Smith *et al.* (1976) suggested that
the deliberately induced clumping of MLO DNA using the somewhat
unconventional Dalton's chrome osmium fixative (Dalton, 1955) could

Table 4.4: Fixation of Plant or Insect Tissues in Buffered Osmium Tetroxide and its Association with the Induction of DNA Clumping in MLO

Tissue Plant	Tissue Insect	OsO$_4$ Conc. %	Duration of Fixation (hr)	Buffer	pH	DNA Clumping	Reference
+	–	2	1	0.2M phosphate	7	+	Cousin et al. (1969a)
+	–	1	2	veronal acetate	7.2	0	Ploaie (1969)
+	–	1	2	0.1M phosphate	7.3	+	Dijkstra & Ie (1969)
+	+	1	0.5	veronal acetate	6.8	+	Nasu et al. (1970)
–	+	1	–	Tyrode's solution	6.8	0	Hibino et al. (1971)
–	+[a]	1	0.5	veronal acetate	6.8	+	Nasu et al. (1974a)
–	+	1	0.5	veronal acetate	6.8	0	Nasu et al. (1974a)
–	+	1	0.5	veronal acetate	6.8	+	Nasu et al. (1974b)
+	–	1	1	0.1M sodium cacodylate	7.2	0	Smith et al. (1976)
+	–	–	–	chrome osmium b	7.2	+	Smith et al. (1976)

Notes: a. Insect cells in organ culture.
b. Prepared according to Dalton (1955).

be used as a diagnostic method to distinguish between MLO and other membrane-bound cellular inclusions such as those described by Esau *et al.* (1976) or cisternae of the endoplasmic reticulum (Florance and Cameron, 1974). The clumping effect of Dalton's fixative was abolished in samples which were post-fixed in uranyl acetate (Smith *et al.*, 1976) and evidence from an unrelated study (Rishi *et al.*, 1973) indicates that primary fixation with glutaraldehyde will also prevent the formation of DNA clumping. Smith *et al.* (1976) concluded that the clumping effect they observed was in part due to the fixative action of the ethanol used for dehydration prior to embedding. Several attempts (Waters, unpublished) to reproduce DNA clumping following the method described by Smith *et al.* (1976) in the MLO associated with coconut lethal yellowing proved unsuccessful.

Whilst osmium tetroxide can provide satisfactory fixation, it suffers from the disadvantage of producing artefacts which appear to be uncontrollable. In addition osmium tetroxide penetrates tissues only very slowly and therefore unless very small tissue pieces are used inadequate fixation will result. This disadvantage is particularly significant in studies of MLO in the sieve elements of plants where for the reasons discussed earlier (see Section 7.A) the primary fixation of large tissue pieces is to be preferred. The use of osmium tetroxide as the sole fixative for MLO cannot be recommended.

D. Potassium Permanganate Fixatives

Potassium permanganate buffered with veronal acetate was introduced as a fixative for electron microscopy by Luft (1956) and for several years after its introduction it was widely used for botanical specimens. In tissues fixed with permanganate, membranes are starkly revealed against a background of cytoplasm from which many components including ribosomes have been extracted. Permanganate also induces swelling of organelles such as mitochondria. Smith *et al.* (1976) examined the suitability of Luft's original method for the preservation of MLO and as might be expected they observed highly contrasted membranes and swollen MLO even after taking precautions to minimise any adverse tonicity effects. In a modification of Luft's method using a formaldehyde/permanganate fixation followed by uranyl acetate block staining Beakbane *et al.* (1971) figured structures thought to be MLO. These appeared as approximately circular profiles without a membrane and contained either one or two centrally located dense circular bodies of unknown origin. This ultrastructure is quite unlike that of mycoplasmas and any suggestion that they are MŁO must be regarded with scepticism.

Potassium permanganate fixation is not suitable for the preservation of MLO or host cells.

E. Specialised Fixation Methods

Apart from the study made by Smith *et al.* (1976) which is discussed in Section 7.C only Chen and Hiruki (1978b) have investigated the use of specialised fixation methods allied to electron microscopic histochemistry to study MLO. In their study Chen and Hiruki used the tannic acid-glutaraldehyde fixation method introduced by Mizuhira and Futaesaku (1972) to enhance the membranes of MLO and associated tubular structures. The use of histochemical methods is to be encouraged and the reader is referred to the range of methods used by Wilson and Collier (1976) in their studies of *M. pneumoniae* and Lewis and Knight's (1977) description of electron microscopic histochemistry.

8. Electron Microscopy of Negatively-stained MLO and Spiroplasmas

The successful use of negative staining to describe the morphology of mycoplasmas during the 1960s (e.g. Anderson and Barile, 1965; Morowitz and Maniloff, 1966; Chu and Horne, 1967) encouraged investigators of MLO to apply similar techniques because the method seemed to offer the possibility of speedier disease diagnosis than the preparation of material for ultrathin sectioning. The expectation was that a method akin to the leaf-dip technique used for the detection of plant viruses would be applicable to MLO. Instead the negative staining of MLO has had a chequered history.

Giannotti *et al.* (1968c, d) using centrifuged extracts of plants affected by clover phyllody and stolbur demonstrated that structures analogous to those described for mycoplasmas could be visualised using phosphotungstic acid (PTA) as a negative stain. No MLO structures were observed in extracts from healthy plants. Similar observations were also reported from vines affected with Flavescence dorée (Giannotti *et al.*, 1969) and rice plants with giallume disease (Belli, 1969; Pellegrini *et al.*, 1969).

A more rigorous study, including infectivity assays of the extracts, of the corn stunt agent demonstrated the presence of polymorphic bodies similar to mycoplasmas in clarified extracts or leaf-dip preparations from diseased plants negatively stained with 2% PTA (Granados, 1969). Similar structures were not present in extracts from healthy plants. Granados (1969) did however show that another group of bodies was present in extracts from both diseased and healthy plants but that these could be confidently identified as mitochondria or chloroplasts.

Hirumi and Maramorosch (1969b) also demonstrated that bodies similar to mycoplasmas could be detected in negatively stained extracts from both infectious insects and plants infected with the aster yellows MLO. They were not as confident as Granados (1969) that the bodies observed by them could always be differentiated as MLO against a background of host cell debris. The suggestion that background debris could be misidentified as MLO was investigated in comparative studies of unclarified and clarified extracts from healthy and diseased plants and HeLa cells (as model MLO cultures) from tissue culture (Wolanski and Maramorosch, 1970; Wolanski, 1973). Samples were negatively stained (2% PTA, pH 7) either with or without prior fixation in osmium tetroxide and irrespective of the conditions of preparation MLO could not be reliably differentiated from cell contents which mimicked the appearance of MLO similarly prepared. These investigations also showed that prior fixation with osmium tetroxide removed, implying lysis, all those structures which bore any resemblance to MLO in extracts from diseased plants and markedly affected the appearance of non-MLO bodies in extracts from both healthy and diseased plants. Wolanski and Maramorosch (1970) and Wolanski (1973) commented unfavourably on the suitability of PTA as a negative stain for MLO and HeLa cells but they did not investigate other negative stains or fixatives despite the suggestion that ammonium molybdate (AMB) was a better negative stain for extracted MLO (Belli, 1969). The effect of these two publications in 1970 and 1973 was, with the exception of an investigation of highly purified extracts of the clover phyllody MLO (Sinha, 1974), to halt any further exploration of negative staining for the detection of MLO in plant or insect extracts.

The unique helical morphology of the MLO (later called spiroplasma) associated with corn stunt was discovered (Davis *et al.*, 1972) in extracts examined by phase-contrast light microscopy and *in vivo* by freeze etching (Davis *et al.*, 1972) and stereo transmission electron microscopy of sectioned sieve elements (Davis and Worley, 1973). The early attempts to demonstrate the same helical morphology by negative staining of either plant extracts (Granados, 1969; Chen and Grenados, 1970; Wolanski and Maramorosch, 1970; Davis *et al.*, 1972; Wolanski, 1973) or primary cultures (Chen and Granados, 1970, Fudl-Allah *et al.*, 1972, Fudl-Allah and Calavan, 1974) all failed. The helical

Table 4.5: Osmolarity and the Stability of Helices of *Spiroplasma citri* during Log Phase Growth

	Suspension Medium	Osmolarity mOsmols kg^{-1}	Helices
SMC culture medium (isotonic)		809	+
deionised water		0	0
1%	osmium tetroxide[a]	–	lysis
2%	PTA	54	0
4%	PTA + 0.004% sucrose	105	0
2%	AMB	331	+
3%	AMB	421	+
6%	AMB	776	+
2%	GA in 0.02M sodium cacodylate	304	0
3.35%	GA in 0.02M sodium cacodylate	420	0
3.35%	GA in SMC culture medium	–	+
10%	formalin in SMC	–	+

Notes and abbreviations: a. Solvent not specified; PTA, phosphotungstic acid; AMB, ammonium molybdate; GA, glutaraldehyde.
Source: after Cole *et al.* (1973).

form was eventually demonstrated in cells from cultures using organisms fixed with glutaraldehyde prior to negative staining (as recommended by Cole *et al.*, 1973) with 0.5% aqueous uranyl acetate (Williamson and Whitcomb, 1975) or 2% PTA (Chen and Liao, 1975).

Many of the previously unexplained responses of MLO and the corn stunt spiroplasmas to the conditions of negative staining were resolved by studies of *S. citri in vitro*. In these studies advantage was taken of the ability to correlate directly the effects of different fixatives and negative stains on wet preparations viewed by dark-field light microscopy with the appearance of similarly treated organisms as visualised by electron microscopy (Cole *et al.*, 1973). *S. citri* in early log phase cultures like the corn stunt spiroplasma from plant extracts or cultures appeared as variously contorted filaments with attached blebs when negatively stained with 2 or 4% PTA. On the other hand AMB at concentrations of 2, 3 and 6% preserved the helices of *S. citri* with the highest concentration being the most efficient. This difference in response to the two negative stains was interpreted as reflecting an improvement in the osmotic environment which in PTA was strongly hypotonic but in 6% AMB was nearly isotonic to the SMC culture medium (Table 4.5). Cole *et al.* (1973)

found that 1% osmium tetroxide lysed cells of *S. citri* confirming the
earlier observations (Wolanski and Maramorosch, 1970; Wolanski,
1973) about the unsuitability of osmium tetroxide as a fixative for
MLO or spiroplasmas in plant extracts.

These observations on *S. citri*, apart from their intrinsic significance,
also emphasise the importance of maintaining the appropriate osmolarity of media used for the negative staining of spiroplasmas and MLO.

All the more recent studies requiring the negative staining of spiroplasmas either in extracts from plants or insects or cells cultivated *in
vitro* have benefitted (Davis, 1979) from the suggestion by Cole *et al.*
(1973) that cells should be fixed with glutaraldehyde before negative
staining taking care to avoid hypotonic conditions. Perhaps the time
is ripe, especially with the recent evidence that some organisms thought
to be MLO might be spiroplasmas (Kondo *et al.*, 1976; Maramorosch
and Phillips, 1978; Giannotti *et al.*, 1979) to re-examine the application of negative staining for the diagnosis of MLO diseases basing the
methods on those described by Cole *et al.* (1973) whilst bearing in mind
the strictures on interpretation discussed by Wolanski and Maramorosch
(1970). It may be that the results to be obtained could be improved
by the use of wetting agents in the staining solutions (Gregory and
Pirie, 1973) and taking precautions to avoid artefacts (Reuss, 1967;
Anderson, 1969; Robertson *et al.*, 1975b).
Serologically Specific Electron Microscopy (SSEM). This technique
using negative staining was introduced by Derrick (1973) and used to
assay the corn stunt spiroplasma from cultures and plant extracts at
antiserum dilutions of 1:1,000 to 1:10,000 by Derrick and Brlansky
(1976). The sensitivity of this method in comparison with immunodiffusion in SDS agar gels or ELISA for detecting the pea-seed-borne
virus has been assessed (Hamilton and Nichols, 1978) and been shown
to be more sensitive than either of the other serological methods.
SSEM may be worthy of consideration for development as a method
for the detection of MLO assuming suitable antisera can be obtained.

9. Scanning Electron Microscopy

Scanning electron microscopy (SEM) was introduced for the study of
mycoplasmal morphology by Biberfeld and Biberfeld (1970) and
Kammer *et al.* (1970) and subsequently its usefulness for the examination of mycoplasmas *in vitro* has been frequently demonstrated
(Boatman, 1979).

To date the application of SEM to the study of MLO and spiroplasmas has been barely explored. Maramorosch and Phillips (1978)
have described the morphology of individual organisms and colonies
identified by them as the aster yellows spiroplasma grown in solid
media.

SEM has also been used to examine MLO in sieve tube elements
(Petzold *et al.*, 1977; Haggis and Sinha, 1978) but comparable *in vivo*
studies of MLO in insects are lacking. Petzold *et al.* (1977) tested four
different methods for the preservation of MLO associated with European yellows diseases artificially transmitted to *Vinca rosea* via
Cuscuta subinclusa. Of the methods the best preservation (and the only
one figured) was obtained after double fixation in buffered glutaraldehyde and osmium tetroxide, dehydration in acetone, embedding in
wax, sectioning at 20 to 40 μm, mounting the sections on cover glasses,
removal of the wax, critical point drying and finally coating. Whilst
this method permitted the detection of MLO in sieve elements the
embedding of tissues in wax to obtain 'fractured cells' seems to be an
unnecessary operation and one which can only increase the chances of
introducing artefacts. Haggis and Sinha (1978) used less draconian
freeze fracturing techniques on tissues doubly fixed in glutaraldehyde
and osmium tetroxide prior to critical point drying, coating and observation. The surfaces of the MLO in freeze-fractured specimens were
smooth and free of surface debris whereas the surfaces of MLO exposed
to wax embedding were rough and often carried what appeared to be
surface debris. The quality of preservation obtained by freeze fracturing
suggests that such methods are to be preferred to those involving
wax embedding. It must be borne in mind that the SEM studies of
MLO so far reported have followed specimen fixation according to
regimes used for TEM and therefore the MLO have been exposed to
all the hazards associated with such treatments.

Acknowledgements

The financial and technical support received from United Kingdom
Overseas Development Administration of the Foreign and Common-
wealth Office under the Lethal Yellowing of Coconuts Research Scheme
(R3098), The Coconut Industry Board, Kingston, Jamaica and The
Government of Jamaica is gratefully acknowledged.

References

Allen, T.C. (1972). Bacilliform particles within asters infected with a western strain of aster yellows. *Virology 47*, 491–3.

Allen, T.C., Stevens, J.O., Florance, E.R. and Hampton, R.O. (1970). Ultrastructure of *Mycoplasma gallisepticum* isolate 1056. *Journal of Ultrastructural Research 33*, 318–31.

Anderson, D.R. (1969). Ultrastructural studies of mycoplasmas and the L-phase of bacteria. In *The Mycoplasmatales and the L-phase of Bacteria*, pp. 365–402, L. Hayflick Jr. (ed). New York: Appleton-Century-Crofts.

Anderson, D.R. and Barile, M.F. (1965). Ultrastructure of *Mycoplasma hominis*. *Journal of Bacteriology 90*, 180–92.

Beakbane, A.B., Mishra, M.D., Posnette, A.F. and Slater, C.H.W. (1971). Mycoplasma-like organisms associated with chat fruit and rubbery wood diseases of apple, *Malus domestica* Borkh, compared with those in strawberry with green petal disease. *Journal of General Microbiology 66*, 55–62.

Begtrup, J. and Lange, L. (1977). Mycoplasma-like organism in phloem elements of *Silene vulgaris* and *Agrostemma githago*. *Phytopathologische Zeitschrift 90*, 164–71.

Begtrup, J. and Thoasen, A. (1975). Mycoplasma-like organisms in phloem elements of *Cirsium, Stellaria* and *Epilobium*. *Phytopathologische Zeitschrift 83*, 119–26.

Belli, G. (1969). Mycoplasma-like particles in clarified extracts of diseased rice plants. *Rivista di Patologia Vegetale 5*, 3–11.

Bernstein-Ziv, R. (1971). The effect of hypotonic solutions on the morphology of cells of *Mycoplasma gallisepticum*. *Canadian Journal of Microbiology 17*, 1203–5.

Biberfeld, G. and Biberfeld, P. (1970). Ultrastructural features of *Mycoplasma pneumoniae*. *Journal of Bacteriology 102*, 855–61.

Boatman, E.S. (1979). Morphology and ultrastructure of the Mycoplasmatales. In *The Mycoplasmas*, Vol. 1, pp. 63–102, M.F. Barile and S. Razin (eds). New York: Academic Press.

Bone, Q. and Denton, E.J. (1971). The osmotic effects of electron microscope fixatives. *Journal of Cell Biology 49*, 571–81.

Borges, M. de L.V. and David-Ferreira, J.F. (1968). Presence of mycoplasma in *Lycopersicon esculentum* Mill. with 'mal azul'. *Bolitim da Sociedade Broteriana 42*, 321–33.

Bowyer, J.W. and Atherton, J.G. (1970). Observations on the relationship between Mycoplasma-like bodies and host cells of legume little leaf-diseased plants. *Australian Journal of Biological Sciences 23*, 115–25.

Bowyer, J.W. and Atherton, J.G. (1971). Mycoplasma-like bodies in french bean, dodder, and the leafhopper vector of the legume little leaf agent. *Australian Journal of Biological Sciences 24*, 717–29.

Braun, E.J. (1977). A freeze-etch and thin-section study of mycoplasmas in *Vinca rosea* phloem. *Journal of Ultrastructural Research 60*, 44–51.

Braun, E.J. and Sinclair, W.A. (1976). Histopathology of phloem necrosis in *Ulmus americana*. *Phytopathology 66*, 598–607.

Brcák, J., Králík, O., Limberk, J. and Ulrychová, M. (1969). Mycoplasma-like bodies in plants infected with potato witches'-broom disease and the response of plants to tetracycline treatment. *Biologia Plantarum* (Praha: Prague) *11*, 470–6.

Bredt, W. (1970). Experimentelle Untersuchungen über morphologie und Vermehrung der beim Menschen verkommenden Mycoplasmen unter besonderer Berucksichtigung von *Mycoplasma hominis*. *Zeitschrift für medizinische*

Mikrobiologie und Immunologie 155, 248–74.

Bredt, W., Heunert, H.H., Höfling, K.H. and Milthaler, B. (1973). Microcinematographic studies of *Mycoplasma hominis* cells. *Journal of Bacteriology 113*, 1223–7.

Cadilhac, B. and Giannotti, J. (1975). Sur la présence d'éléments à structure helicoïdal dans le phloème de *Vinca rosea* atteinte de Stolbur. *Comptes Rendus Hebdomadaires des Séances de l'Académie des Sciences, Paris, Série D 281*, 539–42.

Carle, P. (1965). Fluoroscopie des symptômes histologiques de la flavescence dorée de la vigne. *Annales épiphyties 16*, 73–85.

Cheadle, V.I., Gifford, E.M. and Esau, K. (1953). A staining combination for phloem and contiguous tissues. *Stain Technology 28*, 49–53.

Chen, M.H. and Hiruki, C. (1977). Effects of dark treatment on the ultrastructure of the aster yellows agent *in situ*. *Phytopathology 67*, 321–4.

— (1978a). Occurrence of tubular structures in *Vinca rosea* infected with the Alberta isolate of the aster yellows agent. *Protoplasma 95*, 207–16.

— (1978b). The preservation of membranes of tubular bodies associated with mycoplasmalike organisms by tannic acid. *Canadian Journal of Botany 56*, 2878–82.

Chen, M., Miyakawa, T. and Matsui, C. (1973). Citrus likubin pathogens in salivary glands of *Diaphorina citri*. *Phytopathology 63*, 194–5.

Chen, T.A. (1971). Mycoplasmalike organisms in sieve tube elements of plants infected with blueberry stunt and cranberry false blossom. *Phytopathology 61*, 233–6.

Chen, T.A. and Granados, R.R. (1970). Plant-pathogenic mycoplasma-like organism: maintenance *in vitro* and transmission to *Zea mays* L. *Science 167*, 1633–6.

Chen, T.A. and Liao, C.H. (1975). Corn stunt spiroplasma: isolation, cultivation, and proof of pathogenicity. *Science 188*, 1015–17.

Chu, H.P. and Horne, R.W. (1967). Electron microscopy of *Mycoplasma gallisepticum* and *Mycoplasma mycoides* using the negative staining technique and their comparison with *Myxovirus*. *Annals of the New York Academy of Sciences 143*, 190–203.

Cole, R.M. (1979). Mycoplasma and spiroplasma viruses: Ultrastructure. In *The Mycoplasmas*, Vol. 1, pp. 385–410, M.F. Barile and S. Razin (eds). New York: Academic Press.

Cole, R.M., Tully, J.G., Popkin, T.J. and Bové, J.M. (1973). Morphology, ultrastructure and bacteriophage infection of the helical mycoplasmalike organism (*Spiroplasma citri* gen. nov., sp. nov.) cultured from 'stubborn' disease of citrus. *Journal of Bacteriology 115*, 367–86.

Cousin, M.T. (1975). L'enroulement violacé de la pomme de terre. *Annales de Phytopathologie 7*, 167–73.

Cousin, M.T., Darpoux, H., Faivre-Amiot, A. and Staron, T. (1970). Sur la présence de micro-organismes de type mycoplasme dans le paranchyme cortical de féverolles présentant des symptômes de virescence. *Comptes Rendus Hebdomadaires des Séances de l'Académie des Sciences, Paris, Série D 271*, 1182–4.

Cousin, M.T., Gourret, J.P., Lacote, J.P. and Leclant, F. (1969a). Découverte de particules de type mycoplasme dans le liber de *Convolvulus arvensis* recoltes dans un champ de lavandins attaints de flétrissements. *Annales de Phytopathologie 1*, 297–300.

Cousin, M.T. and Grison, C. (1966). Premières observations concernant une fluorescence anormale dans le liber interne de plusieurs solanées infectées par le virus de Stolbur et d'une apocynacea atteinte de Phyllodie. *Annales épiphyties 17*, 93–8.

Cousin, M.T. and Kartha, K.K. (1975). Electron microscopy and plant mycoplasma-like agents (MLA). *Proceedings of the Indian National Science Academy; Part B Biological Sciences 41*, 343–54.

Cousin, M.T., Maillet, P.L. and Gourret, J.P. (1969b). La virescence du cotonnier *(Gossypium hirsutum* L.) novelle maladie a Mycoplasmas. *Comptes Rendus Hebdomadaires des Séances de l'Académie des Sciences, Paris, Série D 268*, 2382–4.

Cousin, M.T., Moreau, J.P., Kartha, K.K., Staron, T. and Faivre-Amiot, A. (1971b). Polymorphisme des micro-organismes de type mycoplasme recontrés dans les tubes criblés de lavandins 'Abrial' attaints de 'Dépérissement jaune'. *Comptes Rendus Hebdomadaires des Séances de l'Académie des Sciences, Paris, Série D 272*, 2082–5.

Cousin, M.T., Ruegg, E.F. and Kartha, K.K. (1972). Observation d'apex de tabacs *(Nicotiana tabacum* L. var. *Xanthi*) atteints de stolbur: étude de quelques zones a mycoplasmes. *Comptes Rendus Hebdomadaires des Séances de l'Académie des Sciences, Paris, Série D 274*, 538–41.

Cousin, M.T., Schweisguth, B., Faivre-Amiot, A., Kartha, K.K., Staron, T. and Moreau, J. (1971a). Contribution à l'étude du cycle des mycoplasmes chez les végétaux à l'aide d'observations effectuées sur Oignon atteint d'"Aster Yellow'. *Comptes Rendus Hebdomadaires des Séances de l'Académie des Sciences, Paris, Série D 272*, 830–3.

Dabek, A.J. (1977). Electron microscopy of Kaincopé and Cape St. wilt diseased coconut tissue from West Africa. *Phytopathologische Zeitschrift 88*, 341–6.

Dalton, A.J. (1955). A chrome-osmium fixative for electron-microscopy. *Anatomical Record 121*, 281.

Davis, R.E. (1978). Spiroplasma associated with flowers of the tulip tree *(Lirodendron tulipifera* L.). *Canadian Journal of Microbiology 24*, 954–9.

— (1979). Spiroplasmas: newly recognised arthropod-borne pathogens. In *Leafhopper Vectors and Plant Disease*, pp. 451–84., K. Maramorosch and K.F. Harris (eds). New York: Academic Press.

Davis, R.E. and Whitcomb, R.F. (1971). Mycoplasma, rickettsiae and chlamydiae: possible relation to yellows diseases and other disorders of plants and insects. *Annual Review of Phytopathology 9*, 119–54.

Davis, R.E., Worley, J.F., Whitcomb, R.G., Ishijima, T. and Steere, R.L. (1972). Helical filaments produced by a mycoplasma-like organism associated with corn stunt. *Science 176*, 521–3.

Davis, R.E. and Worley, J.F. (1973). Spiroplasma: motile, helical microorganism associated with corn stunt disease. *Phytopathology 63*, 403–8.

Derrick, K.S. (1973). Quantitative assay for plant viruses using serologically specific electronmicroscopy. *Virology 56*, 652–3.

Derrick, K.S. and Brlansky, R.H. (1976). Assay for viruses and mycoplasmas using serologically specific electron microscopy. *Phytopathology 66*, 815–20.

Dijkstra, J. and Hiruki, C. (1974). A histochemical study on sandal *(Santalum album)* affected with spike disease and its diagnostic value. *Netherlands Journal of Plant Pathology 80*, 37–47.

Dijkstra, J. and Ie, T.S. (1969). Presence of mycoplasma-like bodies in the phloem of sandal affected with spike disease. *Netherlands Journal of Plant Pathology 75*, 374–8.

Dijkstra, J. and Lee, P.E. (1972). Transmission by dodder of sandal spike disease and the accompanying mycoplasma-like organisms via *Vinca rosea*. *Netherlands Journal of Plant Pathology 78*, 218–24.

Doi, Y., Teranka, M., Yora, K. and Asuyama, H. (1967). Mycoplasma- or PLT-like microorganisms found in the phloem elements of plants infected with mulberry dwarf, potato witches'-broom, aster yellows or paulowinia witches' broom. *Annals of the Phytopathological Society of Japan 33*. 259- 66. [Translated from the original Japanese in *Review of Plant Protection Research* (1969) *2*, 84-8.]

Dollet, M., Giannotti, J. and Czarnecky. (1976). Maladie de Kaincopé: présence de mycoplasmes dans le phloème des cocotiers malades. *Oléagineux 31*, 169-71.

Eden-Green, S.J. and Tully, J.G. (1979). Isolation of *Acholeplasma* spp. from coconut palms affected by lethal yellowing disease in Jamaica. *Current Microbiology 2*, 311-16.

Edward, D.G. ff. (1954). The pleuropneumonia group of organisms; a review, together with some new observations. *Journal of General Microbiology 10*, 27-64.

Esau, K. (1969). *The Phloem*. Berlin: Gebrüder Borntraeger.

— (1977). Membraneous modifications in sieve element plastids of spinach affected by the aster yellows disease. *Journal of Ultrastructural Research 59*, 87-100.

Esau, K., Magyarosy, A.C. and Breazeale, V. (1976). Studies of the mycoplasma-like organism (MLO) in spinach leaves affected by aster yellows disease. *Protoplasma 90*, 189-203.

Eschrich, W. (1975). Sealing systems in phloem. In *Transport in Plants: Phloem Transport Encyclopedia of Plant Physiology*, Vol. 1, pp. 39-56, M.H. Zimmerman and J.A. Milburn (eds). Berlin: Springer-Verlag

Eschrich, W. and Currier, H.B. (1964). Identification of callose by its diachrome and fluochrome reactions. *Stain Technology 39*, 303-7.

Feder, N. and O'Brien, T.P. (1968). Plant microtechnique: some principles and new methods. *American Journal of Botany 55*, 123-42.

Feder, N. and Wolf, M.K. (1965). Studies on nucleic acid metachromasy. II. Metachromatic and orthochromatic staining by toluidine blue of nucleic acids in tissue sections. *Journal of Cell Biology 27*, 327-36.

Florance, E.R. and Cameron, H.R. (1974). Vesicles in expanded endoplasmic reticulum cisternae structures that resemble mycoplasma-like bodies. *Protoplasma 79*, 337-48.

— (1978). Three-dimensional structure and morphology of mycoplasma-like bodies associated with albino disease of *Prunus avium*. *Phytopathology 68*, 75-80.

Freundt, E.A. (1952). Morphological studies of the peripneumonia organism (*Micromyces peripneumoniae bovis*). *Acta pathologica et microbiologica scandinavica 31*, 508-29.

— (1960). Morphology and classification of the PPLO. *Annals of the New York Academy of Sciences 79*, 312-25.

— (1969). Cellular morphology and the mode of replication of the mycoplasmas. In *The Mycoplasmatales and the L-Phase of Bacteria*, pp. 281-315, L. Hayflick Jr. (ed). New York: Appleton-Century-Crofts.

Freundt, E.A. and Edward, D.G. (1979). Classification and taxonomy. In *The Mycoplasmas*, Vol. 1, pp. 1-41, M.F. Barile and S. Razin (eds). New York: Academic Press.

Fudl-Allah, A.E.A. and Calavan, E.C. (1974). Cellular morphology and reproduction of the mycoplasmalike organism associated with citrus stubborn disease. *Phytopathology 64*, 1309-13.

Fudl-Allah, A.E.A., Calavan, E.C. and Igwegbe, E.C.K. (1972). Culture of a mycoplasmalike organism associated with stubborn disease of citrus. *Phytopathology 62*, 729-31.

Giannotti, J. (1969). Lésions cellulaires chez deux cicadelles vectrices de la phyllodie du Trèfle. *Annales de la Société Entomologique de France* (N.S.) *5*, 155–60.

Giannotti, J., Devauchelle, G. and Vago, C. (1968a). Micro-organismes de type mycoplasme chez une cicadelle et une plante infectées par la phyllodie. *Comptes Rendus Hebdomadaires des Séances de l'Académie des Sciences, Paris, Série D 266*, 2168–70.

Giannotti, J., Morvan, G. and Vago, C. (1968b). Micro-organisms de type mycoplasme dans les cellules libériennes de *Malus sylvestris* L. atteint de la maladie des proliferations. *Comptes Rendus Hebdomadaires des Séances de l'Académie des Sciences, Paris, Série D 267*, 76–7.

Giannotti, J., Vago, C. Devauchelle, G. and Marchoux, G. (1968c). Recherches sur les microorganisms de type mycoplasme dans les cicadelles vectrices et dans les végétaux atteints de jaunisses. *Entomologia experimentalis et applicata 11*, 470–4.

Giannotti, J., Vago, C. and Duthoit, J.L. (1968d). Isolement et purification de microorganismes à structure mycoplasmes à partir de cicadelles et de plantes infectées de jaunisses. *Revue de Zoologie Agricole et Appliquée 4-6*, 69–72.

Giannotti, J., Devauchelle, G., Marchoux, G. and Vago, C. (1969). Recherches sur le pleomorphisme des micro-organismes de type mycoplasme chez les plantes atteintes de jaunisses. *Comptes Rendus Hebdomadaires des Séances de l'Académie des Sciences, Paris, Série D 268*, 1354–6.

Giannotti, J., Devauchelle, G., Vago, C. and Marchoux, G. (1973). Rod-shaped virus-like particles associated with degenerating mycoplasma in plant and insect vector. *Annales de Phytopathologie 5*, 461–5.

Giannotti, J., Vago, C. and Giannotti, D. (1979). Culture *in vitro* d'un mycoplasme agent étiologique de phyllodie chez Trèfle. *Comptes Rendus Hebdomadaires des Séances de l'Académie des Sciences, Paris, Série D 288*, 85–7.

Glauert, A.M. (1974). Fixation, dehydration and embedding of biological specimens. In *Practical Methods in Electron Microscopy*, Vol 3, pp. 1–207, A.M. Glauert (ed). Amsterdam: North-Holland Publishing Company.

Goszdziewski, M. and Petzold, H. (1975). Versuche zum fluoreszenzmikroskopischen Nachweis mykoplasmaähnlicher Organismen in Pflanzen. *Phytopathologische Zeitschrift 82*, 63–9.

Gourret, J.P. (1974). Mycoplasmas as phytopathogenic agents ultrastructural studies and some new problems. *Les Mycoplasmes/Mycoplasmas. Les Colloques de l'Institut National de la Santé et de la Recherche Médicale 33*, 215–22.

Gourret, J.P., Maillet, P.L. and Gouranton, J. (1973). Virus-like particles associated with the mycoplasmas of clover phyllody in the plant and insect vector. *Journal of General Microbiology 74*, 241–9.

Graf, M.E., Ehrenfeld, R. and Davis, R.E. (1978). Stereo electronmicroscopy of mycoplasma-like organisms in *Erodium cicutarium* with yellows disease symptoms. *Plant Disease Reporter 62*, 535–8.

Granados, R.R. (1969). Electron microscopy of plants and insect vectors infected with the corn stunt disease agent. *Contributions of the Boyce Thompson Institute 24*, 173–87.

Granados, R.R., Maramorosch, K. and Shikata, E. (1968). Mycoplasma: suspected etiologic agent of corn stunt. *Proceedings of the National Academy of Sciences of the United States of America 60*, 841–4.

Granados, R.R. and Meehan, D.J. (1975). Pathogenicity of the corn stunt agent to an insect vector, *Dalbulus elimatus. Journal of Invertebrate Pathology 26*, 313–20.

Granett, A.L. and Gilmer, R.M. (1971). Mycoplasmas associated with X-disease in various *Prunus* species. *Phytopathology 61*, 1036–7.

Gregory, D.W. and Pirie, B.J.S. (1973). Wetting agents for biological electron microscopy 1. General considerations and negative staining. *Journal of Microscopy 99*, 261–5.

Haggis, G.H. and Sinha, R.C. (1978). Scanning electron microscopy of mycoplasmalike organisms after freeze fracture of plant tissues affected with clover phyllody and aster yellows. *Phytopathology 68*, 677–80.

Hamilton, R.I. and Nichols, C. (1978). Serological methods for detection of pea seed-borne mosaic virus in leaves and seeds of *Pisum sativum*. *Phytopathology 68*, 539–43.

Hammel, H.T. (1968). Measurement of turgor pressure and its gradient in the phloem of oak. *Plant Physiology 43*, 1042–8.

Hampton, R.O., Florance, E.R., Whitcomb, R.F. and Seidler, R.J. (1976). Evidence suggesting nonassociation of mycoplasma with pea disease. *Phytopathology 66*, 1163–8.

Hampton, R.O., Stevens, J.O. and Allen, T.C. (1969). Mechanically transmissible plant mycoplasma from naturally infected peas. *Plant Disease Reporter 53*, 499–503.

Hearon, S.S., Lawson, R.H., Smith, F.F., McKenzie, J.T. and Rosen, J. (1976). Morphology of filamentous forms of a mycoplasmalike organism associated with Hydrangea virescence. *Phytopathology 66*, 608–16.

Heinze, K., Petzold, H. and Marwitz, R. (1972). Beitrag zur Ätiologie der Tödlichen Vergilbung der Kokospalme (Lethal Yellowing Disease of coconut palm). *Phytopathologische Zeitschrift 74*, 230–7.

Hibben, C.R. and Wolanski, B. (1971). Dodder transmission of a mycoplasma from ash witches' broom. *Phytopathology 61*, 151–6.

Hibino, H., Kaloostian, G.H. and Schneider, H. (1971). Mycoplasma-like bodies in the pear psylla vector of pear decline. *Virology 43*, 34–40.

Hibino, H. and Schneider, H. (1970). Mycoplasma-like bodies in sieve tubes of pear trees affected with pear decline. *Phytopathology 60*, 499–501.

Hiruki, C. and Dijkstra, J. (1973a). Light and electron microscopy of *Vinca* plants infected with mycoplasma-like bodies of the sandal spike disease. *Netherlands Journal of Plant Pathology 79*, 207–17.

— (1973b). An anomalous form of mycoplasma-like bodies in periwinkle infected with the sandal spike agent. *Netherlands Journal of Plant Pathology 79*, 112–21.

Hiruki, C., Giannotti, J. and Dijkstra, J. (1974). A comparative study of fluorescence in stems of *Vinca rosea* infected with mycoplasmas of different plant origins. *Netherlands Journal of Plant Pathology 80*, 145–53.

Hiruki, C. and Shukla, P. (1973). Mycoplasma-like bodies associated with witches'-broom of bleeding heart. *Phytopathology 63*, 88–92.

Hirumi, H. and Maramorosch, K. (1969a). Mycoplasma-like bodies in the salivary glands of insect vectors carrying the aster yellows agent. *Journal of Virology 3*, 82–4.

— (1969b). Further evidence for a mycoplasma etiology of aster yellows. *Phytopathology 59*, 1030–1.

— (1972). Natural degeneration of mycoplasmalike bodies in an aster yellows infected host plant. *Phytopathologische Zeitschrift 75*, 9–26.

— (1973a). Intracytoplasmic mycoplasma-like bodies in phloem parenchyma cells of aster yellows infected *Nicotiana rustica*. *Phytopathologische Zeitschrift 77*, 71–83.

— (1973b). Ultrastructure of the aster yellows agent: mycoplasma-like bodies in sieve tube elements of *Nicotiana rustica*. *Annals of the New York Academy of Sciences 225*, 201–22.

Holmes, F.O., Hirumi, H. and Maramorosch, K. (1972). Witches'-broom of willow: *Salix* yellows. *Phytopathology 62*, 826–8.

Hooper, G.R., Lacy, M.L. and Vest, G. (1971). Mycoplasma-like bodies associated with onion bulbs sprouting in storage. *Plant Disease Reporter 55*, 824–8.

Hopwood, D. (1972). Theoretical and practical aspects of glutaraldehyde fixation. *Histochemical Journal 4*, 267–303.

Hull, R. (1972). Mycoplasma and plant diseases. *Pest Articles and News Summaries 18*, 154–64.

Hummeler, K., Armstrong, D. and Tomassini, N. (1965). Cytopathogenic mycoplasmas associated with two human tumors. II Morphological aspects. *Journal of Bacteriology 90*, 511–16.

Igwegbe, E.C.K. and Calavan, E.C. (1970). Occurrence of mycoplasmalike bodies in phloem of stubborn-infected citrus seedlings. *Phytopathology 60*, 1525–6.

Jacoli, G.G. (1974). Translocation of mycoplasma-like bodies through sieve pores in plant tissue culture infected with aster yellows. *Canadian Journal of Botany 52*, 2085–8.

Jones, A.L., Hooper, G.R., Rosenberger, D.A. and Chevalier, J. (1974). Mycoplasmalike bodies associated with peach and periwinkle exhibiting symptoms of peach yellows. *Phytopathology 64*, 1154–6.

Kahn, R.P., Lawson, R.H., Monroe, R.L. and Hearon, S. (1972). Sweet potato little-leaf (witches'-broom) associated with a mycoplasmalike organism. *Phytopathology 62*, 903–9.

Kammer, G.M., Pollack, J.D. and Klainer, A.S. (1970). Scanning-beam electron microscopy of *Mycoplasma pneumoniae. Journal of Bacteriology 104*, 499–502.

Karnovsky, M.J. (1965). A formaldehyde/glutaraldehyde fixative of high osmolarity for use in electron microscopy. *Journal of Cell Biology 27*, 137A.

Kirkpatrick, H.C., Lowe, S.K. and Nyland, G. (1975). Peach rosette: the morphology of an associated mycoplasmalike organism and chemotherapy of the disease. *Phytopathology 65*, 864–70.

Klieneberger, E. and Smiles, J. (1942). Some new observations on the developmental cycle of the organism of bovine pleuropneumonia and related microbes. *Journal of Hygiene 42*, 110–23.

Kondo, F., McIntosh, A.H., Padhi, S.B. and Maramorosch, K. (1976). Electron microscopy of a new plant-pathogenic spiroplasma isolated from *Opuntia*. In *34th Annual Proceedings of the Electron Microscopy Society of America*, pp. 56–7, G.W. Bailey (ed).

Laflèche, D. and Bové, J.M. (1970). Mycoplasmes dans les agrumes atteintes de 'Greening' de 'Stubborn' ou de maladies similaires. *Fruits (Paris) 25*, 455–65.

Lemcke, R.M. (1971). Sizing small organisms. *Nature 229*, 492–3.

— (1972). Osmolar concentration and fixation of mycoplasmas. *Journal of Bacteriology 110*, 1154–62.

Lemcke, P.A., Kugleman, B., Morimoto, H., Jacobs, E.C. and Ellison, J.R. (1978). Fluorescent staining of fungal nuclei with a benzimidol derivative. *Journal of Cell Science 29*, 77–84.

Lesemann, D. and Casper, R. (1970). 'Mycoplasma-like bodies' in Kakteen mit Hexenbesenwuchs. *Phytopathologische Zeitschrift 67*, 175–9.

Lewis, P.R. and Knight, D.P. (1977). Staining methods for sectioned material. In *Practical Methods in Electron Microscopy*, Vol. 5, pp. 1–311, A.M. Glauert (ed). Amsterdam: North-Holland Publishing Company.

Lillie, R.D. (1954). *Histopathologic Technic and Practical Histochemistry*. New York: Blakiston.

Littau, V.C. and Maramorosch, K. (1956). Cytological effects of aster-yellows virus on its insect vector. *Virology 2*, 128–30.

— (1960). A study of the cytological effects of aster yellows virus on its insect vector. *Virology 10*, 483–500.

Lombardo, G., Bassi, M. and Gerola, F.M. (1970). Mycoplasma development and cell alterations in white clover affected by clover dwarf. An electron microscopy study. *Protoplasma 70*, 61–71.

Lombardo, G. and Pignattelli, P. (1970). Cultivation in a cell-free medium of a mycoplasma-like organism from *Vinca rosea* with phyllody symptoms of the flowers. *Annali de Microbiologica et Enzimologica 20*, 83–8.

Luft, J.H. (1956). Permanganate a new fixative for electron microscopy. *Journal of Biophysical and Biochemical Cytology 2*, 799–801.

MacBeath, J.H., Nyland, G. and Spurr, A.R. (1972). Morphology of mycoplasma-like bodies associated with peach X-disease in *Prunus avium*. *Phytopathology 62*, 935–7.

Maillet, P.L. (1970a). Contribution à l'étude du cycle des mycoplasmes à propos 'pouches a mycoplasmes' dans les glandes salivaires d'*Euscelis plebejus* Brullé, vecteur de la phyllodie du Trèfle. *Comptes Rendus Hebdomadaires des Séances de l'Académie des Sciences, Paris, Série D 270*, 731–3.

— (1970b). Infection simultanée par des particules de type PLT (rickettsiales) et de type PPLO (Mycoplasmatales) chez un insecte vecteur de la phyllodie du Trèfle, *Euscelis lineolatus* Brullé (Homoptera; Jassidae). *Journal de Microscopie 9*, 827–32.

Maillet, P.L. and Gouranton, J.(1970). L'intestin moyen de certains Homoptères, lieu de transit et de multiplication de particules de type mycoplasme. *Comptes Rendus Hebdomadaires des Séances de l'Académie des Sciences, Paris, Série D 270*, 1535–7.

— (1971). Étude du cycle biologique du mycoplasme de la phyllodie du Trèfle dans l'insecte vecteur, *Euscelis lineolatus* Brullé (Homoptera; Jassidae). *Journal de Microscopie 11*, 143–62.

Maniloff, J. and Morowitz, H.J. (1972). Cell biology of the mycoplasmas. *Bacteriological Reviews 36*, 263–90

Maniloff, J.H., Morowitz, H.J. and Barnett, R.J. (1965). Ultrastructure and ribosomes of *Mycoplasma gallisepticum*. *Journal of Bacteriology 90*, 193–204.

Maramorosch, K. (1974). Mycoplasma and rickettsiae in relation to plant diseases. *Annual Review of Microbiology 28*, 301–24.

— (1976). Plant mycoplasma diseases. In *Encyclopedia of Plant Physiology; New Series*, Vol. 4, pp. 150–71, A. Pirson and M.H. Zimmerman (eds). Berlin: Springer-Verlag.

Maramorosch, K., Granados, R.R. and Hirumi, H. (1970). Mycoplasma diseases of plants and insects. *Advances in Virus Research 16*, 135–93.

Maramorosch, K. and Phillips, D.M. (1978). Agar colonies of aster yellows spiroplasma: scanning electron microscopy. *Zentralblatt für Bakteriologie, Parasitenkunde, Infektionskrankheiten und Hygiene, Erste Abteilung Originale, 241*. 224–5.

Maramorosch, K., Shikata, E. and Granados, R.R. (1968a). Mycoplasma-like bodies in leafhoppers and diseased plants. *Phytopathology 58*, 886.

— ((1968b). Structures resembling mycoplasma in diseased plants and insect vectors. *Transactions of the New York Academy of Sciences 30*, 841–55.

Markham, P.G., Townsend, R., Bar-Joseph, M., Daniels, M.J., Plaskitt, A. and Meddins, B.M. (1974). Spiroplasmas are the causal agents of citrus little leaf disease. *Annals of Applied Biology 78*, 49–57.

Markham, P.G., Townsend, R., Plaskitt, K. and Saglio, P. (1977). Transmission of corn stunt to dicotyledonous plants. *Plant Disease Reporter 61*, 342–5.

Marwitz, R. and Petzold, H. (1976). Elektronenmikroskopischer Nachweis mycoplasmaähnlicher Organismen in Delphinium-hybriden mit Blütenvergrünung und verlaubung. *Phytopathologische Zeitschrift 87*, 1–11.

Marwitz, R., Petzold, H. and Kunze, L..(1973). Elektronenmikroskopische

Untersuchungen über das Verkommen mykoplasmaähnlicher Organismen in triebsuchtranken Apfel-bäumen. *Phytopathologische Zeitschrift 77*, 84-8.

McCoy, R.E. (1979). Mycoplasmas and yellows diseases. In *The Mycoplasmas*, Vol. 3, pp. 229-64, R.F. Whitcomb and J.G. Tully (eds). New York: Academic Press.

Metz, J. and Bredt, W. (1971). Elektronenmikroskopische Untersuchungen an *Mycoplasma hominis* (Stamm W 463/69). *Zeitschrift fur medizinische Mikrobiologie und Immunologie 156*, 368-78.

Milburn, J.A. (1975). Pressure flow. In *Transport in Plants I: Phloem Transport. Encyclopedia of Plant Physiology*, Vol. 1, pp. 328-53, M.H. Zimmerman and J.A. Milburn (eds). Berlin: Springer-Verlag.

Miles, P.W. (1972). The saliva of Hemiptera. *Advances in Insect Physiology 9*, 183-255.

Mizuhira, V. and Futaesaku, Y. (1972). New fixation for biological membranes using tannic acid. *Acta Histochemica et Cytochemica 5*, 233-6.

Mollenhauer, H.H. and Totten, C. (1971). Studies on seeds 1. Fixation of seeds. *Journal of Cell Biology 48*, 387-94.

Morowitz, H.J. and Maniloff, J. (1966). Analysis of the life cycle of *Mycoplasma gallisepticum*. *Journal of Bacteriology 91*, 1638-44.

Morowitz, H.J. and Wallace, D.C. (1973). Genome size and life cycle of the mycoplasma. *Annals of the New York Academy of Sciences 225*, 62-73.

Muelas, J.M. and Ales, J.M. (1973). Method for detecting mycoplasma and bacterial L-form colonies in relief with an ordinary light microscope by means of oblique light. *Applied Microbiology 25*, 484-8.

Nasu, S., Jensen, D.D. and Richardson, J. (1970). Electronmicroscopy of mycoplasma-like bodies associated with insect and plant hosts of peach western X-disease. *Virology 41*, 583-95.

— (1974a). Primary culturing of the western X mycoplasmalike organism from *Collandonus montanus* leafhopper vectors. *Applied Entomology and Zoology 9*, 115-26.

Nasu, S., Kono, Y. and Jensen, D.D. (1974b). The multiplication of western X mycoplasmalike organism in the brain of a leafhopper vector, *Collodanus montanus* (Homoptera: Cicadellidae). *Applied Entomology and Zoology 9*, 277-9.

Nienhaus, F. and Steiner, K.G. (1976). Mycoplasmalike organisms associated with Kaincopé disease of coconut palms in Togo. *Plant Disease Reporter 60*, 1000-2.

Okuda, S. and Nishimura, N. (1974). Witches'-broom of *Cryptotaenia japonica* Hassk. *Annals of the Phytopathological Society of Japan 40*, 439-51.

Ørskov, J. (1927) Étude sur la morphologie du virus peripneumoniae. *Annales de l'Institut Pasteur (Paris) 41*, 473-82.

Parthasarathy, M.V. (1974). Mycoplasmalike organisms associated with lethal yellowing disease of palms. *Phytopathology 64*, 667-74.

Pellegrini, S., Belli, G. and Gerola, F.M. (1969). Mycoplasma-like bodies in rice plants infected with a yellows-type disease. *Giornale Botanico Italiano 103*, 395-9.

Pearse, A.G.E. (1968). *Histochemistry Theoretical and Applied*, Vol. 1, 759 pp. London: J. & A. Churchill Ltd.

Pease, D.C. (1964). *Histological Techniques for Electron Microscopy* 2nd Edition, 381 pp. New York: Academic Press.

Petzold, H., Marwitz, R., Özel, M. and Goszdziewski, P. (1977). Versuche zum rasterelektronenmikroscopischen Nachweis von mykoplasmaähnlichen Organismen. *Phytopathologische Zeitschrift 89*, 237-48.

Phatak, H.C., Lundsgaard, T., Verma, V.S. and Singh, S. (1975). Mycoplasma-like bodies associated with *Cannabis* phyllody. *Phytopathologische Zeitschrift 83*, 281–4.

Ploaie, P.G. (1969). Aster yellows agent in Romania. *Revue Romaine de Biologie – Série Botanique 14*, 335–9.

— (1971). Particles resembling viruses associated with mycoplasma-like organism in plants. *Revue Roumaine de Biologie – Série Botanique 16*, 3–6.

Ploaie, P. and Maramorosch, K. (1969). Electron microscopic demonstration of particles resembling mycoplasma or psittacocis – lymphogranuloma–trachoma group in plants infected with European yellow-type diseases. *Phytopathology 59*, 536–44.

Pollard, D.G. (1968). Stylet penetration and feeding damage of *Eupteryx melissae* Curtis (Hemiptera: Cicadellidae) on sage. *Bulletin of Entomological Research 58*, 55–71.

— (1969). Directional control of the stylets in phytophagous Hemiptera. *Proceedings of the Royal Entomological Society, London, Series-A 44*, 173–85.

— (1973). Plant penetration by feeding aphids (Hemiptera: Aphidoidea): a review. *Bulletin of Entomological Research 62*, 631–714.

Poulson, D.F. and Sakaguchi, B. (1961). Nature of 'sex ratio' agent in *Drosophila*. *Science 133*, 1489–90.

Purohit, S.D., Ramawat, K.G. and Arya, H.C. (1978). Light microscopic detection of mycoplasma-like organism (MLO) in *Sesamum* phyllody. *Current Science 47*, 866–7.

Ragozzino, A., Iaccarino, F.M. and Viggiani, G. (1971). Indagini preliminari sulla eziologica della 'Maculatura lineare' del nocciuolo. *Rivista di patologia vegetale 7*, 83–94.

Raine, J. and Forbes, A.R. (1971). The salivary syringe of the leafhopper *Macrosteles facifrons* (Homoptera: Cicadellidae) and the occurrence of mycoplasma-like organisms in its ducts. *The Canadian Entomologist 103*, 110–16.

Raine, J., Forbes, A.R. and Skelton, F.E. (1976). Mycoplasma-like bodies, Rickettsia-like bodies and salivary bodies in the salivary glands and saliva of the leafhopper *Macrosteles fascifrons* (Homoptera: Cicadellidae). *The Canadian Entomologist 108*, 1009–19.

Rasmussen, K.E. (1974). Fixation in aldehydes a study on the influence of the fixative, buffer, and osmolarity upon the fixation of the rat retina. *Journal of Ultrastructural Research 46*, 87–102.

Razin, S. (1963). Osmotic lysis of *Mycoplasma. Journal of General Microbiology 33*, 471–5.

— (1964). Factors influencing the osmotic fragility of Mycoplasma. *Journal of General Microbiology 36*, 451–9.

— (1969). Structure and function in mycoplasma. *Annual Review of Microbiology 23*, 317–56.

— (1978). The mycoplasmas. *Microbiological Reviews 42*, 414–70.

Razin, S. and Cosenza, B.J. (1966). Growth phases of mycoplasma in liquid media observed with phase-contrast microscope. *Journal of Bacteriology 91*, 858–69.

Razin, S., Cosenza, B.J. and Tourtellotte, M.E. (1967). Filamentous growth of mycoplasma. *Annals of the New York Academy of Sciences 143*, 66–72.

Reuss, K. (1967). Influence of fixation on gross morphology of *Mycoplasma. Journal of Bacteriology 93*, 490–2.

Rishi, N., Okuda, S., Arai, K., Doi, Y., Yora, K. and Bhargava, K.S. (1973). Mycoplasmalike bodies, possibly the cause of grassy shoot disease of sugar cane in India. *Annals of the Phytopathological Society of Japan 39*, 429–31.

Robertson, J., Gomersall, M. and Gill, P. (1975a). *Mycoplasma hominis*: growth, reproduction, and isolation of small viable cells. *Journal of Bacteriology 124*, 1007–18.

Robertson, J., Gomersall, M. and Gill, P. (1975b). Effect of preparatory techniques on the gross morphology of *Mycoplasma hominis*. *Journal of Bacteriology 124*, 1019–22.

Rodwell, A.W. (1965). The stability of *Mycoplasma mycoides*. *Journal of General Microbiology 40*, 227–34.

Rodwell, A.W., Peterson, J.E. and Rodwell, E.S. (1973). Nature of striated structures in mycoplasmas. *Annals of the New York Academy of Sciences 225*, 190–200.

Russell, W.C., Newman, C. and Williamson, D.H. (1975). A simple cytochemical technique for demonstration of DNA in cells infected with mycoplasmas and viruses. *Nature 256*, 461–2.

Ryter, A., Kellenberger, E., Birch-Anderson, A. and Maaløe, O. (1958). Étude au microscope électronique de plasmas contenant de l'acide désoxyribonucléique. *Zeitschrift für Naturforschung 13*, 597–605.

Sabatini, D.D., Bensch, K. and Barrnett, R.J. (1963). Cytochemistry and electron microscopy. The preservation of cellular ultrastructure and enzymatic activity by aldehyde fixation. *The Journal of Cell Biology 17*, 19–58.

Saglio, P., L'Hospital, M., Laflèche, D., Dupont, G., Bové, J.M., Tully, J.G. and Freundt, E.A. (1973). *Spiroplasma citri* gen. and sp. n.: a new mycoplasmalike organism associated with 'stubborn' disease of citrus. *International Journal of Systematic Bacteriology 23*, 191–204.

Saglio, P.H.M. and Whitcomb, R.F. (1979). Diversity of wall-less procaryotes in plant vascular tissue, fungi and invertebrate animals. In *The Mycoplasmas*, Vol. 3, pp. 1–36, R.F. Whitcomb and J.G. Tully (eds). New York: Academic Press.

Schneider, H. (1973). Cytological and histological aberrations in woody plants following infection with viruses, mycoplasmas, rickettsias and flagellates. *Annual Review of Phytopathology 11*, 119–46.

Seemüller, E. (1976). Fluoreszenzoptischer Direktnachweis von mykoplasmaähnlichen Organismen in Phloem pear-decline und triebsuchtkranker Bäume. *Phytopathologische Zeitschrift 85*, 368–72.

Seliskar, C.E., Kenknight, G.E. and Bourne, C.E. (1974). Mycoplasmalike organism associated with pecan bunch disease. *Phytopathology 64*, 1269–72.

Seliskar, C.E., Wilson, C.L. and Bourne, C.E. (1973). Mycoplasmalike bodies found in phloem of black locust with witches'-broom. *Phytopathology 63*, 30–4.

Shikata, E. and Maramorosch, K. (1969). Mycoplasma-like bodies in sieve pores of yellows diseased plants and in the fat body cells of two insect vectors. *Phytopathology 59*, 1559.

Shikata, E., Teng, W.S. and Matsumoto, T. (1969). Mycoplasma or PLT like microorganisms detected in leaves of sugarcane plants infected with white leaf disease and suppression of the disease symptoms by the antibiotics of tetracyline group. *Journal of the Faculty of Agriculture Hokkaido University, Sapporo 56*, 79–93.

Sinha, R.C. (1974). Purification of mycoplasma-like organisms from china aster plants affected with clover phyllody. *Phytopathology 64*, 1156–8.

— (1976). Ultrastructure of mycoplasma-like organisms purified from clover phyllody-affected plants. *Journal of Ultrastructural Research 54*, 183–9.

Sinha, R.C. and Black, L.M. (1963). Wound-tumour virus antigens in the internal organs of an insect vector. *Virology 21*, 183–7.

Sinha, R.C. and Paliwal, Y.C. (1969). Association, development and growth cycle of Mycoplasma-like organisms in plants affected with clover phyllody. *Virology 39*, 759–67.

— (1970). Localization of mycoplasma-like organism in tissues of a leafhopper vector carrying clover phyllody agent. *Virology 40*, 665–72.

Sinha, R.C. and Peterson, E.A. (1972). Uptake and persistance of oxytetracycline in aster plants and vector leafhoppers in relation to inhibition of clover phyllody agent. *Phytopathology 62*, 50–6.

Smets, G., Dekegel, D. and Vanderveken, J. (1977). Présence de structures anormales dans les bactériodes de trèfles blancs atteints de phyllodie. *Parasitica 33*, 111–18.

Smith, L.D., Dale, J.L. and Kim, K.S. (1976). A fixation method for demonstrating mycoplasmalike organisms in plants. *Phytopathology 66*, 531–3.

Spurr, A.R. (1969). A low viscosity epoxy resin embedding medium for electron microscopy. *Journal of Ultrastructural Research 26*, 31–43.

Srivastava, L.M. (1975). Structure and differentiation of sieve elements in Angiosperms and Gymnosperms. In *Phloem Transport*, pp. 33–62, S. Aronoff, J. Dainty, P.R. Gorham, L.M. Srivastava and C.A. Swanson (eds). New York: Plenum Press.

Tang, F.G., Wei, H. and Edgar, J. (1936). Further investigations on the causal agent of bovine pleuropneumonia. *Journal of Pathology and Bacteriology 42*, 45–51.

Tang, F.F., Wei, H., McWhirter, D.C. and Edgar, J. (1935). An investigation of the causal agent of bovine pleuropneumonia. *Journal of Pathology and Bacteriology 40*, 391–406.

Thomas, D.L. (1979). Mycoplasmalike bodies associated with lethal declines of palms in Florida. *Phytopathology 69*, 728–34.

Townsend, R., Markham, P.G. and Plaskitt, K.A. (1977). Multiplication and morphology of *Spiroplasma citri* in the leafhopper *Euscelis plebejus*. *Annals of Applied Biology 87*, 307–13.

Tully, J.G. (1978). Biology of the mycoplasmas. In *Mycoplasmal Infection of Cell Cultures*, pp. 1–33, G.J. McGarrity, D.G. Murphy and W.W. Nichols (eds). New York: Plenum Publishing Co.

Turner, A.W. (1935). A study of the morphology and life cycles of the organism of *Pleuropneumonia contagiosa boum* (*Borrelomyces peripneumonia* nov. gen.) by observation in the living state under dark-ground illumination. *Journal of Pathology and Bacteriology 41*, 1–32.

Ushiyama, R., Bullivant, S. and Matthews, R.E.F. (1969). A mycoplasma-like organism associated with phormium yellow leaf disease. *New Zealand Journal of Botany 7*, 363–71.

Waters, H. (1978). A wilt disease of coconuts from Trinidad associated with *Phytomonas* sp., a sieve tube-restricted protozoan flagellate. *Annals of Applied Biology 90*, 293–302.

Waters, H. and Hunt, P. (1978). Serial sectioning to demonstrate the morphology of a plant mycoplasma-like organism. *Zentralblatt für Bakteriologie, Parasitenkunde, Infektionskrankheiten und Hygiene. Erste Abteilung Originale 241*, 225.

— (1980). The *in vivo* three-dimensional form of a plant mycoplasma-like organism by the analysis of serial ultrathin sections. *Journal of General Microbiology 116*, 111–31.

Weatherley, P.E. (1962). The mechanism of sieve tube translocation: observation, experiment and theory. *Advancement of Science 18*, 571–7.

Weatherley, P.E. and Johnson, R.P.C. (1968). The form and function of the sieve tube: A problem in reconciliation. *International Review of Cytology 24*, 149–92.

Welvaert, W., Samyn, G. and Lagasse, A. (1975). Recherches sur les symptomes de la virescence chez l'*Hydrangea macrophylla* Thunb. *Phytopathologische Zeitschrift 83*, 152–8.

Whitcomb, R.F. (1973). Diversity of procaryotic plant pathogens. *Proceedings of the North Central Branch of the Entomological Society of America 28*, 38–60.

Whitcomb., R.F. and Davis, R.E. (1970). Mycoplasma and phytarboviruses as plant pathogens persistently transmitted by insects. *Annual Review of Ento - mology 15*, 405–64.

Whitcomb, R.F., Jensen, D.D. and Richardson, J. (1967). The infection of leafhoppers by western X-disease virus. III. Salivary, neural and adipose histopathology. *Virology 31*, 539–49.

— (1968a). The infection of leafhoppers by western X-disease. VI. Cytopathological interrelationships. *Journal of Invertebrate Pathology 12*, 202–21.

— (1968b). The infection of leafhoppers by western X-disease. IV. Pathology in the alimentary tract. *Virology 34*, 69–78.

Whitcomb, R.F. and Williamson, D.L. (1975). Helical wall-free procaryotes in insects: multiplication and pathogenicity. *Annals of the New York Academy of Sciences 266*, 260–75.

Williamson, D.L. and Whitcomb, R.F. (1974). Helical, wall-free prokaryotes in *Drosophila*, leafhoppers and plants. *Les Mycoplasmes/Mycoplasmas. Les Colloques de l'Institut National de la Santé et de la Recherche Médicale 33*, 283–90.

— (1975). Plant mycoplasmas; a cultivable spiroplasma causes corn stunt disease. *Science 118*, 1018–20.

Wilson, M.H. and Collier, A.M. (1976). Ultrastructural study of *Mycoplasma pneumoniae* in organ culture. *Journal of Bacteriology 125*, 332–9.

Wilson, C.L., Seliskar, C.E. and Krause, C.R. (1972). Mycoplasmalike bodies associated with elm phloem necrosis. *Phytopathology 62*, 140–3.

Wolanski, B.S. (1973). Negative staining of plant agents. *Annals of the New York Academy of Sciences 225*, 223–35.

Wolanski, B.S. and Maramorosch, K. (1970). Negatively stained mycoplasmas: fact or artifact. *Virology 42*, 319–27.

Worley, J.F. (1970). Possible replicative forms of a mycoplasmalike organism and their location in aster yellows diseased *Nicotiana* and aster. *Phytopathology 60*, 284–92.

Zelcer, A., Bar-Joseph, M. and Loebenstein, G. (1971). Mycoplasma-like bodies associated with little-leaf disease of citrus. *Israel Journal of Agricultural Research 21*, 137–42.

Zelcer, A., Loebenstein, G. and Bar-Joseph, M. (1972). Effects of elevated temperature on the ultrastructure of mycoplasmalike organisms in periwinkle. *Phytopathology 62*, 1453–7.

Ziegler, H. (1975). Nature of transported substances. In *Transport in Plants I: Phloem Transport Encyclopedia of Plant Physiology*, Vol 1, pp. 59–100, M.H. Zimmerman and J.A. Milburn (eds). Berlin: Springer-Verlag.

5 CHEMICAL TREATMENT FOR CONTROL OF PLANT MYCOPLASMA DISEASES

Randolph E. McCoy and Donna S. Williams·

1. Introduction
2. Theoretical Considerations
    A.   Effect of Antibiotics on Yellows Diseases
    B.   Transport of Antibiotics in Plants
    C.   Hazards of Environmental Contamination and Selection for
        Resistance
3. Practical Applications
    A.   Methods of Treatment
    B.   Methods for Analysis
    C.   Timing and Dose Rate Studies
4. Summary

1. Introduction

Antibiotic treatment of plant diseases associated with mycoplasma-like organisms (MLO) has been practised as a diagnostic aid since the first report of MLO in plants with yellows diseases. The known susceptibility of mycoplasmas, as a group, to tetracycline antibiotics and their insensitivity to the penicillins, was used by Ishiie *et al.* (1967) as support for the hypothesis of mycoplasmal etiology suggested by Doi and co-workers (1967) when they visualised MLO in the sieve tubes of several plants with yellows diseases. The fact that plants with these diseases, formerly thought to be caused by viruses, produced healthy new growth when treated with tetracycline, indicated the association of a prokaryotic agent with disease expression. Since the pathogens had previously been shown to pass through bacterial filters and the diseases did not respond to penicillin, the mycoplasmas were further implicated as possible etiologic agents. In consequence, the response of plants to differential chemotherapy is considered equally as important as the visualisation of MLO in providing evidence of presumptive mycoplasmal etiologies for the yellows diseases. Of course, the true test for demonstration of pathogenicity is to fulfil Koch's postulates through isolation and culture of the causal agent. Since this has been verified in only two cases, the citrus stubborn and corn stunt diseases, differential chemotherapy remains an important diagnostic aid in identifying diseases of suspected mycoplasmal etiology.

This chapter will discuss the rationale and the methodology of treatment of plants and vector insects with exogenous antibiotics. A recent review by Sinha (1979) covers types of antibiotics, in addition to the tetracyclines, used in plants, as well as susceptibility testing *in vitro*.

2. Theoretical Considerations

Since mycoplasmas are cell wall-free prokaryotes, they are characteristically resistant to antibiotics which block biosynthesis of the bacterial cell wall. This group includes penicillin, cycloserine and bacitracin. Compounds which affect prokaryotes in general by attacking the more basic functions of protein or nucleic acid synthesis are generally inhibitory to mycoplasma growth and reproduction. These include the tetracyclines, chloramphenicol, tylosin, the streptomycins and gentamicin. Certain macrolides, such as filipin and amphotericin B, are also inhibitory to sterol-requiring mycoplasmas (Smith, 1971).

In addition to the antibiotics, a number of other compounds are inhibitory to mycoplasmal growth. These include heavy metal compounds such as the arsenicals and gold-containing materials. Other inhibitory compounds are found among the antiprotozoal agents, such as quinine, atabrine, ethidium, prothidium and antrycide (Smith, 1971).

A. *Effect of Antibiotics on Yellows Diseases*

(1) Suppression of Symptom Development. Treatment of plants affected by yellows diseases with tetracycline antibiotics has resulted in an almost universal improvement in the state of health of the affected plant. The degree of response has varied with plant age, severity of symptoms and method of treatment. The response is also temporary; cessation of treatment results in the initiation of a new cycle of symptom development after a period of time. In a few cases, this remission period is of sufficient duration that antibiotic application has become a practical field control measure (McCoy, 1974a; Nyland and Moller, 1973).

Remission in diseased plants treated with tetracycline usually takes the form of new growth that is free of symptoms. Previously distorted tissues such as witches' brooms and stunted leaves or other organs do not recover their normal shape; however, subsequent flowers, stems and leaves become of normal colour and morphology. Yellowed leaves have been reported to regain their normal green coloration in some instances (Davis and Whitcomb, 1970); however in other cases, such as lethal yellowing, this does not happen (McCoy, 1972, 1975).

(2) Loss of MLO in Antibiotic-treated Tissues. Electron microscopic examination of tetracycline-treated plants and infected vector insects reveals the MLO to degenerate with a loss of cellular content (Delay and Darmanaden, 1977; Sinha and Peterson, 1972). MLO in such tissue often appear broken and many are devoid of ribosomes and the DNA network characteristic of normal mycoplasmal ultrastructure. MLO are not found in new tissues produced during remission; however, the organisms reappear as symptom development resumes at the end of the remission period (Bowyer and Atherton, 1972).

(3) Duration of Remission. The duration of the remission period in tetracycline-treated plants is variable and depends upon dose, duration of exposure, severity of disease at treatment and type of plant. Generally, higher doses and longer exposure to the antibiotics result in a longer period of symptom remission (McCoy, 1975). Also, remission seems to be of much greater duration in woody plants than in herbaceous plants. For example, rice yellow dwarf and aster yellows diseases may only be held in remission for several weeks before symptom progression recurs (Asuyama and Iida, 1973; Davis and Whitcomb, 1970). However, *Opuntia* witches' broom and pear decline symptoms may be repressed for 1–3 years with a single treatment (Maramorosch *et al.*, 1972; Nyland and Moller, 1973). Lethal yellowing in coconut palms may be held in remission for 3–7 months with a single 2 gram dose of oxytetracycline-HCl (McCoy, 1975). Also, remission is less likely to occur and may be of shorter duration in plants expressing severe symptoms at the time of initial treatment.

B. Transport of Antibiotics in Plants

In order to be effective, any applied antibiotic must be transported systemically and uniformly throughout the plant. In addition, the compound must get into the sieve elements of the phloem in which the target MLO reside. The primary pattern of distribution of applied tetracyclines indicates a xylem pathway of transport (McCoy, 1976b). Secondary accumulation in the phloem is requisite for disease remission to occur.

(1) Plant Vascular Anatomy. The vascular system of plants is composed of two radically different transport systems, xylem and phloem. An

understanding of their structure and mechanisms of action is basic to
any chemotherapy programme. Xylem is the water-conducting tissue
of the plant. The conducting tubes or tracheary elements are either
vessels or tracheids. Tracheids are of relatively small diameter, 50 μm,
and up to 3 mm in length (Zimmermann and McDonough, 1978).
Vessels are the major water-conducting units of the angiosperms and
are composed of individual cells up to 500 μm diameter, the vessel
elements, stacked end to end with their cross walls dissolved out to
form a long tube. Vessels are very long, up to 3 m in length, although
most are shorter than 50 cm (Skene and Balodis, 1968). Since the
hydraulic conductivity of a capillary tube increases with the fourth
power of its radius it is seen that the vessels are capable of much
greater conduction (Zimmermann, 1978). However, vessels are also
much more susceptible to injury. Any break in the vessel wall will
result in embolism as air is pulled into the lumen of the tube by the
suction force exerted by transpiration (Zimmermann, 1978). Embolism
breaks the continuity of the water column in the vessel and renders it
nonfunctional. Embolisms are contained within the affected vessels by
the membranes of the bordered pits which connect all tracheary
elements. Water must pass through these membranes to move from
one vessel or tracheid to another. The membranes effectively block the
movement of air and serve as safety valves in limiting the spread of
embolisms within the xylem. The bordered pit membranes may also be
important in limiting the vessel-to-vessel spread of xylem-borne pathogens.

In treatment of dicotyledonous trees a differentiation must be made
between those species with ring-porous and diffuse-porous wood
(Zimmermann, 1978). In temperate ring-porous trees such as elms only
the outer annual ring of xylem is functional. Xylem in the inner rings
is embolised each winter and new vessels must be produced each spring
before conduction can be initiated. In diffuse-porous trees the outer
several annular rings function in transport, but with efficiency decreasing with the age of the vessels. In either case the outer layer of wood is
the most efficient for conduction. Thus, in developing methods for
tree treatment, investigators should strive to make injections or
infusions as shallow as possible. The injection of chemicals into non-
conductive wood in the heart of a stem will greatly reduce the
efficiency of the treatment. Drilling injection holes tangentially rather
than perpendicularly into the trunk will help alleviate this problem.

Whenever an injection is made to a plant, xylem vessels are cut and
embolised. The injured vessels do not serve in transportation of the

injected chemical which must move by alternate pathways until functional xylem is reached. Thus, the initial movement of injected chemicals is in the apoplast, the continuum of cell walls of which the tracheary elements are a part.

Phloem is the food-conducting tissue of the plant. The food conducting tubes of the angiosperms are composed of living cells, the sieve tube elements, stacked end to end to form the sieve tubes. The end walls of each cell, the sieve plates, are perforated, allowing the contents to flow freely from cell to cell (Parthasarathy, 1975). The most readily accepted mechanism for phloem function is the pressure flow hypothesis of Münch (1930). In this proposal, phloem is loaded with photosynthate at its origin, either leaves or storage organs. Specialised transfer cells adjacent to the sieve elements of leaves appear to function in loading specific compounds into the phloem (Geiger, 1976). The specificity of phloem-loading may account for the success of certain antibiotics as chemotherapeutants of yellows diseases. The high carbohydrate content of the sieve elements results in a high turgor pressure induced by osmotic attraction of water into the sieve tubes. Flow in the sieve tubes is directed towards the growing points of root, shoot and fruit where the photosynthate is utilised. As carbohydrate, principally sucrose, is unloaded at the phloem sink areas, the osmotically-driven turgor pressure in the sieve elements is lessened. Thus, a pressure gradient is set up which drives solute flow from sites of manufacture (leaves) to sites of utilisation (growth regions).

(2) Mode of Application. Many means have been employed for the application of exogenous compounds to plants. These include spraying, soaking, infusion or injection, and root dips or soil drenches. While sprays can induce remission of yellows disease symptoms, this method is not very practical because much larger quantities of antibiotic are necessary, and an additional drawback is the widespread environmental contamination evoked by foliar sprays. Soil drenches are for the most part ineffective in that the antibiotics are largely tied up or inactivated in soil and additionally there is still the risk of environmental contamination. Root dips are very effective for obtaining both good uptake and uniform distribution of applied antibiotics in a laboratory or greenhouse, but are impossible for field use. Soaking plant tissues in antibiotic solutions has been used effectively in treating budwood for experimental purposes, but again this is not of commercial value because of the temporary nature of the remission. Infusions or injections may be applied to both herbaceous and woody plants, and have been approved for commercial use on several diseases of woody

plants. Uptake through injection or infusion is quite good, although the uniformity of distribution varies with the type of plant, the method used and the quantity of solution injected. The major advantages of the injection and infusion methods are that a much smaller amount of antibiotic is necessary as compared to spraying or root dips, and that contamination of the environment is minimised because the antibiotic is confined internally to the treated plant.

(3) Transport and Distribution. The pattern of distribution of applied antibiotics follows the transpiration stream, thereby indicating a xylem transport mechanism. Oxytetracycline applied to coconut palms accumulated most in the actively transpiring upper and middle leaves, while lower levels were found in older senescing leaves, in the young, unopened spear leaf, and in trunk, fruits, or roots (McCoy, 1976b). The same pattern has been reported for aster (Sinha and Peterson, 1972) and citrus (Chiu *et al.*, 1979; Igwegbe and Calavan, 1973).

The fact that tetracycline is effective against the yellows diseases indicates that it accumulates, at least passively, in the phloem. A number of antibiotics which have activity against mycoplasma *in vitro* are not effective *in vivo*. This may be related to the translocatability of the antibiotic in the plant. Streptomycin has generally been of little or no value in treating plants with yellows diseases even though it has activity against many mycoplasmas *in vitro*, including the plant pathogen *Spiroplasma citri* (Bowyer and Calavan, 1974). Streptomycin has been shown to move systemically in plant tissue with a xylem pattern of distribution (Goodman, 1962). The fact that it is not effective against the yellows diseases indicates that it probably is not phloem-mobile. Another example is tylosin, which is effective against the aster yellows organism when injected into vector insects (Whitcomb and Davis, 1970); however, tylosin is ineffective against aster yellows in affected plants (Davis and Whitcomb, 1970), again suggesting a lack of transport into the phloem. The phloem mobility of applied antibiotics is a subject which has received very little attention in the past and is deserving of much additional research.

C. Hazards of Environmental Contamination and Selection for Resistance

The public health aspects of antibiotics used for treating plants is an issue which must not be neglected. While the treatment of experimental plants for diagnostic purposes will result in minimal exposure of the environment to antibiotics, the widespread commercial use of these products for treatment of plant diseases must be carefully regulated and monitored to prevent the development of unforeseen side effects.

The potential hazards of widespread antibiotic use are twofold. First are the public health aspects as they relate to the general public and the applicators themselves, and secondly are the potential effects on the pathogen population targeted for control (Logue, 1959). The constant exposure of workers to antibiotics can result in the sensitisation of some individuals to these compounds and this contraindicates the use of these antibiotics for control of future infections in the sensitised persons. Another danger is the potential for selection of antibiotic resistant strains of nontarget bacteria exposed to these chemicals. The proliferation of antibiotic resistance in bacteria has become a limiting factor in the therapeutic treatment of certain human, plant and animal infections. In addition, through the widespread clinical use of antibiotics, there exists a pool of sensitised individuals in the general population. Exposure of these persons to even small amounts of antibiotics can result in severe reactions. To avoid this, the presence of antibiotic residues, particularly in foods, should be minimal.

Finally, one must be aware of the potential for selecting resistant strains of the targeted pathogen. Consequently, one should not depend solely on antibiotic treatment as a control measure. In the case of lethal yellowing disease, oxytetracycline-HCl (OTC) is being applied on a large scale for disease control in existing coconut palms in Florida. However, the ultimate control measure is the development and distribution of resistant cultivars of palms for replanting. The OTC treatment programme is viewed as a holding action to be used for the 5–10 years necessary to complete a replanting programme.

3. Practical Applications

The application of systemic chemotherapeutants to plants with yellows diseases has demonstrated conclusively that tetracycline-group antibiotics are effective in suppressing symptom development. The methods of treatment have varied widely and often have been performed without the benefit of concurrent assays for antibiotic residues. Residue analyses have been used basically as measures of the efficacy of various treatment methods and secondarily to determine antibiotic concentrations in consumable portions of food plants. Studies of the effects of dose and timing on the degree of symptom suppression are necessary to determine the practicality of antibiotic application for disease control.

A. Methods of Treatment

A number of methods have been developed for the application of exogenous compounds to plants. A major dichotomy in the treatment methods utilised involves the size of the plant to be treated and its degree of woody development. This discussion will separately cover methods for treating herbaceous plants and those for treating woody plants. The more successful and practical techniques will be discussed.

(1) Herbaceous Plants. The treatment of herbaceous plants is primarily of diagnostic value. The short remission period and the lack of an environmentally safe method of mass application of antibiotic preclude its practical use in disease control.

The most commonly used treatment method for herbaceous plants and small woody plants has been spraying (Asuyama and Iida, 1973; Chiykowski, 1972, 1973; Davis and Whitcomb, 1970; Davis *et al.*, 1968; Muniyappa and Ramakrishnan, 1976; Tahama, 1973). Other surface applications such as leaf-dips have occasionally been used (Chiykowski, 1972). Most spray trials have used antibiotic concentrations of 100–1000 $\mu g/ml$ sprayed on the leaves until they are thoroughly wet. Applications have been made at intervals of several days to several weeks. To be effective the antibiotic must be absorbed through the cuticle and the epidermis before diffusing through the mesophyll to the vascular system where it will exert its effect. Disease remission can occur with spraying but residue measurements indicate that it is one of the least effective methods for introducing antibiotic into foliage. In some cases, the concentration of antibiotic applied as a spray necessary to induce symptom remission is accompanied by mild to severe phytotoxic effects ranging from foliar chlorosis to severe stunting or distortion of new growth (Chiykowski, 1972).

The most effective method for treating herbaceous plants, or even small woody plants, is by root or shoot immersion (Asuyama and Iida, 1973; Davis and Whitcomb, 1970; Gheorghiu, 1976; Igwegbe and Calavan, 1973; Ishiie *et al.*, 1967; Peterson and Sinha, 1977; Sinha and Peterson, 1972; Tahama *et al.*, 1972) or by the addition of antibiotic to hydroponic culture solutions (Davis and Whitcomb, 1970; Davis *et al.*, 1968; Igwegbe and Calavan, 1973). Uptake in such cases is highly efficient and antibiotic distribution through the plant is more uniform than with any other method. Exposing plant roots to antibiotic concentrations of 10–100 $\mu g/ml$ for periods of several hours to several days has generally given the highest levels of antibiotic in the foliage when compared to other treatment methods. For root immersion tests, the soil is gently washed from the roots of potted plants prior to being placed in the treatment solutions. Care should be taken to remove as much soil and organic matter as possible since most antibiotics, particularly the tetracyclines, rapidly lose activity in soil or are adsorbed to clay complexes (Gonsalves and Tucker, 1977; Martin and Gottlieb, 1952). It is for this reason that soil drenches, another tested treatment method, have by and large been ineffective in inducing symptom remission in the yellows diseases (Igwegbe and Calavan, 1973; Ishiie *et al.*, 1967; McCoy, 1974b), with rare exceptions (Delay and Darmanaden, 1977). The shoot immersion technique is basically the same as the root immersion treatment except that cut ends of shoots from diseased plants, rather than roots, are immersed in the antibiotic solutions, and are then grafted on to healthy plants to observe symptom expression in new growth.

Tissue infusion methods have been used with herbaceous plants by several investigators. These include the use of wicks, vacuum infiltration (Davis and Whitcomb, 1970), and uptake through cut leaves. In the wick method, several folds of cotton thread are drawn through the stem of the plant to be treated with one or both ends of the thread placed in small containers of 50–500 μg/ml antibiotic solutions, (Brčák *et al.*, 1969; Muniyappa and Ramakrishnan, 1976), or one end of a wick can be sealed into a slit in the blade of a leaf (May, 1941). Because tetracycline solutions are unstable at normal plant growing temperatures, solutions must be replaced every 1–2 days and treatment continued for periods of several days to several weeks. Although the immersion of a leaf with the tip cut off has never been tested with antibiotics, it has been used to diagnose mineral deficiencies rapidly by observing the response of a nutrient solution-treated leaf (May, 1941) and would seem to be a viable technique for the absorption of antibiotic solutions through the leaves.

(2) Woody Plants. The most effective treatment methods, such as root or shoot immersion and addition of antibiotic to hydroponic culture solutions applied to herbaceous plants, are impractical in field situations with large woody plants. In some cases, budwood has been treated by the immersion method and subsequently grafted on to root stock (Asuyama and Iida, 1973; Gheorghiu, 1976; Su and Leu, 1972). However, because of the temporary nature of tetracycline remission, this method brings no enduring benefit. Spraying has been used in several instances with varying degrees of success (Capoor and Thirumalachar, 1973; Jones and Rosenberger, 1979; McCoy, 1974b).

Tremendous quantities of antibiotic are required for a large-scale spray programme to be instituted and the equipment necessary for such a programme is costly. Concentrations of 100-1000 μg/ml have been tested by spraying the foliage until the leaves are thoroughly wet. Spraying must be done on a regular basis for disease control because the remission periods achieved with this method have, for the most part, been of short duration. The environmental implications of a massive spray programme must also be taken into consideration. Spraying, too, is considerably more sensitive to deleterious effects of weather conditions than are other methods.

To date the most effective methods for treating yellows diseases in woody plants have comprised the introduction of antibiotic directly into the xylem transport system. Wilson (1979) draws a distinction between infusion methods which depend exclusively on the water transport system to translocate the antibiotic from the introduction site or sites to the rest of the plant, and injection methods which utilise some outside pressure source to introduce and initiate translocation of the antibiotic. Infusion methods transport the antibiotic upwards from the introduction site or sites and depend on movement of the antibiotic into the phloem for distribution to points below the introduction sites. Tetracycline compounds have conclusively demonstrated their phloem-mobility by their ability to induce remission in diseases of suspected mycoplasmal etiology. Limited lateral movement in the xylem of woody dicotyledonous plants necessitates the even spacing of several infusion or injection sites around the trunk or placement of infusion/injection sites under each main branch in order to achieve an even distribution of the antibiotic (Rogers, 1975). Experience with the treatment of elm trees with fungicides for Dutch elm disease control indicates that best distribution occurs when injections are made into the flares of major roots at the base of the trunk (Kondo, 1979). Healing of the wound is also more readily accomplished at these sites. Because woody monocotyledonous plants have vascular bundles spread throughout the plant interior, with many lateral connections, these plants require only a single infusion/injection site for even distribution of the antibiotic, as in the treatment of lethal yellowing of coconut palms (Hunt *et al.*, 1974; McCoy, 1974b).

Acidic tetracycline formulations are most effective with infusion/injection treatment methods because neutral or acidic compounds are more readily transported by the xylem (Dimond, 1965). Basic substances tend to be adsorbed by the negative charges on xylem walls (Marsh, 1977). The tree injection formulation of oxytetracycline-HC1,

Terramycin[R] (Pfizer, Inc.), which has been registered for use in the
control of lethal yellowing in coconut palm by the United States
Environmental Protection Agency, is stabilised and solubilised by the
addition of citric acid, as were the tetracycline compounds tested in
treatment of eastern-X disease of peach (Sands, 1974; Sands and
Walton, 1975).

The most commonly used infusion treatment method has been the
gravity feed technique (Chiu *et al.*, 1978; Filer, 1973; Hunt *et al.*,
1974; La *et al.*, 1976; McCoy, 1974a; Nyland, 1979; Nyland and
Moller, 1973; Rogers, 1975; Schwarz and Van Vuuren, 1971). An
inverted 1-4 litre reservoir containing the antibiotic solution at 100-
1000 μg/ml is suspended above one or more 4-5 cm deep, 4-6 mm
diameter holes drilled or bored at a slight downward angle into the
trunk. Plastic tubing terminating in metal or plastic connectors inserted
into these holes is attached to the reservoir. A small air-hole in the top
of the reservoir allows a free flow of the solution. Uptake is improved
if the hole in the trunk is cleaned of sawdust, and if both the hole and
tubing are flushed of trapped air. Uptake is variable among plant
species and among individual plants of the same species depending on
plant size, disease severity, and environmental conditions. Especially
for this treatment method, uptake can be improved by treating during
times of maximum transpiration activity. Uptake decreases with time
and, because of the instability of tetracycline compounds, any un-
assimilated solution can be removed between 24-72 hr after treatment.
As much as 7.5 ℓ of tetracycline solution has been infused into a single
tree by this method; however, any single hole in a mature tree will
generally take up a maximum of 1.0-1.5 ℓ.

Another infusion method, used in the treatment of eastern-X
disease of peach, involves filling 5-6 mm diameter, 3.4-4.0 cm deep
holes drilled or bored into the trunk at a slight downward angle with
approximately 2.0 ml of a concentrated, 7.5% or 10% (w/v), tetracycline solution in 1.0-2.7% citric acid (Pearson, 1977; Sands, 1974;
Sands and Walton, 1975). The concentrated solution is absorbed in
30 s-2 min and the holes are either sealed with modelling clay or a
fungicidal tree sealant, or are left unsealed. This method greatly reduces
treatment time but the high concentration of the antibiotic often
caused damage to the bark and wood which prevented healing of the
wound (Pearson, 1977). Concentrations of approximately 15% have
been tested also but damage to the trunk was severe (Rosenberger and
Jones, 1977). Solid tablets of oxytetracycline-HCl have similarly been
implanted into holes drilled in the trunk as a preventive treatment for

Veitchia merillii palms in lethal yellowing disease foci and the holes sealed with corks (McCoy and Gwin, 1977).

Because the gravity feed method required a minimum of 24 hours for uptake of the quantities of antibiotic necessary to achieve remission in yellows diseases, and infusion of concentrated antibiotic often caused severe damage to the trunks of treated plants, several injection methods which rely on applied pressure to achieve more rapid uptake of dilute antibiotic solutions have been tested. Many different means of providing pressure for injection have been devised. Most high-pressure injection systems utilise compressed air or nitrogen as the pressure source (Himelick, 1972; McCoy, 1974a; Sachs *et al.*, 1977). Drilled-out lag bolts modified with brass tubing fittings serve as injection posts which can be removed and reused. This injection technique has been elaborated upon by Reil and Beutel (1976) to include a hydraulic cylinder for rapid injection into several posts at a time. One-way valves may be attached between the lag bolt and tubing fitting to prevent back-flow of antibiotic. Pressure-rated nylon tubing connects the pressure tank to a solution reservoir. This type of system is used at pressures up to 200 psi. Uptake is variable but in most tests 0.5–1.0 ℓ of solution was absorbed in a matter of minutes.

Low-pressure injection methods have utilised modified bicycle pumps or blow-torches as pressure sources (Chiu *et al.*, 1978; Llácer, *et al.*, 1976; Schwarz, 1974; Schwarz and Van Vuuren, 1971). These low pressure techniques can force 0.5–1.0 ℓ of solution into a tree in a few hours. A method that should work well with ring porous trees is that developed by Aubert (1979). Injections are made just beneath the bark on opposite sides of the trunk by hollow probes attached to a clamping device. The probes are connected by tubing to an antibiotic reservoir pressurized by a tyre pump.

Another relatively simple and inexpensive low-pressure technique (Heffernan, 1968) has been used in the treatment of lethal yellowing of coconut palms (McCoy, 1974a), X-disease of peach (Pearson, 1977) and pear decline (McIntyre and Lacy, 1979). Developed by the J.J. Mauget Co., this treatment method consists of an aluminium feeder tube, either tapped into the trunk by means of a special insertion tool, or inserted into a drilled or bored hole, 4–5 cm deep, 4.5–5.0 mm diameter. The plastic reservoir unit, which is filled with 14–15 ml concentrated antibiotic solution, 1.0 to 6.0 g ai (active ingredient)/tree, is pressurised to 5–8 psi by compression of the top and bottom portions and is then tapped on to the feeder tube until the diaphragm in the reservoir is broken, allowing the solution to pass through the tube and into the tree. When emptied (approximately 24 hr), both the injector unit and feeder tube can be removed and discarded.

(3) Application to Insects. Tetracycline antibiotics and tylosin tartrate have been demonstrated to reduce the ability of vector leafhoppers to acquire and transmit the agents of several yellows diseases when administered pre-acquisition (Sinha and Peterson, 1972; Whitcomb and Davis, 1970). Post-acquisition administration of antibiotic has on occasion reduced transmission ability (Whitcomb and Davis, 1970), but in most cases has only prolonged the incubation period (Asuyama and Iida, 1973).

Several methods of administering antibiotics to vector leafhoppers have been tested. One method involves direct feeding of leafhoppers through a stretched parafilm membrane containing antibiotic at concentrations up to 1600 μg/ml in 10% sucrose solutions (Amin and Jensen, 1971; Freitag and Smith, 1969).

The most effective method of reducing ability of vector leafhoppers to transmit yellows diseases has been the pre-acquisition feeding of the insects on plants grown in hydroponic culture solutions containing antibiotic (Whitcomb and Davis, 1970) or on plants whose roots have been washed of soil and immersed in antibiotic solutions (Asuyama and Iida, 1973). Insects are allowed to feed on treated plants for 1–7 days. After feeding on treated asters for two days, antibiotic could be detected in the insects for at least seven days and, as a side effect, increased the longevity of treated leafhoppers relative to untreated leafhoppers (Sinha and Peterson, 1972).

Another method of treating vector leafhoppers is the injection of antibiotic directly into the abdomen of the insect with a capillary needle. Asuyama and Iida (1973) injected the vector of mulberry dwarf disease with 0.001 ml/insect of 5000 μg/ml tetracycline. Whitcomb and Davis (1970) injected both a mixture of aster yellows inocula prepared from infected *Macrosteles fascifrons* (Stål) and antibiotics (1000 μg/ml final concentration) into healthy adult insects, and also buffered antibiotics (1000 μg/ml) into AY-infected adults. Ability to transmit was reduced with both methods.

B. Methods for Analysis

Several methods have been investigated to measure tetracycline residues in plants as an indication of the degree of uptake, distribution and persistence after treatment. The most commonly used method for analysis has been the microbiological assay which measures levels of antimicrobial activity of the antibiotic (Chiu *et al.*, 1979; Dudek *et al.*,

1977; Frederick *et al.*, 1971; Igwegbe and Calavan, 1973; McCoy, 1976b; Peterson and Sinha, 1977; Rosenberger and Jones, 1977; Sinha and Peterson, 1972). This procedure is highly efficient, relatively simple to perform, and does not require the use of elaborate chemical analyses. There are many variations on this technique. Basically, samples from different parts of a treated plant (roots, stems, leaves, fruits) are either weighed fresh and ground in a mortar and pestle, or dried (air dried or freeze dried), weighed, powdered and rehydrated in phosphate buffer or distilled water. The ground plant material is then squeezed through several layers of cheese cloth and the extract centrifuged at 1500 to 30,000 g for approximately 10 minutes. Treated leafhoppers are ground in a tissue grinder with 0.85%NaCl at a 1/5 dilution (w/v) and centrifuged (Sinha and Peterson, 1972). The supernatant from the centrifuged extracts is used for the assay. In addition, expressed xylem or phloem sap, coconut milk (McCoy, 1976a), treatment solutions, and standard solutions of the antibiotic being assayed can be sampled directly on sterile paper discs (12.5 mm diameter). The discs are placed on petri dishes containing any of several types of nutrient agar freshly seeded with *Bacillus cereus* var. *mycoides, Arthrobacter globiformis*, or *Bacillus subtilis* when the agar was sufficiently cool (50°C) but not solidified. In some cases, 1 cm diameter holes have been cut in the agar and a small amount of extract pipetted directly into the holes (Hunt *et al.*, 1974). The plates are incubated at 28-34°C for 8-18 hr and the diameters or radii of inhibition zones measured. The antibiotic concentration of the samples is estimated by comparison with a standard curve of the activity of antibiotic solutions of known concentrations assayed concurrently. The minimum detectable level ranges from 0.2-1.0 μg/ml. Activity is expressed as μg/g fresh weight or μg/ml extract. Controls of crude tissue extracts should be run to demonstrate any natural antimicrobial activity.

Thin-layer chromatography (TLC) (Ascione *et al.*, 1967; Aszalos *et al.*, 1968; Willekens, 1977) is a relatively new method for the detection of antibiotic residues in plants. Silica gel TLC plates are spotted with extracts prepared as for the paper disc microbiological assay. The R_F values of spots from the extracts are compared to those for pure antibiotic solutions (Igwegbe and Calavan, 1973; Wilhelm and Knösel, 1976). Bioautography is a variation on this technique whereby agar seeded with an assay organism and supplemented with tetrazolium dye is placed under a glass TLC plate, allowing identification, not only of inhibition zones around the biologically active portions of the antibiotic on the chromatogram, but also of the non-active degradation products (Hamilton and Cook, 1968; Meyers and Erickson, 1967).

Analyses of residues in various parts of antibiotic-treated plants are invaluable aids in determining transport pathways of applied chemo-therapeutants. Intervallic sampling and analysis can demonstrate the persistence of antibiotic activity in treated plants and leafhopper vectors (McCoy, 1976b; Peterson and Sinha, 1977). The persistence of antibiotic activity can be used as an indication of how often a plant would need to be treated to achieve disease control. McCoy (1974a) found that a single treatment of early-stage lethal yellowing-diseased coconut palms with oxytetracycline-HC1 maintained remission of symptoms from 4–7 months, even though the oxytetracycline was detectable in foliage for 2 months or less. Analysis of persistence of antibiotic residues in consumable portions of food plants is essential in any control programme.

C. Timing and Dose Rate Studies

Studies on the influence of timing and dose rate on symptom remission in yellows diseases are important components in achieving disease control through the use of antibiotics. Timing of antibiotic application is especially critical with food crops where residues in consumable products are undesirable (e.g. apple proliferation, X-disease of peach and cherry, pear decline, citrus stubborn and greening, lethal yellowing of coconut palm). Timing of application can be influenced by seasonal considerations such as the seasonal presence of an insect vector making the plant susceptible to inoculation, and the effects of seasonal differences in metabolic activity on phytotoxicity and on uptake of antibiotic. In general, antibiotic treatment has been most effective when applied during seasons of high metabolic activity. In the cases of X-disease of peach (Pearson, 1977; Rosenberger and Jones, 1977) and of pear decline (Nyland and Moller, 1973), applications are best made between the time of harvest and leaf fall, both to avoid possible residues in fruit, and the phytotoxicity that can occur in new growth when applied after leaf fall. Filer (1976) has determined that at least two-monthly treatments of tetracycline antibiotics applied after bud-break each year would give acceptable control of American elm phloem necrosis. Schwarz *et al.* (1974) found that uptake of antibiotic was greatly improved by treating citrus greening-affected Valencia orange trees in September when fruits were developing as compared with treating in July or November; however, antibiotic residues in fruit were not studied.

In other cases, seasonality of applications is less important than the time interval between applications and its effect on disease control through antibiotic treatment. McCoy (1975) has determined the remission period in lethal yellowing (LY) diseased coconut palms to last from 4–7 months after antibiotic treatment and McCoy and Gwin (1977) have found a remission period of 3–5 months in lethal decline-affected *Pritchardia thurstonii, P. pacifica*, and *Trachycarpus fortunei*. Thus, the maximum effective interval between treatments for LY disease control is 4 months, and for lethal decline control is 3 months.

Relatively few dose rate studies have been conducted to date. The relationship between dose and tree size has not been well established in most cases. Likewise, concentration of antibiotic in tissue, as determined by bioassay, has not been reliably related to the degree of symptom remission. Filer (1976) has set a dosage standard for treatment of elm phloem necrosis of 100 mg of tetracycline per inch of diameter of trunk. Rosenberger and Jones (1977) have related trunk size to dose in the control of X-disease in peach, 1.25 g oxytetracycline per tree for less than 17 cm trunk diameter and 2.5 g per tree for trunk diameter greater than 17 cm; doses below 1.2 g per tree (0.5 g and 0.9 g) only delayed onset of symptoms for several weeks whereas 1.25 g or 2.5 g prevented symptom development for a year. Llácer *et al*. (1976) have determined minimum dose rates of 0.6 g per apricot tree and 1.2 g per Japanese plum tree to control apricot chlorotic leaf roll. Pearson (1977) has related dose to per cent remission, increase in yield, and phytotoxicity at the infusion site in oxytetracycline treated X-diseased peach trees.

In practice, the rule for applying antibiotics has often been to use the highest concentration that will not produce damaging phytotoxicity. However, beyond a certain level, increasing the dose of antibiotic applied loses its benefit. Schwarz and Van Vuuren (1971) found little difference in per cent remission between tetracycline applied at 250 μg/ml and at 500 μg/ml. McCoy (1975) has shown a response to doses from 0.5 g to 20.0 g per tree in controlling lethal yellowing of coconut palm. The lower doses showed a response but the higher doses had longer-lasting effects and demonstrated responses in trees with more advanced symptoms of disease. McCoy and Gwin (1977) found no difference in response between doses of 1.0 or 3.0 g per tree in the treatment of lethal decline-affected *Pritchardia thurstonii*. In any large scale treatment program, the benefit of increased dose rate must be weighed against the increased financial cost.

4. Summary

Differential chemotherapy of plants has become an important diagnostic tool in the implication of mycoplasmal etiologies for the yellows diseases. Tetracycline antibiotics, which act on the most basic functions of the cell, protein or nucleic acid synthesis, have been demonstrated to induce temporary remission of symptom expression in the yellows diseases. The length of the remission period varies with the plant species, disease severity, antibiotic concentration and treatment method. Tetracycline treatment follows a xylem transport pathway and depends on secondary accumulation in the phloem for remission to occur. During the remission period MLO appear to degenerate with a loss of cellular content, and MLO of normal ultrastructure reappear at the end of the remission period.

Many means of applying exogenous compounds to both herbaceous and woody plants have been devised. These methods include spraying, drenching, root or shoot immersion, and infusion or injection. Important factors in choosing a treatment method are plant type, uptake , distribution, persistence and risk of environmental contamination. The application of antibiotic to herbaceous plants is mainly of diagnostic value because remission is generally of short duration. The most efficient methods of application to woody plants involve the introduction of antibiotic directly into the internal tissues of the plant. Infusion methods depend solely on transpirational activity for distribution while injection methods utilise some type of pressure source for introduction and initial translocation of applied antibiotics. Several methods have also been devised for the administration of antibiotics to vector insects, either by feeding on treated plants, by direct injection, or by membrane feeding of antibiotic-sucrose solutions.

Analyses of tetracycline residues in plants are important in determinations of the efficacy of different treatment methods, and also in the determination of residue levels in consumable portions of food plants. The microbiological assay, thin-layer chromatography and bioautography have been used in residue analysis studies. These analyses can also identify the transport pathways and persistence of applied antibiotics, and are useful tools in studies on dose rate and timing of treatment.

References

Amin, P.W. and Jensen, D.D. (1971). Effects of tetracycline on the transmission and pathogenicity of the Western X disease agent in its insect and plant hosts. *Phytopathology 61*, 696-702.

Ascione, P.P., Zagar, J.B. and Chrekian, G.P. (1967). Tetracyclines I. Separation and examination by thin-layer chromatography. *Journal of Pharmaceutical Sciences 56*, 1393-5.

Asuyama, H. and Iida, T.T. (1973). Effects of tetracycline compounds on plant diseases caused by mycoplasma-like agents. *Annals of the New York Academy of Sciences 225*, 509-21.

Aszalos, A., Davis, S. and Frost, D. (1968). Classification of crude antibiotics by instant thin-layer chromatography (ITLC). *Journal of Chromatography 37*, 487-98.

Aubert, B. (1979). Une technique d'injection sous pression dans le tronc des arbres. *Fruits 34*, 195-8.

Bowyer, J.W. and Atherton, J.G. (1972). Effect of tetracycline antibiotics on plants affected by legume little leaf disease. *Australian Journal of Biological Science 25*, 43-51.

Bowyer, J.W. and Calavan, E.C. (1974). Antibiotic sensitivity of the mycoplasma-like organism associated with citrus stubborn disease. *Phytopathology 64*, 346-9.

Brčák, J., Králík, O., Limberk, J., and Ulrychová, M. (1969). Mycoplasma-like bodies in plants infected with potato witches' broom disease and the response of plants to tetracycline treatment. *Biologia Plantarum 11*, 470-6.

Capoor, S.P. and Thirumalachar, M.J. (1973). Cure of greening affected citrus plants by chemotherapeutic agents. *Plant Disease Reporter 57*, 160-3.

Chiu, R.J., Tsai, M.Y. and Huang, C.H. (1978). Tree transfusion with tetracyclines as a measure for citrus likubin control. In *Plant Diseases due to Mycoplasma-like Organisms: Proceedings Symposium*, 30 November – 3 December 1977. Tokyo, Japan, pp. 91-103. Taipei: Food and Fertilizer Technology Center Book Series no. 13.

— (1979). Distribution and retention of tetracyclines in healthy and likubin-affected citrus trees following trunk transfusion. In *Proceedings of ROC-United States Cooperative Science Seminar on Mycoplasma Diseases of Plants*, 1978, pp. 143-52. Taipei, Taiwan: National Science Council.

Chiykowski, L.N. (1972). Effects of three tetracyclines and their method of application on the development of clover phyllody and aster yellows symptoms in aster. *Canadian Journal of Plant Science 52*, 29-33.

— (1973). Effectiveness of antibiotics applied as postinoculation sprays against clover phyllody and aster yellows. *Canadian Journal of Plant Science 53*, 87-91.

Davis, R.E. and Whitcomb, R.F. (1970). Evidence on possible mycoplasma etiology of aster yellows disease I. Suppression of symptom development in plants by antibiotics. *Infection and Immunity 2*, 201-8.

Davis, R.E. , Whitcomb, R.F. and Steere, R.L. (1968). Remission of aster yellows disease by antibiotics. *Science 161*, 793-5.

Delay, C. and Darmanaden, J. (1977). Nouvelles observations sur les organismes de type mycoplasme associés a la forme horticole "minor" d'*Opuntia subulata*. Action du chlorhydrate de tétracycline. *Annales des Sciences Naturelles, Botanique et Biologie Végétale 12*, 275-300.

Dimond, A.E. (1965). Natural models for plant chemotherapy. *Advances in Pest Control Research 6*, 127-69.

Doi, Y., Teranaka, M., Yora, K. and Asuyama, H. (1967). Mycoplasma or PLT group-like microorganisms found in phloem elements of plants infected with mulberry dwarf, potato witches broom, aster yellows, or paulownia witches broom. *Annals Phytopathological Society of Japan 33*, 259–66.

Dudek, M., Zawadzka, B. and Burkovicz, A. (1977). The use of oxytetracycline in control of apple proliferation disease. *Proceedings of a Symposium held at the Hungarian Academy of Sciences*, 405–13.

Filer, Jr., T.H. (1973). Suppression of elm phloem necrosis symptoms with tetracycline antibiotics. *Plant Disease Reporter 57*, 341–3.

— (1976). Antibiotic injections control elm phloem necrosis in the urban ecosystem. In *Proceedings of Symposium on Trees and Forests for Human Settlements*, Vancouver, British Columbia, pp. 327–33. University of Toronto Press.

Frederick, R.J., Klein, M. and Maramorosch, K. (1971). Acquisition and retention of tetracycline-hydrochloride by plants. *Plant Disease Reporter 55*, 223–6.

Freitag, J.H. and Smith, S.H. (1969). Effects of tetracyclines on symptom expression and leafhopper transmission of aster yellows. *Phytopathology 59*, 1820–3.

Geiger, D.B. (1976). Phloem loading in source leaves. In *Transport and Transfer Processes in Plants*, pp. 167–83, I.F. Wardlow and J.B. Passioura (eds). New York: Academic Press.

Gheorghiu, E. (1976). Studies on the physical and chemical control of apple proliferation in tree nurseries and bearing orchards. *Acta Horticulturae 67*, 149–57.

Gonsalves, D. and Tucker, D.P.H. (1977). Behavior of oxytetracycline in Florida citrus and soils. *Archives of Environmental Contamination and Toxicology 6*, 515–23.

Goodman, R.N. (1962). The impact of antibiotics upon plant disease control. *Advances in Pest Control Research 5*, 1–46.

Hamilton, P.B. and Cook, C.E. (1968). Some techniques for bioautography of antimicrobial substances on thin-layer chromatograms. *Journal of Chromatography 35*, 295–6.

Heffernan, T. (1968). Advances in tree implantation. *Agrichemical West*, 1–4.

Himelick, E.B. (1972). High pressure injection of chemicals into trees. *Arborist's News 37*, 97–103.

Hunt, P., Dabek, A.J. and Schuiling, M. (1974). Remission of symptoms following tetracycline treatment of lethal yellowing-infected coconut palms. *Phytopathology 64*, 307–12.

Igwegbe, E.C.K. and Calavan, E.C. (1973). Effect of tetracycline antibiotics on symptom development of stubborn disease and infectious variegation of citrus seedlings. *Phytopathology 63*, 1044–8.

Ishiie, T., Doi, Y., Yora, K. and Asuyama, H. (1967). Suppressive effects of antibiotics of tetracycline group on symptom development of mulberry dwarf disease. *Annals of the Phytopathological Society of Japan 33*, 267–75.

Jones, A.L. and Rosenberger, D.A. (1979). Progress on the use of systemic injections and sprays of terramycin for control of peach X-disease. In *Proceedings of the Symposium on Systemic Chemical Treatments in Tree Culture*, 1978, pp. 247–54. Ann Arbor, Michigan: Braun-Brumfield, Inc.

Kondo, E.S. (1979). Root flare and root injection techniques. In *Proceedings of the Symposium on Systemic Chemical Treatments in Tree Culture*, 1978, pp. 133–40. Ann Arbor, Michigan: Braun-Brumfield, Inc.

La, Y.J., Brown, Jr., W.M. and Moon, D.S. (1976). Control of witches'-broom disease of jujube with oxytetracycline injection. *Korean Journal of Plant Protection 15*, 107–10.

Llácer, G., Sánchez-Capuchino, J.A., Forner, J.B., Bono, R. and Casanova, R.

(1976). Tetracycline treatments of stone fruit trees affected by apricot chlorotic leaf roll. *Acta Horticulturae 67*, 141-8.

Logue, J.T. (1959). The public health significance of non-medical uses of antibiotics, In *Antibiotics, Their Chemistry and Non-Medical Uses*, pp. 561-93, H.S. Goldberg (ed). Princeton, New Jersey: D. Van Nostrand Co.

Maramorosch, K., Klein, M. and Wolanski, B.S. (1972). The etiology of witches'-broom of *Opuntia*. *Phytopathology 62*, 497.

Marsh, R.W. (1977). *Systemic fungicides*, 2nd edition, R.W. Marsh (ed). London and New York: Longman Group Ltd, 401 pp.

Martin, N. and Gottlieb, D. (1952). The production and role of antibiotics in the soil III. Terramycin and aureomycin. *Phytopathology 42*, 294-6.

May, C. (1941). Methods of tree injection. *Trees 4*, 7-16.

McCoy, R.E. (1972). Remission of lethal yellowing in coconut palm treated with tetracycline antibiotics. *Plant Disease Reporter 56*, 1019-21.

— (1974a). How to treat your palm with antibiotic. *Florida Agricultural Experiment Station Circular S-228*, 7 pp.

— (1974b). Techniques for treatment of palm trees with antibiotics. *Proceedings of the Florida State Horticultural Society, 1974 87*, 537-40.

— (1975). Effect of oxytetracycline dose and stage of disease development on remission of lethal yellowing in coconut palm. *Plant Disease Reporter 59*, 717-20.

— (1976a). Accumulation of antibiotic residues in the fruit of coconut palms treated with oxytetracycline for the control of lethal yellowing. *Oléagineux 31*, 215-17.

— (1976b). Uptake, translocation, and persistence of oxytetracycline in coconut palm. *Phytopathology 66*, 1038-42.

McCoy, R.E. and Gwin, G.H. (1977). Response of mycoplasmalike organism-infected *Pritchardia, Trachycarpus* and *Veitchia* palms to oxytetracycline. *Plant Disease Reporter 61*, 154-8.

McIntyre, J.L. and Lacy, G.H. (1979). Pear decline in Connecticut: assessment of symptom remission after treatment with oxytetracycline. In *Proceedings of the Symposium on Systemic Chemical Treatments in Tree Culture, 1978*, pp. 223-7. Ann Arbor, Michigan: Braun-Brumfield, Inc.

Meyers, E. and Erickson, R.C. (1967). Bioautography of antibiotics on thin layer chromatograms. *Journal of Chromatography 26*, 531-2.

Münch, E. (1930). *Die Stoffbewegungen in der pflanze*. Jena: Gustav Fischer.

Muniyappa, V. and Ramakrishnan, K. (1976). Chemotherapy of yellow dwarf disease of rice. *Mysore Journal of Agricultural Sciences 10*, 431-9.

Nyland, G. (1979). Chemotherapy of diseases of deciduous trees associated with mycoplasma and rickettsialike organisms. In *Proceedings of ROC-United States Cooperative Science Seminar on Mycoplasma Diseases of Plants, 1978*, pp. 139-42. Taipei, Taiwan: National Science Council.

Nyland, G. and Moller, W.J. (1973). Control of pear decline with a tetracycline. *Plant Disease Reporter 57*, 634-7.

Parthasarathy, M.V. (1975). Sieve element structure. In *Transport in Plants* Vol. 1, *Phloem Transport*, pp. 3-38, M.H. Zimmermann and J.A. Milburn (eds). Berlin, Heidelberg, New York: Springer-Verlag.

Pearson, R.C. (1977). Control of X-disease of peach. *Proceedings New York State Horticultural Society 122*, 176-83.

Peterson, E.A. and Sinha, R.C. (1977). Uptake, distribution and persistence of tetracycline antibiotics in various plant species susceptible to mycoplasma infection. *Phytopathologische Zeitschrift 90*, 250-6.

Reil, W.O. and Beutel, J.A. (1976). A pressure machine for injecting trees. *California Agriculture 30*, 4-5.

Rogers, H.T. (1975). Tree injection. *Fruit Grower*, 13–15.

Rosenberger, D.A. and Jones, A.L. (1977). Symptom remission in X-diseased peach trees as affected by date, method, and rate of application of oxytetracycline-HCl. *Phytopathology 67*, 277–82.

Sachs, R.M., Nyland, G., Hackett, W.P., Coffelt, J., Debie, J. and Giannini, G. (1977). Pressurized injection of aqueous solutions into tree trunks. *Scientia Horticulturae 6*, 297–310.

Sands, D.C. (1974). Tetracycline concentrate treatment for X-disease of peach (Abstr.) *Phytopathology 64*, 585.

Sands, D.C. and Walton, G.S. (1975). Tetracycline injections for control of Eastern X-disease and bacterial spot of peach. *Plant Disease Reporter 59*, 573–6.

Schwarz, R.E. (1974). Injection of mycoplasmacides and insecticides into woody plants: a possible method of controlling mycoplasma-associated diseases and their vectors. *FAO Plant Protection Bulletin 22*, 1–6.

Schwarz, R.E., Moll, J.N. and Van Vuuren, S.P. (1974). Control of citrus greening and its Psylla vector by trunk injections of tetracyclines and insecticides. *Proceedings of the Sixth Conference of the International Organization of Citrus Virologists*, University of California, 26–9.

Schwarz, R.E. and Van Vuuren, S.P. (1971). Decrease in fruit greening of sweet orange by trunk injection of tetracyclines. *Plant Disease Reporter 55*, 747–50.

Sinha, R.C. (1979). Chemotherapy of mycoplasmal plant diseases. In *The Mycoplasmas*, Vol. III, pp. 309–35, R.F. Whitcomb and J.G. Tully (eds). New York: Academic Press.

Sinha, R.C. and Peterson, E.A. (1972). Uptake and persistence of oxytetracycline in aster plants and vector leafhoppers in relation to inhibition of clover phyllody agent. *Phytopathology 62*, 377–83.

Skene, D.S. and Balodis, V. (1968). A study of vessel length in *Eucalyptus obliqua* L'Hérit. *Journal of Experimental Botany 19*, 825–30.

Smith, P.F. (1971). *The Biology of Mycoplasmas*. New York: Academic Press.

Su, H.J. and Leu, S.C. (1972). Study on the pathogen complex causing Likubin of citrus in Taiwan. I. Nature of mycoplasmalike organism associated with the disease. *Proceedings of the National Science Council* (Taiwan) *5*, 109–26.

Tahama, Y. (1973). Studies on the mulberry dwarf disease (XXI). Recovery from the disease with oxytetracycline (Part 2). *Bulletin of the Hiroshima Agricultural College 4*, 283–93.

Tahama, Y., Shikata, E. and Murayama, D. (1972). Studies on the mulberry dwarf disease XX. Recovery from the disease by oxytetracycline. (Part 1). *Bulletin of the Hiroshima Agricultural College 4*, 198–207.

Whitcomb, R.F. and Davis, R.E. (1970). Evidence on possible mycoplasma etiology of aster yellows disease II. Suppression of aster yellows in insect vectors. *Infection and Immunity 2*, 209–15.

Wilhelm, H. and Knösel, D. (1976). Penetration and translocation of tetracycline-^{3}H-hydrochloride in plant tissue. *Journal of Plant Diseases and Protection 83*, 241–52.

Willekens, G.J. (1977). Rapid and sensitive direct TLC fluorometric method for evaluation of impurities in oxytetracycline. *Journal of Pharmaceutical Sciences 66*, 1419–22.

Wilson, C.L. (1979). Injection and infusion of trees. In *Proceedings of the Symposium on Systemic Chemical Treatments in Tree Culture*, 1978, pp. 1–6. Ann Arbor, Michigan: Braun-Brumfield, Inc.

Zimmermann, M.H. (1978). Structural requirements for optimal water conduction in tree stems. In *Tropical Trees as Living Systems*, pp. 517–32, M.H. Zimmermann and P.B. Tomlinson (eds). London, New York: Cambridge University

Press.
Zimmermann, M.H. and McDonough, J. (1978). Dysfunction in the flow of food. In *Plant Disease*, Vol. III, pp. 117–40, J.G. Horsfall (ed). New York: Academic Press.

6 MEDIA AND METHODS FOR CULTURE OF SPIROPLASMAS

C.H. Liao and T.A. Chen

1. Introduction

Spiroplasmas (Davis *et al.*, 1972; Davis and Worley, 1973) are of special interest for their unique helical cell shape and motility, and also for their economic importance and medical interest as pathogens of plants (Chen and Liao, 1975; Williamson and Whitcomb, 1975), insects (Clark, 1977; Tully *et al*, 1977; Whitcomb *et al.*, 1974), and vertebrates (Tully *et al.*, 1977). The frequency of their recent isolations and the

174

discovery of their new habitats suggests that this distinct group of microorganisms is widespread in nature, and we expect many more to be recovered in the future – some from unexpected sources.

The objective of this chapter is to generalise the techniques and methods which have been used in isolation, cultivation and maintenance of spiroplasmas. Historical developments and theoretical discussions on the culturing of spiroplasmas have been reviewed elsewhere (Chen and Davis, 1979; Bové and Saillard, 1979; Davis, 1979). In certain aspects, spiroplasmas resemble animal and human mycoplasmas. For general methods used in the cultivation of the class Mollicutes, readers may be referred to Fallon and Whittlestone (1969).

2. Media

A. Formulation

More than 20 artificial media have been formulated for primary isolation and routine cultivation of spiroplasmas. Different media have been used by different investigators, and generally it is not known to what extent the differences between the different media used are significant. Spiroplasmas are usually thought to require certain nutrients that are not normally contained in the conventional mycoplasma media of Chanock *et al.* (1962) and Hayflick and Chanock (1965). Media that were originally devised to cultivate pathogenic spiroplasmas were all enriched with several complex ingredients (Table 6.1). In addition to the basal components (PPLO broth base, animal serum and yeast extract) used in most mycoplasma media, three other ingredients (tryptone, peptone and animal tissue culture media) are often included. These complex media (Table 6.1) are still being used in many laboratories for primary isolation and routine cultivation of spiroplasmas. Nevertheless, they are being gradually supplanted by several media with simpler formulations (Table 6.2).

All spiroplasmas so far cultivated have been shown to grow in media containing only PPLO broth, horse serum and sugars. The first simple medium for spiroplasmas was formulated in 1975 (Liao and Chen). This medium, C–3G, (containing 1.5% PPLO broth [Difco], 15% agamma horse serum and 12% sucrose) has been used to isolate corn stunt spiroplasmas, *S. citri* (Liao and Chen, 1977) and the green leaf bug spiroplasma (Lei *et al.*, 1979). The medium C-3G and a medium slightly modified from C-3G are also satisfactory for isolation and cultivation of honey bee spiroplasmas (Davis *et al.*, 1976) and flower

Table 6.1: Composition of Complex Media for Culture of Spiroplasmas

| Ingredients (% w/v or v/v) | *S. citri* | | Corn stunt spiroplasma | | | SMCA |
	A	B	C	D	E	F
PPLO broth (Difco)	3.4	2.1	1.5	1.5	1.1	
Mycoplasma broth (BBL)						0.35
Tryptone (Difco)	1.0				3.3	1.0
Peptone (Difco)					0.3	0.53
Glucose	0.1	0.1			0.3	0.5
Fructose	0.1	0.1			0.3	
Sucrose	1.0	0.1	8.5	16.0	3.3	
Sorbitol	7.0	5.0			2.3	
Medium 199 (1X) (v/v)			5.0	1.0		
CMRL 1066 with glutamine (10X) (v/v)			2.5	0.5		5.0
Schneider's *Drosophila* medium (1X) (v/v)			2.5	0.5	66.0	
Fresh yeast extract (25%) (v/v)	10.0	10.0		10.0	3.3	0.35
a-ketoglutaric acid						0.02
Yeastolate			0.1			0.2
Fetal bovine serum (v/v)					20.0	17.0
Horse serum (v/v)	20.0	20.0	20.0	20.0		

Sources: column A, Saglio *et al.* (1973); B, Fudl-Allah *et al.* (1972); C, Chen and Granados (1970); D, Chen and Liao (1975); E, Williamson and Whitcomb (1975); F, Tully *et al.* (1977).

spiroplasmas (Davis, 1978; Su *et al.*, unpublished). The honey bee spiroplasma can also be grown in the standard mycoplasma medium (Grand Island Biological Lab.) and in the Singh's Mosquito Tissue Culture medium plus 20% fetal bovine serum (Clark, 1977). The suckling mouse cataract agent (spiroplasma) (SMCA) fails to grow in most spiroplasma media. A simple medium containing PPLO broth (Difco) 2.1%, agamma horse serum 20%, and glucose 0.4–0.6% has been devised for SMCA (Liao and Chen, 1979).

B. Basal Ingredients and Supplements

(1) PPLO (or Mycoplasma) Broth, Tryptone, Peptone. The ingredient PPLO (Mycoplasma) broth has been used in almost every medium formulated for spiroplasma cultivation. The PPLO broth (or agar) and

Table 6.2: Composition of Simple Media for Culture of Spiroplasmas

Ingredients (% w/v or v/v)	*S. citri*, corn stunt spiroplasma, honey bee spiroplasma, flower spiroplasma, and green leaf bug spiroplasma			Corn stunt spiroplasma and *S. citri*	SMCA	*S. citri*
	A	B	C	D	E	F
PPLO broth (Difco)	1.5	1.5	1.5	1.5	2.1	
Sucrose	12.0	10.0	8.0	16.0		1.0
Horse serum (v/v)	15.0	15.0	10.0	5.0[b]	20.0	10.0
Fresh yeast extract (25%) (v/v)			(10.0)[a]			
Glucose					0.4	0.1
Fructose						0.1
Sorbitol						7.0
Heart infusion broth						2.25

Notes: a. Primary isolations were occasionally made in medium supplemented with 10% fresh yeast extract.
b. In our laboratory, both *S. citri* and corn stunt spiroplasma grow very little in media containing 5% horse serum.
Sources: Column A, Liao and Chen (1975b, 1977), Lei *et al.* (1979); B, Liao and Chen (unpublished); C, Davis *et al.* (1976), Davis (1978); D, Igwegbe (1978b); E, Liao and Chen (1979); F, Bové and Saillard (1979).

Mycoplasma broth (or agar) are, respectively, available from Difco Laboratory (Detroit, Michigan) and Baltimore Biologicals Ltd. (BBL, Maryland). The chemical composition of neither product has been defined, but some differences between them are expected. Although both products are prepared from the same ingredients (beef heart infusion, peptone and sodium chloride), the compositions of beef heart infusion and peptone are not specified. The use of either PPLO broth (Difco) or Mycoplasma broth (BBL) for culturing spiroplasmas has been reported (Tables 6.1, 6.2).

The PPLO (or Mycoplasma) broth is often added at concentrations ranging from 1.1 to 3.5%. The concentrations higher than 4.0% are inhibitory for the growth of corn stunt spiroplasma and SMCA (Liao and Chen, unpublished). Several ingredients may be used to replace the PPLO (or Mycoplasma) broth in spiroplasma media. Chang and Chen (1979) reported that *S. citri* can be grown in a medium containing horse serum, sucrose, and a combination of CMRL 1066 and

Schneider's *Drosophila* medium. Clark (1977) reported growth of
honey bee spiroplasma in a medium containing lactalbumin hydro-
lysate, yeastolate, glucose, balanced salts and fetal bovine serum.
Davis (1979) has cultivated several spiroplasmas in a medium containing
tryptose instead of PPLO broth. The SMC medium of Saglio *et al.*
(1971) has also been simplified by replacing PPLO broth and tryptone
with heart infusion broth and by omitting fresh yeast extract and
lowering the amount of horse serum from 20% to 10% (Bové and
Saillard, 1979).

Besides PPLO (Mycoplasma) broth, tryptone and peptone have
been added occasionally to enrich the spiroplasma medium. Although
these two ingredients have been proven nonessential (see Table 6.2),
they may improve the buffer capacity of the culture media and consequently promote or prolong the growth of organisms. No experimental data, however, have been presented to verify such a possibility.
(2) Animal Sera. Spiroplasmas require certain components present in
animal sera for growth. In culture media, horse serum or fetal bovine
serum is usually added. The use of other serum such as porcine and
avian serum has never been reported. In most cases, serum is added at
a final concentration of 20% (v/v), although 10-15% has been used
successfully (Tables 6.1, 6.2). Nevertheless, Igwegbe (1978a, b)
reported that corn stunt spiroplasma grows best in medium containing
5% horse serum, and grows poorly in medium containing 20%. In our
laboratory, both corn stunt spiroplasma and *S. citri* have been shown to
grow equally well in media in which 10-20% horse serum or fetal
bovine serum is used. In a medium containing 5% serum, we observed
very little growth. Furthermore, we have found no significant difference
between sera purchased, respectively, from GIBCO (Grand Island Biological Lab.), Microbiological Associates, and Flow Lab. Recently, *S.
citri* has been shown to grow in a medium containing 40-50% horse
serum without any detrimental effects (P.J. Cotty and T.A. Chen,
unpublished). Since low-density serum proteins have been shown to be
inhibitory for growth of *Mycoplasma* sp. (Slutzky *et al.*, 1977), the
observations of Igwegbe (1978a, b) are interesting and need to be
further clarified.

A wide variety of natural antibodies (immunoglobulins) are present
in animal sera. The agamma form of horse serum is recommended for
use because a possible interaction berween natural antibodies with
spiroplasmas in culture media may be prevented. Before using, animal
serum is often heated at $56°C$ for 30-40 min. Such a step may not be
necessary, but would inactivate complements that might lyse

spiroplasmas and would kill mycoplasmas that might contaminate the serum.

Animal serum may be replaced by PPLO serum fraction or a combination of cholesterol, albumin, palmitic acid and Tween 80 (Saglio *et al.*, 1973; Freeman *et al.*, 1976; Mudd *et al.*, 1977; Lee, 1977). Very little is known about the role of animal serum in spiroplasma growth. Presumably, animal serum provides such essential nutrients as cholesterol, fatty acids and other components. Meanwhile, it may also protect spiroplasmas from certain toxic actions that are exerted by other compounds naturally present in culture medium. Animal serum has been well-known as a source of cholesterol, phospholipid, fatty acids and proteins for some *Mycoplasma* spp. (Edwards and Fitzgerald, 1951; Rodwell and Abbot, 1961; Smith and Boughton, 1960). The serum protein is to detoxify and to regulate the cholesterol uptake. The phospholipids, acting as surface active agents, function in the aqueous solubilisation of cholesterol (Smith and Boughton, 1960).

(3) Energy Sources. Several spiroplasma isolates including *S. citri* (Saglio *et al.*, 1973; Hawthorne and Van Demark, 1979), corn stunt spiroplasma (Malloy and Chen, unpublished), flower spiroplasma (Davis, 1978), honey bee spiroplasma (Davis *et al.*, 1976), and SMCA (Liao and Chen, 1979) have been shown to ferment glucose and/or fructose. Glucose and/or fructose are usually added to the medium at a final concentration of 0.4-0.6%. Since monosaccharides are often destroyed by prolonged heating, it is desirable to sterilise them by filtration or by a short period of autoclaving (121°C, 5 min). In addition to glucose and fructose, a large quantity of sucrose or sorbitol (at a final concentration of 8-16%) is also often added into the spiroplasma medium to raise the osmotic pressure. The use of sucrose or sorbitol as osmotic pressure adjustants will be discussed in Section 2.B (6).

Failure to utilise sucrose as an energy source by spiroplasmas has been described in several recent reports (Malloy and Chen, unpublished; Liao and Chen, 1979; Saglio *et al.*, 1973; Hawthorne and Van Demark, 1979; Davis, 1978; Lei *et al.*, 1979). It would be interesting to learn how spiroplasmas can grow in simple media (Table 6.2) containing only PPLO broth, horse serum and a large quantity of sucrose. It is likely that sucrose is converted into a degradable form of sugar during the autoclaving process (T.A. Chen; R.E. Davis, unpublished). This possiblity is strengthened by the observation (K. Malloy and T.A. Chen, unpublished) that spiroplasmas can grown in media containing autoclaved sucrose, but not in media containing filtered sucrose as the energy source.

The degradation of arginine by some spiroplasmas has been disputed for some time. Positive results have been reported with *S. citri* (Townsend, 1976) and flower spiroplasmas (Davis, 1978). McCoy (1978) found that the addition of arginine to spiroplasma culture broth particularly in the 20–40mM range, greatly increased the duration of viability of the cultures and induced a secondary peak of growth. It is now believed that utilisation of arginine by *S. citri* only occurs when glucose or fructose is present to encourage growth (Townsend, 1976).

Active fermentation of sugars by spiroplasmas is always accompanied by a rapid acid production (presumably lactic acid and acetic acid). A pH indicator, usually phenol red, is included in culture media at a final concentration of about 20 μg per ml. The decrease of pH in culture media as a result of spiroplasma growth is indicated by the colour change of indicator from red to yellow. The phenol red is usually added before autoclaving. A stock solution of phenol red dissolved in 0.01N NaOH is often used.

(4) Fresh Yeast Extract and Yeastolate. These two ingredients are often used in conventional mycoplasma media to supply vitamins. They have been used in some spiroplasma media, presumably for the same purpose. Although it has become clear (Table 6.2) that all spiroplasmas do not require either fresh yeast extract or yeastolate for growth, the yeast products greatly improve spiroplasma growth in media containing PPLO serum fraction instead of whole serum (Chang and Chen, 1979). Fresh yeast extract also promotes the growth of *S. citri*, but not of corn stunt spiroplasma (Igwegbe, 1978b). A 25% solution of fresh yeast extract is commercially available and is usually added to spiroplasma media at concentrations of 0.3–10%, v/v. Yeastolate at a final concentration of 0.1–0.2% may be used to replace fresh yeast extract.

(5) Animal Tissue Culture Media, Amino Acids, and Nucleotides. Spiroplasmas were previously thought to require some metabolic precursors which are not regularly contained in conventional mycoplasma media. Three animal tissue culture media (Medium 199, Schneider's *Drosophila* medium, and CMRL 1066) are often added (0.5–5.1%, v/v) to provide the needs of amino acids, nucleotides, fatty acids and vitamins (Chen and Granados, 1970). Lately, all spiroplasmas except SMCA have been successfully isolated and cultivated in simple media (Table 6.2) containing only PPLO broth, horse serum and sugar; the necessity of adding tissue culture media is now in doubt.

Additional amounts of various amino acids promote or prolong the growth of spiroplasmas. Lee and Davis (1978) found that *S. citri* divides rapidly, producing short, helical filaments, in the presence of added arginine, asparagine, cysteine, glutamine and methionine. Jones *et al.* (1977) observed that amino acid components from Schneider's *Drosophila* medium stimulated growth of *S. citri* but not of corn stunt spiroplasma. Also, McCoy (1978) reported that arginine prolonged the growth of *S. citri* and corn stunt spiroplasma. The mechanism explaining the effect of these amino acids on growth of spiroplasmas remains to be elucidated.

(6) Osmotic Pressure Adjustants. Plant-pathogenic spiroplasmas (*S. citri* and corn stunt spiroplasma) inhabit sieve tubes, where relatively high osmotic pressures (600–700 mOsm) prevail. When a culture medium for plant spiroplasmas is devised, the osmotic pressure is deliberately raised with certain compounds such as sorbitol and sucrose. Ionic compounds may be used, but spiroplasmas seem to respond differently to NaCl. A cystine-tryptone medium using NaCl as osmotic pressure adjustant has been employed for culture of *S. citri* (Davis *et al.*, 1975). A medium containing 1.5% PPLO broth, 15% horse serum, and 0.5% NaCl has been used in our laboratory to study the sugar catabolism of *S. citri*, honey bee spiroplasmas, flower spiroplasmas, and the green leaf bug spiroplasma (LB-12). Corn stunt spiroplasmas grow poorly in media using NaCl to replace sucrose. Apparently, the NaCl concentration in this medium is detrimental to corn stunt spiroplasmas. A balanced ion ratio appears to be especially important, at least in the case of corn stunt spiroplasmas (Liao and Chen, unpublished).

Flower spiroplasmas (23-6), green leaf bug spiroplasmas (LB-12) and SMCA exhibit good growth in media with low osmotic pressures (300–400 mOsm) (Table 6.3), and the use of osmotic pressure adjustants is not necessary. They can be easily cultured in a medium that contains only 1.5% PPLO broth, 15% horse serum and 0.4–0.8% of glucose or fructose (Liao and Chen, 1979).

(7) Antibacterial Agents. To protect the spiroplasma cultures from contamination with bacteria, especially in primary isolation, some chemicals that specifically inhibit growth of bacteria but not of spiroplasmas may be added. One of the compounds most often used is penicillin G. Penicillin, which blocks the synthesis of bacterial cell walls, is usually added at a concentration of 1,000–10,000 units per ml of medium. Thallium acetate may also be added into the medium at a final concentration of 0.1–0.2%, w/v.

Table 6.3: Physical and Chemical Environments for Growth of Spiroplasmas

	Temperature (°C)[b]	pH	Osmolality[a] (mOsm)	Gaseous Environments	References
S. citri	22-35 (32)[b]	7.0-8.2 (7.6)	310-1450 (500-610)	facultative aerobic	Lee (1977); Saglio et al. (1973)
Corn stunt spiroplasma (Strain 2-747)	15-35 (30-32)	6.8-8.0 (7.2)	310-1300 (610-840)	"	Liao and Chen (1978)
Honey bee spiroplasma (Strain AS 576)	30-37	7.5	310-1450 (500-610)	"	Davis et al. (1976)
Flower spiroplasma (Strain 23-6)	22-37 (34-35)	7.5	310-1450 (310-360)	"	Davis (1978)
SMCA	30-37	7.0-7.4	310-610 (310-360)	"	Tully et al. (1977)
Leaf bug spiroplasma (Strain LB-12)	23-35 (30)	6.0-7.8	310-1300 (310-1300)	"	Lei et al. (1979)

Notes: a. Data were obtained from Liao and Chen (1978, 1979), Liao et al. (1979b) and Cotty et al. (1980).
b. Numbers in brackets indicate optimal range for growth.
c. (Partially) anaerobic conditions may promote the growth in solid medium: (i) corn stunt spiroplasma (95% N_2 + 4.75% CO_2 + 0.25% O_2), (ii) SMCA (95% N_2 + 5% CO_2), (iii) S. citri (95% N_2 + 5% CO_2).

C. Preparation

Ingredients of spiroplasma media can be grouped into two categories, heat-stable and heat-labile. The heat stable category includes PPLO (or Mycoplasma) broth, tryptone, peptone, sorbitol, sucrose, HEPES buffer and phenol red. The heat-labile category includes animal sera, fresh yeast extract, yeastolate, sugars, amino acids, organic acids, animal tissue culture media and penicillin. The heat-stable ingredients are usually added to distilled water and autoclaved at 121°C (15 psi) for 15 minutes, while the heat-labile ingredients are usually sterilised by filtration through 0.22–0.45 μm membrane filters. The heat-labile ingredients are added when the autoclaved portion has cooled to 50°C or lower. The pH of medium may be adjusted using 1N NaOH or HCl before or after autoclaving. Most heat-labile ingredients are normally furnished in sterile containers by manufacturers.

3. Isolation and Cultivation

A. Inoculum Sources

Plant-pathogenic spiroplasmas are distributed systemically, but not uniformly, in sieve tubes of the entire diseased plants. For primary isolation, any part of a diseased plant could serve as the source of inoculum. Both *S. citri* and corn stunt spiroplasmas have been successfully isolated from different organs of infected citrus or corn plants, including leaf, stem, root and reproductive organs (Table 6.2). Practically, the young and succulent tissues having severe disease symptoms are usually chosen for three reasons: (1) they normally contain the disease agent at a relatively higher concentration; (2) they are less exposed to the environment and contamination of their surface with other microbes is minimal; and (3) the juice expressed from these tissues has a lower degree of anti-spiroplasma activity, which is detectable shortly after the tissue is crushed (Liao and Chen, 1975a, 1979, 1980). In order to avoid a possible anti-spiroplasma action of plant tissue homogenates, plant-pathogenic spiroplasmas may be isolated indirectly from leafhopper vectors. Sources of materials which have been used to isolate spiroplasmas are summarised in Table 6.4.

B. Isolation Methods

(1) Diseased Plants. A piece of diseased tissue (0.2–0.3 x 1.0–1.5 cm), preferably the young and succulent portion, is surface-sterilised with

Table 6.4: Sources of Materials Used for Isolation and *in vitro* Culture of Spiroplasmas

Spiroplasma strains	Plant or Vertebrate Animal Host	Arthropod Host	References
S. citri	Leaf, stem, root, seed and fruit axis of citrus; cabbage; broccoli; brussel sprouts; Chinese cabbage; pak-choi; turnip; radish; periwinkle; *Pisum sativum; Trifolium repens; Vicia faba; Chrysanthemum carinatum; Trifolium pratense;* London rocket; mustard	*Circulifer tenellus; Scaphytopius nitridus; S. acutus delongi; Euscelis plebejus*	Saglio et al. (1971); Fudl-Allah et al. (1971); Markham et al. (1974); Markham and Townsend (1974); Sparr et al. (1974); Townsend et al. (1977a); Allen (1975); Granett et al. (1976); Calavan et al. (1976); Lee et al. (1973); Oldfield and Kaloostian (1979); Kaloostian et al. (1975)
Corn stunt spiroplasma	Leaf vein, stem, root of corn plant; periwinkles (*Vinca rosea* and *V. faba*)	*Dalbulus elimatus; D. maidis; Euscelidius variegatus*	Chen and Liao (1975); Williamson and Whitcomb (1975); Liao and Chen (1977); Markham et al. (1977)
Honey bee spiroplasma		honey bee (*Apis mellifera*)	Davis et al. (1976); Clark (1977); H.J. Su et al. (unpublished)
Flower spiroplasmas	Nectars of tulip tree (*Liriodendron tulipifera* L.); Spanish needles, (*Bidens pilosa* L.); *Magnolia grandiflora* L; Powder puff (*Calliandra haematocephala*); citrus, rose and azalea		Davis (1978); Davis (1979); Clark (1978); McCoy et al. (1979); Su et al. (unpublished)
SMCA and GT 48	Infected chicken embryo	rabbit tick, (*Haemaphysalis leporispalustris*)	Tully et al. (1977); Stiller et al. (1978)
277F agent	Infected chicken embryo		Brinton and Burgdorfer (1976); Stalheim et al. (1978)
Green leaf bug spiroplasma (LB-12)		*Trigonotylus ruficornis*	Lei et al. (1979)

0.1% $HgCl_2$ or 0.25–1.0% sodium hypochlorite for 2–5 min. After rinsing in sterile water 2–3 times, the piece of tissue may be dipped in 75% ethyl alcohol for 30–50 seconds and then flamed quickly. The surface-sterilised tissue thus obtained is subsequently placed in a petri dish and cut into small pieces in the presence of culture medium (0.5–1.5 ml). The inoculum is immediately released into the medium when the tissue is squeezed by using forceps. The inoculum source thus prepared may be added directly into another portion of fresh medium at the ratio of 1/20. The inoculum may be filtered through 0.45 μm membrane filters to remove possible contamination of bacteria before being added to fresh medium. Growth of spiroplasmas in the primary culture is usually limited because of the presence of anti-spiroplasma factors in the inoculum source (Chen and Liao, 1975; Liao and Chen, 1975a; Calavan, 1979).

An anti-spiroplasma factor has been demonstrated in a wide variety of plant tissue extracts including corn, periwinkle, lettuce and celery. The corn and periwinkle extracts at dilutions up to 1/640 or 1/2560, respectively, are inhibitory for the growth of *S. citri* and corn stunt spiroplasmas when the spiroplasma concentration of 10^4 cells/ml is used for testing. The anti-spiroplasma action of plant extracts is static. The spiroplasma concentration remains constant in a medium containing plant extracts, but immediate multiplication of spiroplasmas is observed after plant extracts are removed (Liao and Chen, 1975a, 1979, 1980).

In order to prevent the anti-spiroplasma action of plant tissue extracts in the primary cultures, two steps may be taken. The primary cultures can be subcultured at 1–2 day intervals (Chen and Liao, 1975; Liao and Chen, 1977; Calavan, 1979) or may be serially tenfold-diluted in the fresh medium. Spiroplasmas often grow at a faster rate in the secondary or the diluted cultures. The inoculum source or the primary cultures as prepared above may also be centrifuged at 16,000 g for 30 minutes (Williamson and Whitcomb, 1975) to remove the plant juice which is presumably inhibitory to spiroplasma growth. Generally, both *S. citri* and corn stunt spiroplasmas exhibit growth in the secondary subcultures 1–2 weeks after incubation at 30°C.

(2) Insects. Hemolymphs are collected from naturally diseased vectors or from insects infected with spiroplasmas and are immediately dispensed in a small volume (1–2 ml) of culture medium. After filtration (0.45 μm membrane), the filtrate may be transferred into fresh medium or directly incubated at 30°C. Alternatively, 1–5 insects after surface sterilisation in 1% sodium hypochlorite may be gound in a

tissue grinder or in a mortar containing 2–3 ml of broth medium. The homogenate is either centrifuged at low speed to remove tissue debris or directly filtered through 0.45 μm membrane filters. The filtrate may be serially diluted in fresh medium or directly placed in an incubator (30°C). Spiroplasma growth is indicated by the colour change and also by the increase of helices visible under the dark-field microscope. Various arthropods from which spiroplasmas have been isolated are listed in Table 6.4 (Lei *et al.*, 1979; Stiller *et al.*, 1978; Lee *et al.*, 1973; Davis *et al.*, 1976; Clark, 1977).

(3) Flowers. Techniques for the successful isolation of flower spiroplasmas have been described in detail in the reports of Davis (1978) and McCoy *et al.* (1979). Briefly, healthy flowers are cut from plants and placed in plastic bags without touching by hand. Flower spiroplasmas presumably reside on the surface of flowers, and surface sterilisation of the flowers should be avoided. When nectar is abundant, the floral surfaces are simply rinsed with sterile broth medium. When flowers appear dry, they are soaked in medium for 15 to 30 minutes. The medium used to rinse or to soak the flower parts is filtered through 0.45 μm filter membranes to eliminate bacteria. The filtrate and dilutions of the filtrate are incubated at 27–32°C and are monitored for growth at 1–3 day intervals.

C. Cultivation in Broth Media

Primary isolations of spiroplasmas are usually made in broth medium, and established cultures are often maintained in liquid medium for routine tests in the laboratory. Based on growth rate, spiroplasmas may be grouped into three categories: the fast-growing, the moderate-growing and the slow-growing. The fast-growing isolates include flower spiroplasmas (strains 23–6 and SR-3). The moderate-growing isolates include honey bee spiroplasma (strain AS576 and others) and *S. citri* strains. Other spiroplasma isolates including SMCA, corn stunt spiroplasma and green leaf bug spiroplasma belong to the slow-growing category. When spiroplasmas are grown in broth medium, subculturing has to be made within a period of 1–8 days depending on the isolate, medium and temperature of incubation. Normally, subculturing is done when the colour of a culture medium containing phenol red is about to turn yellow. The slow-growing isolates may be subcultured at 6–8 day intervals. For the moderate-growing isolates, a serial passage at 2–3 day intervals is adequate. The fast-growing isolates are usually subcultured daily. The inoculum size used for each passage is about 1/10–1/20 of the volume of fresh sterile medium.

The growth pattern of spiroplasmas in broth medium is similar to that of other microorganisms. Four phases (lag, exponential, stationary and death phases) are observed in a growth cycle. The short stationary and death phases are probably due to the production of large quantities of acids in the culture medium. The helicity and motility of the organisms are greatly distorted when the pH of culture medium drops to 5.5 or lower. To offset the acid production by spiroplasmas, medium may be supplemented with HEPES buffer (0.06M, Liao and Chen, 1977). In HEPES-buffered medium, the yield of spiroplasmas is often increased and the stationary phase is usually prolonged.

Factors affecting spiroplasma growth have been previously reviewed (Chen and Davis, 1979; Bové and Saillard, 1979). Some physical and chemical environments that are suitable for growth of various spiroplasma are summarised in Table 6.3. All spiroplasmas so far cultivated tend to grow better at a slightly alkaline pH. The initial pH of culture medium is adjusted to 7.0-7.5. The detrimental effect of low pH (6.0 or lower) has been examined (Liao and Chen, 1977; Lee, 1977; Patel *et al.*, 1978). Some spiroplasmas grow best at 29-32°C. Plant pathogenic spiroplasmas and green leaf bug spiroplasmas exhibit no (or very little) growth at 37°C. The honey bee spiroplasmas, flower spiroplasmas and SMCA grow equally well at 30°C and at 37°C. The optimum for honey bee spiroplasmas is close to 34-35°C. In spite of the lack of cell wall, spiroplasmas can be cultured at a wide range of osmotic pressures. All spiroplasmas thus far studied, except SMCA, multiply in media containing 1.5% PPLO broth (Difco), 15% horse serum, and 0-0.65M sucrose. The SMCA grows best in a medium without added sucrose, although slight growth may be detected in a medium that contains 4-6% sucrose. The requirement of low osmotic pressure for growth is one of the characteristics by which SMCA differs from other spiroplasmas (Liao and Chen, 1979, unpublished).

D. Colony Formation in Agar Media

Solid medium may be prepared by using PPLO (or Mycoplasma) agar base to substitute for PPLO (or Mycoplasma) broth base or by supplementing broth medium with agar. If agar is added separately, a concentration of 0.8-1.5% is usually used. Although Ionagar and Noble agar are favoured because of their purity, no detrimental effect of ordinary agar on spiroplasma growth has ever been reported. Occasionally, the normal agar and agar purified of Difco and the granulated agar of BBL at a concentration of 1.0-1.7% are used in our laboratory.

Spiroplasma cultures may be seeded on to agar medium by spreading on the surface of the medium or by mixing with agar medium when the medium is cool but not solidified. If the spiroplasma concentration in broth culture is high, it is diluted in a tenfold series in broth medium. Aliquots of 30–50 μl of each dilution are seeded on to the agar. Seal-tightened culture dishes (0.5 x 5 cm, Falcon) have at least two advantages over the ordinary Petri dishes (1.5 x 10 cm). The former take less medium (2.5–3.5 ml) and would reduce the evaporation of medium especially when weeks of incubation are needed. Seeded plates may be incubated aerobically or placed in a BBL Gas Pak (CO_2 + H_2) or incubated in other gaseous environments (Table 6.3).

Spiroplasmas often form typical 'fried-egg'-shaped colonies, but Davis *et al.* (unpublished data) suggest that 'fried-egg' colonies may tend to form in media unfavourable for spiroplasma growth. Granular colonies are frequently observed. The size of colonies varies from 0.05 to 3 mm depending on culture conditions and spiroplasma concentrations. Several reports (Williamson and Whitcomb, 1975; Tully *et al.*, 1977; Saglio *et al.*, 1973) show that anaerobic or partially anaerobic conditions (Table 6.3) promote the colony formation, but no comparative data or statistical analyses are included. Variations in medium composition and agar concentration also affect the ability of spiroplasmas to form colonies (Whitcomb, 1980). The growth rate of spiroplasmas in solid medium generally corresponds to that in broth media. For the fast-growing (flower spiroplasmas 23–6 and SR 3), colonies can be observed under the dissecting microscope or by the naked eye within 3–4 days. For the moderate-growing (honey bee spiroplasma and *S. citri*), colonies become visible in 7–10 days or less. For the slow-growing (corn stunt spiroplasma, green leaf bug spiroplasma and SMCA), it usually takes 14–18 days to form visible colonies. When enhanced contrast is desired, colonies may be stained with Dienes stain (Davis, 1978).

Variations of colony morphology reflecting biochemical or structural changes have not been carefully studied. It has been demonstrated (Townsend *et al.*, 1977), however, that nonhelical mutants of *S. citri* form smooth and relatively small (< 0.05 mm) colonies. The nonhelical strain also fails to form tiny satellite colonies, that often appear in the vicinity of primary colonies of the helical strain. Helical spiroplasma strains, even of *S. citri* (Davis, 1974; Townsend *et al.*, 1977b), contain abundant helical cells in colonies, in contrast to earlier reports (Cole *et al.*, 1973).

E. Cloning Procedures

The Subcommittee on the Taxonomy of Mollicutes (1979) recommended that all newly isolated spiroplasmas should be triple-cloned before any deposition or study is made. Such a procedure is important for it ensures an isolate consisting of a homogeneous population. The broth culture is filtered through the smallest pore diameter (normally 0.3 or 0.22 μm) to remove any clumps of cells. The filtrate is then serially diluted in broth medium; aliquots of 30–50 μl are seeded on to agar plates. An isolated colony supposedly originating from a single cell is transferred to the broth medium, and the cloning procedure is repeated at least twice more. The cloned cultures are finally examined by light and electron microscopy to verify the characteristics of spiroplasma morphology and ultrastructure.

F. Alternative Methods for Propagation of Spiroplasmas

There exist at least two recognised spiroplasmas which are unable to be cultivated by using the methods just described. One of them inhabits natural populations of the sharpshooter (*Oncometopia nigricans*) (McCoy *et al.*, 1978). Another known as 'sex ratio organism' (SRO) is inherited maternally and associated with the absence of males in the progeny of infected female *Drosophila* (Williamson and Whitcomb, 1974). For those spiroplasmas which are difficult to cultivate axenically, a number of alternative methods may be applied.

(1) Cultivation in Embryonated Hen's Eggs. The strains SMCA, GT–48 and 277F agent have been isolated from different pools of rabbit ticks and maintained in embryonated eggs for indefinite passages (Pickens *et al.*, 1968; Clark, 1964; Tully *et al.*, 1976). A high titre of spiroplasma was observed in allantoic and amniotic fluids of the inoculated eggs (Tully *et al.*, 1976). All embryos receiving SMCA and GT 48 die between 6 and 7 days.

Recently, *S. citri*, honey bee spiroplasmas and flower spiroplasmas have also been shown to multiply in chick embryos (Rose *et al.*, 1979; T.A. Chen and C.J. Chang; H.J. Su; unpublished). Both honey bee spiroplasmas and flower spiroplasmas are pathogenic to embryonated eggs (Rose *et al.*, 1979), but corn stunt spiroplasma and *S. citri* do not exert obvious pathogenicity for vertebrates.

To cultivate spiroplasmas in chick embryos, the eggs are inoculated by injecting the spiroplasma suspension via the yolk sac route into 7-day incubated hen's egg. The developing chick embryos may also be inoculated via the amniotic or allantoic cavity route or via the chorioallantoic membranes. The spiroplasma cultures may be serially transferred in embryonated eggs at 5–7 day intervals.

(2) Cultivation in Organ and Cell Cultures. Successful cultivation of SMCA in cottontail rabbit whole-lens organ culture has been previously reported by Fabiyi *et al.* (1971). Infective titres of spiroplasma in culture fluids and in lens tissue reach a peak 5 days after inoculation. Serial passage of other spiroplasmas in animal or plant organ culture systems has never been tried. A recent observation by G.J. McGarrity (personal communication) indicates that both plant and insect spiroplasmas may be grown in a mammalian or invertebrate cell culture system as well.

(3) Multiplication in Non-vector Insects. The ability of spiroplasmas to grow in atypical hosts especially in nonvector insects has been extensively studied. In 1973, the Moroccan isolate of *S. citri* was first shown to multiply in the leafhopper vector of corn stunt (*Dalbulus elimatus*), in the vector of aster yellows (*Macrosteles fascifrons*), and also in *Draeculacephala* spp. (Whitcomb *et al.*, 1973). Corn stunt spiroplasma was also shown to adapt and grow through at least nine passages in *Drosophila pseudoobscura* females. Recently, McCoy and Davis (1980) reported that larvae of the greater wax moth (*Galleria mellonella*) supported extensive multiplication of *S. citri* and flower spiroplasmas. Spiroplasmas were observed in adult moths after pupation. Cultivation of spiroplasmas in non-vector insects or in other atypical hosts, however, poses at least one problem, i.e. the pathogenicity or other biochemical characters of a spiroplasma may be altered after serial passages in such an unnatural environment. The corn stunt spiroplasma is no longer virulent after the fifth passage in *D. pseudoobscura* (Williamson and Whitcomb, 1974, 1975).

4. Quantitation

A. Turbidity

Measurement of tubidity as a function of growth has not been well-adapted to spiroplasma research for several reasons. The growth of spiroplasmas in broth media generally does not give high turbidity even under the most favourable conditions. The tendency of spiroplasmas to clump in most broth media also makes it impossible to interpret the turbidity measurement correctly. In addition, precipitates are often formed in cultures after several days of incubation. This phenomenon is especially marked when the pH of culture media drops to 5.5 or lower. Nevertheless, Lee (1977) estimated the growth of *S. citri* in his complex medium by measurement of absorption at 660 nm. Absorbence reached 0.094 after three days of incubation.

B. Protein and Nucleic Acid Concentrations

Direct measurement of protein or nucleic acid concentrations as a function of growth has been applied in spiroplasma research with very limited success. Because of the relatively slow growth rate and the minute size of cells, the yield of spiroplasmas in broth medium is small (0.1–0.3 g fresh weight/l, culture). It is practically impossible to analyse the protein or nucleic acid content by chemical means. The complex components of culture medium, if not removed completely, can also interfere with the result.

A more sensitive method that measures the incorporation of radio-active materials into cells may be applied. Carrier-free [^{32}P]-phosphate can be added to the medium at a concentration of 1–4 μCi/ml. The quantity of phosphate incorporated into DNA as a function of spiroplasma growth is determined from the radioactivity of TCA-insoluble precipitate. The [^{32}P]-phosphate technique has been used to study the effect of temperature and horse serum concentration on the growth of *S. citri* (Bové *et al.*, 1973; Saglio *et al.*, 1973). [^{14}C]-thymidine at a concentration of 0.1–0.5 μCi per ml of medium may be used to replace [^{32}P]-phosphate. Townsend *et al.* (1977b) applied [^{14}C]-thymidine to compare the growth of helical and non-helical strains of *S. citri*. The radioactivity of TCA-insoluble precipitate is normally measured after the removal of phospholipid by ethanol and ether. Growth of *S. citri* may also be estimated by measuring the content of ATP (Saglio *et al.*, 1979).

C. Colour-Changing-Unit (CCU)

Growth of spiroplasmas in broth medium is often indicated by a colour change of the phenol red indicator from red to yellow. The use of titrations involving dilution series has been used by Whitcomb and Williamson (1975) and later by Liao *et al.* (1979) and Cotty *et al.* (1980) to quantitate the concentration of spiroplasmas. Spiroplasma cultures are serially tenfold-diluted in medium containing 20 μg/ml of phenol red. The colour change in each tube is recorded after a given period (2–3 weeks) of incubation at 30°C or 37°C. The highest dilution at which the colour change occurs is defined as containing 1 CCU. The cell titre of the undiluted culture is then the reciprocal of the dilution at the endpoint. The CCU method is very time- and material-consuming. When measurement of cell viability and concentration is equally important in some experiments, this method or the CFU method (Section D) may be performed. The statistical validity of the CCU procedures has been recently discussed (Whitcomb, 1980). An alternative method by measuring the acid production by spiroplasmas in broth medium has been employed by Jones *et al.* (1977).

D. Colony-Forming-Unit (CFU)

Methods to cultivate spiroplasmas in agar media have been described in Section 2.D. Quantitation of spiroplasma cells by the CFU method is probably the most useful and reliable, especially in experiments where the viability of cells has to be taken into account. Cultures are usually diluted in a tenfold series in broth medium. Aliquots of 30-50 μl are then spread over the surface of agar plates which have been previously dried at 30°C for 2 hours. The numbers of colonies are counted with the aid of a dissecting microscope. Only those plates having the 50-150 colonies are counted and used for calculation of the CFU. In our experience, all spiroplasmas form colonies consistently in agar media as listed in Table 6.2.

E. Direct Cell Counting

The most distinctive properties of spiroplasmas are their helical morphology and contractile motility. These two valuable characteristics make it easy to evaluate cell numbers in the light microscope with dark-field optics. Light microscopy was first used to enumerate the helical bodies to study spiroplasma pathogenicity in insects (Whitcomb and Williamson, 1975), and was later extended by Liao and Chen (1977, 1978, 1979) to study various aspects of spiroplasma growth. Five μl aliquots of culture are deposited on a microslide. Care is taken to distribute the sample under the exact area of one cover slip (18 x 18 mm). The area of one visual field is determined using a grid ocular micrometer. Five visual fields for each sample are randomly selected and counted under dark-field (1,500 x). The cell number in 5 μl of culture is calculated by multiplying the average cell number per visual field by a constant (18 mm x 18 mm/area of one visual field). Cell aggregates may be dispersed by vortexing (2 min). When the cell concentration is high, a tenfold dilution of culture is made before counting. When the dark-field micrographs are desired, spiroplasma cells may be fixed at 4°C by directly adding glutaraldehyde into the culture at a final concentration of 2% (Cole *et al.*, 1973; Lee, 1977).

F. Measurement by Electron Microscopy

Quantitation of spiroplasma cells in the electron microscope has been described recently by Bové and Saillard (1979). The cells are fixed with glutaraldehyde at a final concentration of 1% in culture medium. A known amount of calibrated polystyrene is added at the same time. Twenty μl of the fixed culture is deposited on a 2% agar block. The spiroplasmas and the beads remain on the surface, while the liquid phase is absorbed by the agar. Collodion is then spread over the agar. The collodion film containing absorbed spiroplasmas and beads is removed by floating on water and collected on a carbon-sprayed grid. The specimen is then examined in the electron microscope. The number of helices per unit volume can be calculated from the number of beads present. By using this technique, large numbers of helices can be observed in the electron microscope, and the helicity can be well preserved (A. Rodwell, M. Garnier, M.T. Clerc and J.M. Bové, unpublished).

5. Preservation

A. Subculturing

Spiroplasmas may be preserved in the laboratory by continuous subculturing. The growth rates of spiroplasmas differ from one isolate to another; the duration of days and the amount of inoculum required for each transfer has been described in Section 2.C. In each transfer two tubes are prepared; one tube is used only for the next transfer and the second tube is used for other purposes. This method may be useful for laboratories that handle only one or two spiroplasma isolates. For those laboratories that deal with more than two spiroplasmas, it is fairly easy to contaminate one isolate with others. Since subculturing is a frequent event, much care must also be taken to prevent contamination by bacteria or mycoplasmas. Spiroplasmas are usually cultured in broth medium, and the homogeneity of the cell population is theoretically impossible to maintain as the numbers of passages increase. The method is tedious, especially for flower spiroplasmas, which require transfer daily.

B. Freezing (−20°C or −70°C)

All spiroplasmas can be readily preserved in the frozen state for a period of months or years. At low temperatures the metabolic rate of cells is depressed and the available energy for biochemical reactions is limited. Cultures at the mid- or the late-log phase are best for storage.

They can be directly placed in the freezer without changing the suspending medium. The osmotic pressure in SMCA media is relatively low (300-400 mOsm). More sugar (6-8%) may be added to the SMCA cultures immediately before storage. For other spiroplasmas which have been grown in media containing high concentrations of sucrose, this step is not required. The rate of cooling and the rate of rewarming should be as rapid as possible. For this purpose, it is preferable to freeze a small volume (0.5-1.0 ml) of cultures rather than 5 or 10 ml. Although storage at $-70°C$ is preferable to that at $-20°C$, some loss of viability is expected. Damage caused by the freezing process largely results from the formation of ice crystals and from the presence of electrolytes in high concentrations, which often remove water from proteins and DNA.

C. Freeze-drying (Lyophilisation)

Freeze-drying has been in use for preservation of spiroplasmas in some laboratories. The principle of this method is simple. The organism is first frozen, and then water is removed by sublimation from the ice as vapour. Therefore, the damage caused by the freezing and thawing process (Section 4.b) can be prevented. It has been shown that the addition to the culture medium of sucrose at a final concentration of 12%, as an additive in freeze-drying of *Mycoplasma* spp. enhances the recovery of freeze-dried mycoplasmas (Norman *et al.*, 1970). Spiroplasma cells for freeze-drying are usually suspended in a medium containing 12% sucrose. Log-phase cultures can be readily pre-frozen in liquid nitrogen, dry ice, or other ultracool solvents. The frozen ampoules that contain spiroplasmas are immediately connected to the vacuum system of a lyophiliser for further drying. For more details about practical aspects of freeze-drying, readers are referred to Lapage *et al.*, 1970.

D. Drying (Paper Disc Method)

An easy method of drying cultures on paper discs was originally developed by Coe and Clark (1966) to preserve *Staphylococcus aureus* and other bacteria. This method was recently adopted by H.J. Su and T.A. Chen (unpublished) to preserve spiroplasmas. The filter paper is cut into discs (about 3-4 mm in diameter) and autoclaved at $121°C$ for 15 minutes. A drop of log-phase culture is deposited on each disc. When the discs are air-dried, they are placed in a dessicator without a vacuum. Spiroplasmas can be recovered from the discs 6 weeks after storage at room temperature and 3 months after storage at $4°C$. This method is convenient and is suited for the inexpensive transport of large numbers of spiroplasma cultures by post. The same method may also be used for the preservation of animal mycoplasmas. Vogelzang (1975) has demonstrated that *Mycoplasma pulmonis* (R-1) remains viable on dried filter paper strips (1 x 4 cm, Whatman paper no. 1) for at least 4 days.

References

Allen, R.M. (1975). Spiroplasma organism found in naturally infected periwinkle. *Citrograph 60*, 426–46.

Barile, M.F. and Kern, J. (1971). Isolation of *Mycoplasma arginini* from commercial bovine sera and its implication in contaminated cell cultures. *Proceedings of the Society for Experimental Biology and Medicine 138*, 432-7.

Bové, J.M. and Saillard, C. (1979). Cell Biology of spiroplasmas. In *The Mycoplasmas*, Vol. III, pp. 85–153, R.F. Whitcomb and J.G. Tully (eds). New York: Academic Press.

Bové, J.M., Saglio, P., Tully, J.G., Freundt, E.A., Lund, Z., Pillot, J. and Taylor-Robinson, D. (1973). Characterization of the mycoplasma-like organism associated with 'stubborn' disease of citrus. *Annals of the New York Academy of Sciences 225*, 462-70.

Brinton, L.P. and Burgdorfer, W. (1976). Cellular and subcellular organiztion of the 277 F agent, a mycoplasma from the rabbit tick (*Haemaphysalis leporispalustris* [*Acari: Ixodidae*]). *International Journal of Systematic Bacteriology 26*, 545–60.

Calavan, E.C. (1979). Symptoms of stubborn disease and the culture of *Spiroplasma citri*. In *Proceedings of ROC-United States Cooperative Science Seminar on Mycoplasma Diseases of Plants*, pp. 67–73, H.J. Su and R.E. McCoy (eds). National Science Council, Taiwan.

Calavan, E.C., Oldfield, G.N. and Blue, R.L. (1976). Stubborn pathogen found in London rocket. *Citrograph 61*, 389.

Chang, C.J. and Chen, T.A. (1979). A PPLO broth base-free medium for the cultivation of *Spiroplasma citri. Abstracts of the 71st Annual Meeting of the American Phytopathological Society*, 647.

Chanock, R.M., Hayflick, L. and Barile, M.F. (1962). Growth on artificial medium of an agent associated with atypical pneumonia and its identification as a PPLO. *Proceedings of the National Academy of Sciences of the United States of America 48*, 41-9.

Chen, T.A. and Davis, R.E. (1979). Cultivation of spiroplasmas. In *The Mycoplasmas*, Vol. III, pp. 65–82, R.F. Whitcomb and J.G. Tully (eds). New York: Academic Press.

Chen, T.A. and Granados, R.R. (1970). Plant pathogenic mycoplasma-like organism: Maintenance *in vitro* and transmission to *Zea mays* L. *Science 167*, 1633-6.

Chen, T.A. and Liao, C.H. (1975). Corn stunt spiroplasma: Isolation, cultivation, and proof of pathogenicity. *Science 188*, 1015-17.

Clark, H.F. (1964). Suckling mouse cataract agent. *Journal of Infectious Diseases 114*, 476-87.

Clark, T.B. (1977). *Spiroplasma* sp., a new pathogen in honey bees. *Journal of Invertebrate Pathology 29*, 112-13.

— (1978). Honey bee spiroplasmosis: a new problem for beekeepers. *American Bee Journal 29*, 112-13.

Coe, A.W. and Clark, S.P. (1966). Preservation of bacteria by paper discs. *Monthly Bulletin of Ministry of Health 25*, 97–100.

Cole, R.M., Tully, J.G., Popkin, T.J. and Bové, J.M. (1973). Morphology, ultra-structure, and bacteriophage infection of the helical mycoplasma-like organism (*Spiroplasma citri* gen. nov., sp. nov.) cultured from 'stubborn' disease of citrus. *Journal of Bacteriology 115*, 367–86.

Cotty, P.J., Liao, C.H. and Chen, T.A. (1980). Osmotic parameters of the growth and viability of spiroplasmas. *Abstracts of the 3rd Meeting of International Organization of Mycoplasmology.* Custer, South Dakota, p. 139.

Daniels, M.J., Markham, P.G., Meddins, B.M., Plaskitt, A.K., Townsend, R. and Bar-Joseph, M. (1973). Axenic culture of a plant pathogenic spiroplasma. *Nature (London) 244*, 523–4.

Davis, R.E. (1978). Spiroplasma associated with flowers of the tulip tree (*Liriodendron tulipfera* L.). *Canadian Journal of Microbiology 24*, 954–9.

— (1979). Spiroplasmas: helical cell wall-free prokaryotes in diverse habitats. *Proceedings of ROC-United States Cooperative Science Seminar on Mycoplasma Diseases of Plants*, 59-64.

Davis, R.E. and Worley, J.F. (1973). Spiroplasma: motile, helical microorganism associated with corn stunt disease. *Phytopathology 63*, 403–8.

Davis, R.E., Worley, J.F., Clark, T.B. and Moseley, M. (1976). New spiroplasma in diseased honey bee *Apis mellifera*: Isolation, pure culture, and partial characterization *in vitro. Proceedings of American Phytopathological Society 3*, 304.

Davis, R.E., Worley, J.F. and Moseley, M. (1975). Spiroplasmas: primary isolation and cultivation in cystine-tryptone media, and translational locomotion in semi-solid versions. *Proceedings of American Phytopathological Society 2*, 56.

Davis, R.E., Worley, J.F., Whitcomb, R.F., Ishijima, T. and Steere, R.L. (1972). Helical filaments produced by a mycoplasma-like organism associated with corn stunt disease. *Science 176*, 521–3.

Edwards, D.G. and Fitzgerald, W.A. (1951). Cholesterol in the growth of organisms of the pleuropneumonia group. *Journal of General Microbiology 5*, 576–86.

Fabiyi, A., Elizan, T.S. and Pounds, J.E. (1971). Cultivation of suckling mouse cataract agent in rabbit whole-lens organ culture. *Proceedings of the Society of Experimental Biology and Medicine 136*, 88–91.

Fallon, R.J. and Whittlestone, P. (1969). Isolation, cultivation, and maintenance of mycoplasmas. In *Methods in Microbiology*, Vol. 3B, pp. 211–67, J.R. Norris and D.W. Ribbons (eds). New York: Academic Press.

Fudl-Allah, A.E.A. and Calavan, E.C. (1973). Effect of temperature and pH on growth *in vitro* of a mycoplasmalike organism associated with stubborn disease of citrus. *Phytopathology 63*, 256–9.

Fudl-Allah, A.E.A., Calavan, E.C. and Igwegbe, E.C.K. (1971). Culture of a mycoplasmalike organism associated with stubborn disease of citrus. *Phytopathology 61*, 1321.

—(1972). Culture of a mycoplasmalike organism associated with stubborn disease. *Phytopathology 62*, 729–31.

Freeman, B.A., Sissenstein, R., McManus, T.T., Woodward, J.K., Lee, I.M. and Mudd, J.B. (1976). Lipid composition and lipid metabolism of *Spiroplasma citri. Journal of Bacteriology 125*, 946–54.

Granett, A.L., Blue, R.I., Harjung, M.K., Calavan, E.C. and Gumpf, D.J. (1976). Occurrence of *Spiroplasma citri* in periwinkle in California. *California Agriculture 30*, 18–19.

Hawthorne, J.D. and Van Demark, P.J. (1979). Metabolic studies of *Spiroplasma citri. Abstracts of the Annual Meeting of the American Society for*

Microbiology 1979, G4.

Hayflick, L. and Chanock, R.M. (1965). *Mycoplasma* species of man. *Bacteriological Reviews 29*, 185–221.

Igwegbe, E.C.K. (1978a). High concentrations of horse serum inhibit growth of corn stunt spiroplasma. *Applied and Environmental Microbiology 35*, 146–8.

— (1978b). Contrasting effects of horse serum and fresh yeast extract on growth of *Spiroplasma citri* and corn stunt spiroplasma. *Phytopathology 68*, 1530–4.

Jones, A.L., Whitcomb, R.F., Williamson, D.L. and Coan, M.E. (1977). Comparative growth and primary isolation of spiroplasmas in media based on insect tissue culture formulation. *Phytopathology 67*, 738–46.

Kaloostian, G.H., Oldfield, G.N., Calavan, E.C. and Blue, R.L. (1976). Leafhoppers transmit citrus stubborn disease to weed host. *Citrograph 61*, 389–90.

Kaloostian, G.H., Oldfield, G.N., Pierce, H.D., Calavan, E.C., Granett, A.L., Rana, G.L. and Gumpf, D.J. (1975). Leafhopper–natural vector of citrus stubborn disease? *California Agriculture 29*, 14–15.

Lapage, S.P., Shelton, J.E., Mitchell, T.G. and MacKenzie, A.R. (1970). Culture collections and the preservation of bacteria. In *Methods in Microbiology*, Vol. 3A, pp. 135–228, J.R. Norris and D.W. Ribbons (eds). New York: Academic Press.

Lee, I.M. (1977). The *in vitro* life cycle, morphology, and ultrastructure of the citrus stubborn organism, *Spiroplasma citri*. PhD Thesis, University of California, Riverside, Ca., USA.

Lee, I.M., Cartia, C., Calavan, E.C. and Kaloostian, G.H. (1973). Citrus stubborn disease organism cultured from beet leafhopper. *California Agriculture 27*, 14–15.

Lee, I.M. and Davis, R.E. (1978). Identification of some growth-promoting components in an enriched cell-free medium for cultivation of *Spiroplasma citri*. *Phytopathology News 12(9)*, 215.

Lei, J.D., Su, H.J. and Chen, T.A. (1979). Spiroplasmas isolated from green leaf bug, *Trigonotylus ruficornis* Geoffroy. In *Proceedings of ROC-United States Cooperative Science Seminar of Mycoplasma Diseases of Plants*, pp. 89–98, H.J. Su and R.E. McCoy (eds). National Science Council, Taiwan.

Liao, C.H. and Chen, T.A. (1975a). Inhibitory effect of corn stem extract on the growth of corn stunt spiroplasma. *Proceedings of American Phytopathological Society 2*, 53

— (1975b). A simple medium for isolation and cultivation of corn stunt spiroplasma. *Proceedings of American Phytopathological Society 2*, 100.

— (1977). Culture of corn stunt spiroplasma in a simple medium. *Phytopathology 67*, 802–7.

— (1978). Effects of osmotic potentials, pH, and temperature on the growth of a helical, motile mycoplasma causing corn stunt disease. *Canadian Journal of Microbiology 24*, 325–9.

— (1979). Cultivation of suckling mouse cataract spiroplasma in a simple medium. *Abstracts of the Annual Meeting of the American Society for Microbiology (1979)*, 82 (G2).

— (1980). Presence of spiroplasma-inhibitory substances in plant tissue extracts. *Canadian Journal of Microbiology 26*, 807–11.

Liao, C.H., Chang, C.J. and Chen, T.A. (1979a). Spiroplasmostatic action of plant tissue extracts. In *Proceedings of ROC-United States Cooperative Science Seminar on Mycoplasma Diseases of Plants*, pp. 99–103, H.J. Su and R.E. McCoy (eds). National Science Council, Taiwan.

Liao, C.H., Cotty, P.J. and Chen, T.A. (1979b). Osmostability of plant and insect spiroplasmas. In *Proceedings of ROC-United States Cooperative Science*

Seminar on Mycoplasma Diseases of Plants, pp. 83–7, H.J. Su and R.E. McCoy (eds). National Science Council, Taiwan.

Markham, P.G. and Townsend, R. (1974). Transmissions of *Spiroplasma citri* to plants. *Les Mycoplasmes/Mycoplasmas. Les Colloques de l'Institut Nationale de la Santé et de la Recherche Médicale 33*, 201–6.

Markham, P.G., Townsend, R., Bar-Joseph, M., Daniels, M.J., Plaskitt, A. and Meddins, B.M. (1974). Spiroplasmas are the causal agents of citrus little-leaf disease. *Annals of Applied Biology 78*, 49–57.

Markham, P.G., Townsend, R., Plaskitt, K. and Saglio, P. (1977). Transmission of corn stunt to dicotyledonous plants. *Plant Disease Reporter 61*, 342.

McCoy, R.E. (1978). Use of arginine to prolong longevity of spiroplasmas in culture media. *Zentralblatt für Bakteriologie, Parasitenkunde, Infektions-Krankheiten und Hygiene, Erste Abteilung Originale 241*, 231.

McCoy, R.E. and Davis, M.J. (1980). Multiplication of spiroplasmas in larvae of the wax moth, *Gelleria mellonella* (L.). *Proceedings of the Fourth Meeting of the International Council on Lethal Yellowing, p. 12*. University of Florida Publication FL-80-1.

McCoy, R.E., Tsai, J.H. and Thomas, D.L. (1978). Occurrence of a spiroplasma in natural populations of the sharpshooter *Oncometopia nigricans*. *Phytopathology News 12(9)*, 217.

McCoy, R.E., Williams, D.S. and Thomas, D.L. (1979). Isolation of mycoplasmas from flowers. In *Proceedings of ROC-United States Cooperative Science Seminar on Mycoplasma Diseases of Plants*, pp. 75–81, H.J. Su and R.E. McCoy (eds). National Science Council, Taiwan.

Mudd, J.B., Ittig, M., Roy, B., Latrille, J. and Bové, J.M. (1977). Composition and enzyme activities of *Spiroplasma citri* membranes. *Journal of Bacteriology 129*, 1250–6.

Norman, M.C., French, E.B. and Choate, R.V. (1970). Preservation of *Mycoplasma* strains by freezing in liquid nitrogen and by lyophilization with sucrose. *Applied Microbiology 20*, 69–71.

Oldfield, G.N. and Kaloostian, G.H. (1979). Vectors and host range of the citrus stubborn disease pathogen, *Spiroplasma citri*. In *Proceedings of ROC-United States Cooperative Science Seminar on Mycoplasma Disease of Plants*, pp. 119–25, H.J. Su and R.E. McCoy (eds). National Science Council, Taiwan.

Oldfield, G.N., Kaloostian, G.H., Pierce, H.D., Calavan, E.C., Granett, A.L., Blue, R.L., Rana, G.L. and Gumpf, D.J. (1977a). Transmission of *Spiroplasma citri* from citrus to citrus by *Scaphytopius nitridus*. *Phytopathology 67*, 763–5.

Oldfield, G.N., Kaloostian, G.H., Pierce, H.D., Sullivan, D.A., Calavan, E.C. and Blue, R.L. (1977b). New hosts of citrus stubborn disease. *Citrograph 62*, 309–12.

Patel, K.R., Mayberry-Carson, K.J. and Smith, P.F. (1978). Effect of external environmental factors on the morphology of *Spiroplasma citri*. *Journal of Bacteriology 133*, 925–31.

Pickens, E.G., Gerloff, R.K. and Burgdorfer, W. (1968). Spirochete from the rabbit tick *Haemaphysalis leporispalustris* (Packard). *Journal of Bacteriology 95*, 291–9.

Rana, G.L., Kaloostian, G.H., Oldfield, G.N., Granett, A.L., Calavan, E.C., Pierce, H.D., Lee, I.M. and Gumpf, D.J. (1975). Acquisition of *Spiroplasma citri* through membranes by homopterous insects. *Phytopathology 65*, 1143–5.

Razin, S., Hasin, M., Ne'Eman, Z. and Rottem, S. (1973). Isolation, chemical composition, and ultrastructural features of the cell membrane of the mycoplasma-like organism, *Spiroplasma citri*. *Journal of Bacteriology 116*, 1421–5.

Rodwell, A.W. and Abbot, A. (1961). The function of glycerol, cholesterol, and long-chain fatty acids in the nutrition of *Mycoplasma mycoides*. *Journal of General Microbiology 25*, 201-4.

Rose, D.L., Tully, J.G. and Whitcomb, R.F. (1979). Experimental pathogenicity of spiroplasmas for vertebrates. *Abstracts of the Annual Meeting of the American Society for Microbiology (1979)*, G10.

Saglio, P. (1979). Motility and improvement in selective isolation of spiroplasmas. *Plant Disease Reporter 63*, 293-6.

Saglio, P., Daniels, M.J. and Pradet, A. (1979). ATP and energy charge as criteria of growth and metabolic activity of Mollicutes: application to *Spiroplasma citri*. *Journal of General Microbiology 110*, 13-20.

Saglio, P., L'Hospital, M., Laflèche, D., Dupont, G., Bové, J.M., Tully, J.G. and Freundt, E.A. (1973). *Spiroplasma citri* gen. and sp. n.: mycoplasmalike organism associated with 'stubborn' disease of citrus. *International Journal of Systematic Bacteriology 23*, 191-204.

Saglio, P., Laflèche, D., Bonissol, C. and Bové, J.M. (1971). Isolement et culture *in vitro* des mycoplasmes associés au 'stubborn' des agrumes et leur observation au microscope electronique. *Comptes Rendus des Séances Hebdomadaires de l'Academie des Sciences, Paris, Série D 272*, 1387-90.

Saglio, P., Lafleche, D., L'Hospital, M., Dupont, G. and Bové, J.M. (1972). Isolation and growth of citrus mycoplasmas. In *Pathogenic Mycoplasmas*, pp. 187-203, K. Elliott and J. Birth (eds). CIBA Foundation Symposium.

Slutzky, G.M., Razin, S., Kahane, I. and Eisenberg, S. (1977). Inhibition of mycoplasma growth by human very-low-density lipoproteins. *FEMS Microbiology Letters 2*, 185-7.

Smith, P.F. and Boughton, J.E. (1960). The role of protein and phospholipid in the growth of pleuropneumonia-like organisms. *Journal of Bacteriology 80*, 851-60.

Spaar, D., Kleinhempel, H., Müller, H.M., Stanarius, A. and Schimmel, D. (1974). Culturing mycoplasmas from plants. *Les Mycoplasmes/Mycoplasmas. Les Colloques de l'Institut National de La Santé et de la Recherche Médicale 33*, 207-13.

Stalheim, O.H.V., Ritchie, A.E. and Whitcomb, R.F. (1978). Cultivation, serology, ultrastructure, and virus-like particles of spiroplasma 277F. *Current Microbiology 1*, 365-70.

Stiller, D., Whitcomb, R.F. and Coan, M.E. (1978). Direct isolation of the suckling mouse cataract spiroplasma from ticks in cell-free medium. *Abstracts of the Annual Meeting of the American Society for Microbiology (1979)*, G7.

Subcommittee on the Taxonomy of Mollicutes (1979). Proposal for minimal standards for description of new species of the class *Mollicutes*. *International Journal of Systematic Bacteriology 29*, 172-80.

Townsend, R. (1976). Arginine metabolism by *Spiroplasma citri*. *Journal of General Microbiology 94*, 417-20.

Townsend, R., Markham, P.G. and Plaskitt, K.A. (1977a). Multiplication and morphology of *Spiroplasma citri* in the leafhopper *Euscelis plebejus*. *Annals of Applied Biology 87*, 307-13.

Townsend, R., Markham, P.G., Plaskitt, K.A. and Daniels, M.J. (1977b). Isolation and characterization of a non-helical strain of *Spiroplasma citri*. *Journal of General Microbiology 100*, 15-21.

Tully, J.G., Whitcomb, R.F., Clark, H.F. and Williamson, D.L. (1977). Pathogenic mycoplasmas: cultivation and vertebrate pathogenicity of a new spiroplasma. *Science 195*, 892-4.

Tully, J.G., Whitcomb, R.F., Williamson, D.L. and Clark, H.F. (1976). Suckling mouse cataract agent is a helical wall-free prokaryote. *Nature (London)*

259, 117–20.

Vogelzang, A.A. (1975). The survival of *Mycoplasmas pulmonis* in drinking water and in other materials. *Zeitschrift für Versuchstierkunde 17*, 240–6.

Whitcomb, R.F. (1980). The genus *Spiroplasma. Annual Review of Microbiology 34*, 677–709.

Whitcomb, R.F., Tylly, J.G., Bové, J.M. and Saglio, P. (1973). Spiroplasmas and acholeplasmas: Multiplication in insects. *Science 182*, 1251–3.

Whitcomb, R.F. and Williamson, D.L. (1975). Helical wall-free prokaryotes in insects: Multiplication and pathogenicity. *Annals of the New York Academy of Sciences 266*, 260–75.

Whitcomb, R.F., Williamson, D.L., Rosen, J. and Coan, M. (1974). Relationship of infection and pathogenicity in the infection of insects by wall-free prokaryotes. *Les Mycoplasmes/Mycoplasmas. Less Colloques de l'Institut Nationale de la Santé et de la Recherche Médicale 33*, 275–82.

Williamson, D.L. and Whitcomb, R.F. (1974). Helical, wall-free prokaryotes in *Drosophila*, leafhoppers, and plants. *Les Mycoplasmes/Mycoplasmas. Les Colloques de l'Institut National de la Santé et de la Recherche Médicale 33*, 283–90.

— (1975). Plant mycoplasmas: a cultivable spiroplasma causes corn stunt disease. *Science 188*, 1018–20.

7 CULTURE OF OTHER MICROORGANISMS FROM YELLOWS-DISEASED PLANTS

S.J. Eden-Green

1. Introduction

The recognition that plant diseases of the yellows group were associated with structures resembling classical mycoplasmas (Doi *et al.*, 1967; Ishie *et al.*, 1967) raised early hopes that the disease agents would be cultured and their etiological role confirmed. In the rush of reports that followed, several laboratories described the successful isolation of mycoplasmas from diseased plants, and demonstration of pathogenicity (Hampton *et al.*, 1969; Lin *et al.*, 1970; Ghosh *et al.*, 1971; Giannotti and Vago, 1971); in fact, an examination of scientific literature from the early 1970s might suggest that the isolation of mycoplasmas from plants presented few difficulties (Giannotti *et al.*, 1972). In other instances, however, isolation attempts were unsuccessful (Hayflick and Arai, 1973; Caudwell *et al.*, 1974; Cousin *et al.*, 1974) or could not be repeated (Hampton *et al.*, 1976), and an early note of caution was sounded by Maramorosch (1972).

Amidst these claims, the only mycoplasmas that have been repeatedly isolated from plants or insects, made accessible through type culture collections and shown independently to be plant-pathogenic, belong to an entirely new and distinctive family, the spiroplasmas, which are dealt with elsewhere in this volume. Other isolates that have been characterised include representatives of the genus *Acholeplasma*, which may be epiphytic or saprophytic on plants (see below), and *Mycoplasma* strains related to species of bovine (Saglio and Whitcomb, 1979) or avian (Hampton *et al.*, 1976) origin. A diversity of mycoplasmas and spiroplasmas has recently been isolated from floral surfaces (R.E. Davis *et al.*, 1977; McCoy and Basham, 1980); these include spiroplasmas pathogenic to insects but there has been no suggestion that any isolate is pathogenic to plants (R.E. Davis, 1979).

Associations between yellows diseases and previously unsuspected agents have not been limited to mycoplasmas. Small bacteria, distinguishable by the presence of cell walls that are often reminiscent of rickettsias, and apparently sensitive to penicillin, have been found in xylem or phloem tissues in over thirty plant diseases (Hopkins, 1977; Nienhaus and Sikora, 1979). A yet more dramatic consequence of the new awareness of the diversity of intravascular agents associated with plant diseases came with rediscovery of phloem-inhabiting flagellate protozoa of the genus *Phytomonas* (Parthasarathy *et al.*, 1976; Waters 1978).

The majority of the agents covered by this chapter have not been cultured. The diverse organisms, mycoplasmas, bacteria and protozoa, are linked by their restriction to the specialised vascular environments of plant phloem or xylem and, where known, by similar transmission characteristics involving multiplication in hemipteran vectors. One may suppose that the eventual requirements for successful isolation and culture of these agents will be similar and that techniques used for handling specific organisms will find a wider application.

2. Cultivable and Noncultivable Agents

A. *Spiroplasmas and Mycoplasma-like Organisms (MLOs)*

The ultrastructural features and *in vivo* antibiotic sensitivity spectra of plant mycoplasmas are insufficient characteristics to classify them in the class Mollicutes, for which the trivial term 'mycoplasma' is reserved in this account. Culture in cell-free media, or at least the demonstration of a very close serological relationship to a cultured species, is central to the definitive characterisation of mycoplasmas and the term 'mycoplasma-like organism' (MLO) has thus been widely used to describe non-cultivable agents associated with yellows diseases. In contrast, the distinctive helical morphology of spiroplasmas provides a reliable means to identification, even when an organism cannot be cultured (R.E. Davis, 1979). This characteristic is not always maintained *in vivo*, however (Markham and Townsend, 1979), and it is thus possible that an MLO may prove on culturing to be a spiroplasma.

This view has been expanded by Maramorosch (1978) into a working hypothesis that other plant MLOs are spiroplasmas, and several recent reports have described the isolation of spiroplasmas from yellows diseases which were earlier the subject of intensive unsuccessful culturing efforts (Kondo *et al.*, 1977; Raju and Nyland, 1978; Charbonneau *et al.*, 1979; Giannotti *et al.*, 1979). Although differences in host range and transmission characteristics are claimed, some of these isolates are closely related to *Spiroplasma citri* (McIntosh *et al.*, 1977; Raju *et al.*, 1980) and these preliminary results should be interpreted with caution: *S. citri* is known to infect a broad range of plant and insect hosts in nature (Kaloostian *et al.*, 1979; Bové *et al.*, 1979), and instances of dual infections involving both spiroplasmas and noncultivable MLO are known or suspected (Section 3.F, below). McCoy (1980) has drawn a further distinction between spiroplasmas and nonhelical MLO, or virescence agents, on the grounds of differences in host plant symptomatology. The term MLO is thus retained here to describe wall-free prokaryotes associated with yellows diseases, for which general acceptance of morphological, serological or biochemical similarities to the genus *Spiroplasma* has not yet been achieved.

B. *Acholeplasmas*

Representatives of the sterol-nonrequiring family *Acholeplasmataceae* were originally isolated from sewage (Laidlaw and Elford, 1936), soil, compost and manure (Seiffert, 1937a, b) and were thought to be saprophytes (Sabin, 1941). More recent isolates of the type species,

Acholeplasma laidlawii (originally isolated from sewage) and other *Acholeplasma* species have been found as parasites, and possibly pathogens, in a variety of mammalian and avian tissues, and as contaminants in animal tissue cultures, commercial sera and serum-free culture media. The ecology of these organisms has thus been open to question (Tully, 1979).

Sporadic isolations of *A. laidlawii* were reported in the course of earlier attempts to culture mycoplasmas from plants (Daniels and Meddins, 1972; Kleinhempel *et al.*, 1972) and contamination by this easily cultured organism may account for some of the initial claims of success. Recently, over thirty isolates of *A. axanthum, A. oculi* and possibly another *Acholeplasma* species have been repeatedly recovered from coconut palms affected by lethal yellowing disease in Jamaica (Eden-Green and Tully, 1979; Townsend *et al.*, 1980). Tissues sampled in the course of this work included secondary rots, plant debris, surface and symptomless tissues, but these organisms were largely associated with decaying tissues or surfaces that may have been contaminated from that source. Recent isolations from palms affected by bud-rot disease (Eden-Green, unpublished results), caused by the fungus *Phytophthora palmivora*, support the conclusion that these organisms are epiphytic or saprophytic on plants.

So far, acholeplasmas have not been shown to be phytopathogenic, although they may persist for several days following mechanical inoculation and are reportedly translocated in plants (McIntosh and Maramorosch, 1973; Sethi and Nienhaus, 1974). The acquisition and transmission of acholeplasmas by leafhoppers following natural feeding has not been demonstrated (Eden-Green *et al.*, 1980) but these and other authors (Whitcomb *et al.*, 1973) have shown that these organisms are well-adapted to multiplication in leafhoppers, and could thus be disseminated by insects.

C. Other Agents

'Rickettsia-like' Organisms (RLO). A malformation of dodder (*Cuscuta subinclusa*) provided the first example of a phloem-inhabiting rickettsia-like bacterium (Giannotti *et al.*, 1970), but a more dramatic discovery was the demonstration of an association between similar organisms and clover club leaf disease, one of the classical diseases of the yellows group (Windsor and Black, 1972, 1973). Subsequently, RLO were detected in the xylem vessels of plants affected by phony peach (Hopkins *et al.*, 1973) and Pierce's diseases (Goheen *et al.*, 1973) and these agents have since been associated with an increasing number of plant maladies.

Diseases associated with either phloem or xylem agents show some consistent differences in respect of symptomatology and range of vectors. In the former, symptoms are closer to the yellows type (for example, growth malformations, phyllody and virescence) whilst the latter tend to be typified by progressive chlorosis and wilting. It is not at present known whether these differences reflect fundamental dissimilarities in the suspected causal agents, or are merely consequences of the adaptation of similar organisms to different vascular tissues of plants. Both groups of agents are small bacterial rods bounded by two trilaminar membranes, or an inner membrane and outer cell wall, with a combined width of 20–40 nm. The outer layer is often convoluted or rippled and this feature, together with the small size and apparent non-cultivability of these organisms and their association with insects, has led to their comparison with certain rickettsias. Phloem-inhabiting agents are reported in the range of 0.2–0.4 μm wide by 1–3 μm long (Windsor and Black, 1973; Markham *et al.*, 1975), which is slightly smaller than RLO in xylem (0.25–0.5 μm by 1–4 μm; Nyland *et al.*, 1973; Mollenhauer and Hopkins, 1974). The phloem-restricted agent associated with citrus greening disease was thought exceptionally to be bounded by a single but unusually wide (20 nm) trilaminar membrane (Saglio *et al.*, 1971; Moll and Martin, 1973), but later investigations (Moll and Martin, 1974; Garnier and Bové, 1978) have demonstrated a typical bacterial wall structure. Ultrastructural features of xylem-limited bacteria associated with sugarcane ratoon-stunting disease differ from those of RLO and suggest closer affinities to corynebacteria (Teakle *et al.*, 1973) or filamentous actinomycetes (Kao and Damann, 1978).

Phytomonas. Trypanosomatid protozoa classified as the genus *Phytomonas* (Donovan, 1909) have long been known to inhabit the laticiferous tissues of many species of plants, especially within the Euphorbiaceae and Asclepiadaceae (Nieschulz, 1931), but phyto-pathogenic effects have rarely been attributed to these organisms. Stahel (1931) described a flagellate (*Phytomonas leptovasorum*) in the sieve elements of coffee affected by a disease in Suriname, South America, which he termed phloem necrosis, but this work received little attention for over 30 years and the etiology of the disease remains unproven (Vermeulen, 1968). In 1975, similar protozoa were found in phloem elements of coconut palms affected by a sudden wilt disease ('Hartrot') in the same region (Parthasarathy *et al.*, 1976) and reports followed of similar conditions affecting coconut, African oil palm and maripa palm (*Maximiliana maripa*) in several South American countries (Dollet and Lopez, 1978; Waters, 1978).

Symptomatologically, diseases associated with protozoa are not typical of the yellows group, although coconut Hartrot was at first confused with lethal yellowing. Phloem-inhabiting phytomonads have not been maintained in culture, but indications that their growth requirements *in vitro* can be at least partly met by mycoplasma media (Section 5.B, below) further justifies their inclusion in this account.

3. General Approaches to the Isolation of Mycoplasmas from Plants

A. The Value of 'Blind' Isolation Attempts

The early stages of growth of a mycoplasma inoculum are difficult to monitor; thus primary isolations and the first subcultures of an unknown organism are usually carried through 'blind', until sufficient growth occurs to cause detectable metabolic changes, or visible colonies. Reasons for the failure of the isolation procedure will not usually be apparent and this approach to the isolation of MLO from plants and insects has not been rewarding in the past. An outstanding exception was the isolation of *Spiroplasma citri*, but culture of the corn stunt spiroplasma was greatly facilitated by direct observations on its characteristic spiral morphology (Chen and Liao, 1975; Williamson and Whitcomb, 1975). What, then, is the present role of conventional mycoplasma isolation techniques in the study of yellows disease agents?

In the case of a newly identified disease, the answer may be clear: isolations may succeed either because the MLO are more amenable to culture or are more readily extracted from that particular host. Clearly, there is also scope for testing new culture media and innovatory techniques on well-researched diseases and, although blind isolation attempts seem unlikely to isolate yellows disease agents at present, conventional techniques for handling mycoplasmas are relevant to the development and application of techniques for handling mycoplasma-like agents that cannot yet be cultured.

The techniques that follow are drawn from experience with classical mycoplasmas, largely of vertebrate origin and, to a lesser extent, with spiroplasmas. More comprehensive reviews on isolation and culture of these agents will be found in Hayflick (1965), Fallon and Whittlestone (1969), Frey *et al.* (1973) and Liao and Chen (this volume, Chapter 6).

B. Choice of Inoculum

Host tissues used as a starting point for the isolation of mycoplasmas must obviously be shown to contain MLO and an initial electron microscope survey of different parts of the host, at various stages of infection, may provide valuable information on their quantity and quality. The type of host material may itself influence the release and viability of MLO in a culture medium: plant organs that are richer in phloem, such as petioles, flower stalks or the stele of roots, and developing tissues that are active 'sinks' for photosynthates, may be preferable to predominantly photosynthetic or mature storage tissues. It is a fairly common experience that MLO are more readily extracted from infective insects than from plant tissues (Section 4.B, below); the proportion of tissues invaded by MLO is usually lower in plant than in insect inocula, and mechanical release of the contents of phloem sieve elements requires more drastic extraction techniques. Inhibitory compounds, such as phenolics or highly reactive quinones produced on oxidation, are widely distributed in plant tissues and may be toxic to mycoplasmas (Teranaka *et al.*, 1976; Liao *et al.*, 1978).

Extracellular animal or tissue culture mycoplasmas are commonly isolated by incubating blocks of excised tissues or intact cells in culture medium (Barile, 1974), and MLO in insects, which circulate in the hemolymph in at least some stages of infection, may be amenable to isolation by similarly nondisruptive techniques. The infection of other insect organs by MLO may be intracellular, however, and whole insects or the head capsule containing the salivary glands should be extracted. Surface-sterilisation of leafhoppers prior to maceration may not be a practical proposition and is usually unnecessary. Townsend *et al.* (1977) advocated immersion for one minute in 70% ethanol followed by two rinses in sterile distilled water, but a more rigorous technique suggested for the isolation of entomogenous bacteria is as follows (Poinar and Thomas, 1978). Dip in 70% or 95% ethanol (wetting agent) for 2 seconds, transfer to sodium hypochlorite (household bleach, 5.25%) for 3–5 minutes, follow by an equal period in 10% sodium thiosulphate (to remove free chlorine), and three rinses in sterile distilled water.

Microhomogenisers for macerating individual leafhoppers in 0.1– 0.2 ml of suspending medium (usually basal or complete culture medium) have been described (Townsend *et al.*, 1977) but a simple and effective alternative consists of a micropestle and mortar, comprising a 20–30 mm diameter solid watch glass with a 6–8 mm diameter glass rod, rounded at the 'business' end. This can be conveniently rinsed and sterilised by flushing with 70% ethanol and flamed off for re-use almost immediately. Plant tissues can be surface-sterilised and homogenised by more vigorous application of the same techniques but a series of transverse cuts, 0.5 mm or less, across vascular tissues placed in culture medium should effectively release the contents of phloem elements, which are under positive hydrostatic pressure. Plant sap expressed from intact tissues by squeezing with pliers was an effective source of inoculum for corn stunt spiroplasma from maize (Eden-Green and Waters, 1981) and also gave good preparations of *Phytomonas* from cocunut phloem (Waters, 1978) and RLO from periwinkle xylem (McCoy *et al.,* 1978). A single cycle of slow freezing and thawing ruptures plant cells and greatly increases the yield of sap, but with unknown effects on the viability of MLO.

Selective isolation of MLO from plant or insect tissues takes advantage of the ability of mycoplasmas to pass through 'sterility grade' filters (0.45 μm apd or less). Pressure filtration, using disposable syringes and 'Swinnex'-type filter holders with appropriate grade filters (for example, Millipore MF series, with pre-filters if necessary) is a convenient technique for isolating from several specimens. Excessive pressure should be avoided and vacuum filtration may increase the titre of organisms extracted (Saglio, 1979). This can be arranged by attaching a sterile syringe to the outlet of the filter holder, using a male-to-male luer adaptor made from a 10 mm length of suitable PVC tubing and fitted to the filter holder before autoclaving. Filtration of mycoplasmas may cause a large drop in titre in the filtrate, and a larger pore size, used in conjunction with selective antibacterial agents in the initial isolation medium, may be preferable to 0.22 μm or 0.45 μm sterility grade filters. Crude extracts can be clarified by a coarse filtration, through, for instance, glass fibre filters, and MLO can be concentrated and washed by cycles of differential centrifugation; data on the filtration and sedimentation properties of *A. laidlawii* (Figures 7.1 and 7.2) may serve as a guide. Operations should be carried out at low temperature, and exclusion of air, by, for instance, filtering under nitrogen and centrifuging beneath a layer of liquid paraffin, will reduce oxidation of the extract.

C. Isolation Media and Conditions of Culture

Whilst it is doubtful whether media given in earlier reports of successful isolation of plant mycoplasmas have any special value, it is significant that most were based on slight variations of conventional mycoplasma media developed by Edwards (Hayflick, 1965). A typical formula (Fallon and Whittlestone, 1969) is:

Figures 7.1 and 7.2: Effects of Centrifugation (7.1) and Membrane Filtration (7.2) on a Suspension of *Acholeplasma laidlawii* in Coconut Phloem Sap. Colony counts ($\log_{10}$ cfu/ml) of organisms remaining in suspension were determined after 20 min centrifugation at increasing relative centrifugal force (rcf), or after serial low positive pressure filtration through Millipore MF filters of decreasing average pore diameter (apd). Points X and Y (Figure 7.2) are respective counts on the original suspension before and after filtration through a Whatman GF/A glass fibre filter.

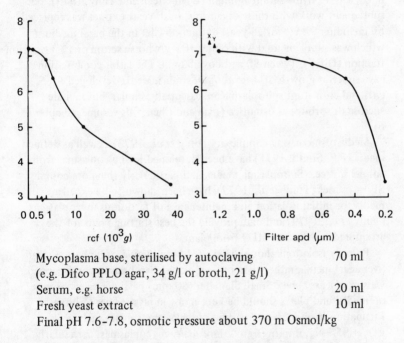

Mycoplasma base, sterilised by autoclaving	70 ml
(e.g. Difco PPLO agar, 34 g/l or broth, 21 g/l)	
Serum, e.g. horse	20 ml
Fresh yeast extract	10 ml
Final pH 7.6–7.8, osmotic pressure about 370 m Osmol/kg	

Sterile serum and fresh yeast extract can be obtained from commercial sources or alternatively the latter can be prepared as described by these authors. Sera, in particular, are a well-known source of contaminating mycoplasmas and should be heat-inactivated for 0.5–1 hr at 55°C before use. Media are commonly supplemented with 20 µg/ml calf thymus DNA, energy sources, such as 0.5% w/v glucose and/or 0.1% w/v L-arginine HCl, and phenol red may be included at 20 µg/ml as a pH indicator. Bacterial inhibitors, such as penicillin G (1000 IUs/ml) and thallous acetate (up to 500 µg/ml) are often employed, but the latter is inhibitory to some mycoplasmas (notably the ureaplasmas) and *S. citri* is sensitive to only slightly higher concentrations. Antifungal agents, such as cycloheximide ('Actidione') may be included at 100-200 μg/ml, and solidified media containing a 'cocktail' of these antibiotics are usually sufficiently selective for direct isolation and enumeration of acholeplasmas and spiroplasmas from experimentally infected insects.

The medium given above was used to isolate acholeplasmas from coconut palm tissues, with the serum content reduced to 10% and addition of 0.01% v/v Tween 80 (polyoxethylene sorbitan monooleate) in 0.1% w/v bovine serum albumin (Eden-Green and Tully, 1979). For subsequent work with these organisms, fresh yeast extract was replaced by including 5% w/v dried yeast extract powder in the basal medium, which was supplemented with either 10% v/v horse serum or 1% v/v serum fraction (Difco), Tween 80 and bovalbumin. The latter combination gave superior growth of *A. axanthum* strains. Media developed for *S. citri* and corn stunt spiroplasma are essentially similar, but include sucrose or sorbitol as osmotica (Liao and Chen; this volume, Chapter 6).

Media of increasing complexity (Frey *et al.*, 1973) as well as defined media (P.F. Smith, 1971) have been developed for mycoplasmas from animal sources. Spiroplasma media, and particularly the more complex SP 1-4 series (Tully *et al.*, 1977), have been shown to be excellent media for initial isolation and maintenance of fastidious mycoplasmas (Tully *et al.*, 1979) and may provide the best starting point for the attempted isolation of MLO from plants.

Primary isolations should be carried out in liquid or biphasic (liquid over agar) media, rather than on agar alone, dispensed in screw-capped vials or culture tubes. Small diameter (50 mm) petri dishes economise on media, and plates should be kept moist in plastic bags or boxes. Incubation in an increased carbon dioxide atmosphere, such as 5% CO_2 + 95% N_2, improves growth of many mycoplasmas, particularly on primary isolation (Barile, 1974), but additional buffering, with 0.01-0.05M sodium bicarbonate or N-2-hydroxyethylpiperazine-N'-2-ethanesulphonic acid (HEPES), may be required. A suitable range of incubation temperatures may be inferred from growth temperature optima of *S. citri* and corn stunt spiroplasma (30-32°C), although lower temperatures might be selected for temperate disease agents. Most acholeplasma isolates obtained from coconut palms grew equally well at 25° and 29°C on agar media, but many showed marked inhibition at 37°C (Figure 7.3). Cultures should be observed for at least three weeks, but several serial blind passages to fresh media should be

Figure 7.3: Effects of Incubation Temperature on Variation in the Colony Morphology of *Acholeplasma* spp. isolated from Coconut Palms (Eden-Green and Tully, 1979). Typical 'fried-egg' colonies of *A. oculi* isolate G363 grown on 10% serum medium at 29°C [A] compared with minute colonies (cl) and extensive pseudocolonies (ps) on identical plates incubated at 37°C [B]; absence of central downgrowth into agar on 1% serum fraction plates of *A. axanthum* isolate G381 grown at both 29°C [C] and 37°C [D]; and *A. axanthum* isolate B117 grown at 25°C [E] showing extensive downgrowth into agar at 29°C [F] on 1% serum fraction medium. All plates were incubated under the same conditions and photographed 14 days after inoculation. Unstained, oblique transmitted light, same magnification throughout.

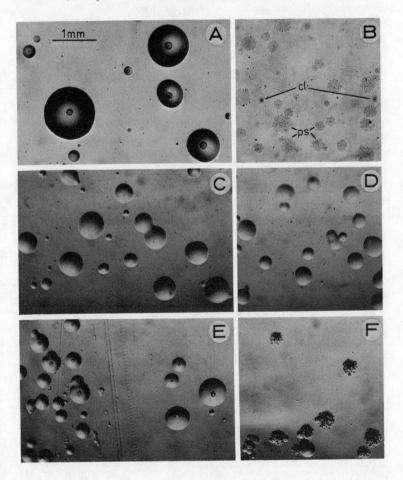

Figure 7.4: Colonies of Acholeplasma Isolate E847 Showing Gross Morphology [A] and Detail of Peripheral Zone [B] after Dienes' Staining. Bright field, transmitted light.

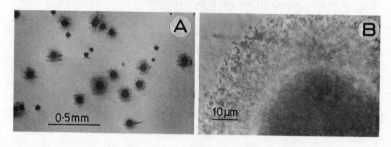

carried out at intervals of a few days, particularly where inhibitors are suspected in the original inoculum (Chen and Liao, 1975). At least ten blind passages, at 2 or 3 day intervals, were recently suggested for isolation of spiroplasmas from aster yellows, pear decline and western X diseases (Raju and Nyland, 1978; Raju *et al.*, 1980).

Growth in liquid media is frequently detected by indicators of metabolic activities such as acid production by fermentative organisms, elevation of pH as a result of the hydrolysis of arginine or urea, or reduction of tetrazolium salts. Some mycoplasmas possess none of these metabolic capabilities, however, and relatively large amounts of growth may be required to produce detectable metabolic changes or classical 'fried-egg' colonies on agar media. More sensitive techniques, such as incorporation of radioactive precursors (for instance inorganic phosphate, amino acids or DNA bases; Schneider, 1975; Schneider and Stanbridge, 1975) or detection of ATP and energy charge by a luciferase/luciferin assay (Saglio *et al.*, 1979) might be utilised to detect the growth of plant MLO.

Light microscopy may indicate early stages of growth in liquid media and is useful to distinguish mycoplasma colonies from artefacts or pseudocolonies on agar (Figures 7.3 and 7.4). Careful comparison with control media, both uninoculated and inoculated with healthy or heat-inactivated specimens, is particularly important, as serum-containing media tend to develop finely suspended precipitates which can be confused with mycoplasmas in unstained preparations viewed by phase contrast or dark-field microscopy. Air-dried films can be stained by Giemsa (Fallon and Whittlestone, 1969) but a rapid technique for staining fresh preparations is to mix a drop of culture with Dienes'

stain, diluted to about 2% in saline or culture medium. Mycoplasmas
stain quite rapidly against a sufficiently light background for viewing
with a 100x oil immersion objective. Mycoplasma colonies stain a deep
greenish-blue, against a pale blue background, on plates flooded with
the same strength stain (Figure 7.4). One formula for Dienes' stain
(Hayflick, 1965) is: 2.5 g methylene blue, 1.25 g azur II, 10 g maltose
and 0.25 g sodium carbonate per 100 ml water.

In the absence of effective positive or negative staining procedures
for mycoplasmas (Wolanski, 1973), it is rarely practicable to monitor
the growth of cultures routinely by electron microscopy. Where
sufficient cell yield is obtained, cultures can be centrifuged and ultrastructural features examined by embedding pellets in agar for
sectioning by conventional techniques (Waters; this volume, Chapter
4). An alternative technique, applicable to small volumes of culture
where only limited growth has occurred, is to filter through a 0.1 or
0.22 μm membrane filter and examine ultrathin sections of the filter.
Cellulose ester (Millipore MF) filters can be embedded and sectioned
following dehydration in ethanol.

D. Purification and Characterisation of Cultures

Primary or early subcultures of a putative mycoplasma should be subcultured to antibiotic-free media to detect low levels of bacterial
contaminants, but additional tests may be required to exclude bacterial
L forms. Purification of contaminated cultures is simplified if the
organism grows on solid media, so that discrete colonies can be picked
or cut out and subcultured. Broth cultures contaminated by bacteria
can be purified by subculturing in media containing selective antibiotics
or by filtration via 0.3 μm or 0.45 μm filters.

Procedures for further purification and characterisation of mycoplasmas are summarised by the International Committee on Systematic
Bacteriology (ICSB, 1979) and in Chapters 8 and 9 of this volume.
Identification to species, and the description of new species in particular,
require comparison of a variety of metabolic, serological and biochemical
properties that will usually involve more than one specialist centre;
unilateral nomination of a new species is to be deprecated. Initial
characterisation should establish that a newly isolated organism belongs
to the class Mollicutes, and indicate its affinities with any specific
family. The ICSB recommendations can be summarised as follows.
Preliminary Cloning. The organism should be cloned at least three
times by filtering through the smallest pore diameter membrane filter
(0.22 μm to 0.45 μm) on to a solid medium, incubating, and subculturing

an isolated colony to fresh broth medium. Filtration is repeated at least three times in the hope that the final clone derives from a single organism. At least two clones should be selected for comparison, and it should be borne in mind that cloning does not guarantee the purity of a stain and that clones may not be representative of components of a mixed culture. Essential features, such as pathogenicity, may be lost on passaging (Williamson and Whitcomb, 1975) and adequate stocks of early passage cultures should be maintained for comparison. Other essential characteristics of the organism, notably *colony form* and *filterability* will be demonstrated during filter cloning, and organisms retained on filters can be fixed and embedded for electron microscopy. Typical 'fried-egg' colonies may not always be produced, particularly by motile organisms, or by cultures grown under suboptimal conditions or on excessively dry media, when central down-growth may occur into the medium without formation of a peripheral surface zone.

Morphology. Logarithmic phase cultures should be examined by dark-field or phase-contrast light microscopy or by staining. Electron microscopy of thin sections is essential to demonstrate that the organism lacks a cell wall and is bounded only by a unit membrane.

Absence of Reversion. At least five consecutive subcultures should be carried out in media free of antibiotics or other L-phase inducing agents, to establish that the organism does not revert to a bacterial form. The isolate should be tested at early passage to avoid selection of stable L-phase variants.

Sterol Dependence. An absolute requirement for sterols is a fundamental characteristic of the *Mycoplasmataceae, Spiroplasmataceae* and *Anaeroplasma*, and growth in sterol-free media distinguishes members of the *Acholeplasmataceae* and *Thermoplasma*. Direct determination of sterol requirements should be carried out in serum-free media containing fatty acids (for example Tween 80), albumin, and increasing concentrations of cholesterol (solubilised in ethanol) and should be carried through sufficient passages to dilute out sterols from the original inoculum. The growth of most *Acholeplasma* spp. on solidified serum-free medium is usually as good or better than *Mycoplasma* spp. grown under optimal conditions. Acholeplasmas are also relatively insensitive to digitonin on media containing at least 10% serum, but not on serum-free media, and to sodium polyanethol sulphonate. A simple test is to apply blank antibiotic assay discs impregnated with 1.5% w/v digitonin (in ethanol) and 5% w/v sodium polyanethol sulphonate to freshly inoculated plates of the test organism, on media with and without serum, incubate, and compare inhibition zones with control plates inoculated with *Acholeplasma, Mycoplasma* and *Spiroplasma* test species.

Classification to Genus and Species. Current ICSB proposals suggest the following minimal generic criteria for members of the class Mollicutes. Sterol nonrequiring, facultative anaerobes: *Acholeplasma* or *Thermoplasma* (the latter distinguished by growth optima at very high temperatures, 55–60°C, and low pH, 1–3). Sterol-dependent, obligate anaerobes: *Anaeroplasma*. Sterol-dependent, hydrolyse urea: *Ureaplasma*. Sterol-dependent, form helical motile filaments: *Spiroplasma*. All other sterol-dependent organisms: *Mycoplasma*. The species concept in the Mollicutes, as in other prokaryotic taxa, is arbitrary and serves as a convenience for the designation of isolates. It is usually necessary to establish patterns of relatedness by alternative techniques, such as serology and physicochemical properties (this volume, Chapters 8 and 9). The immunological properties of plant mycoplasmas cannot be expected to have the same ecological significance as in animal infections, and it seems likely that the future taxonomic criteria for plant MLOs will have to take into account biological characteristics, such as plant pathogenicity and host range, as with bacterial plant pathogens.

E. Preservation of Isolates

Mycoplasma cultures frequently lose viability rapidly if incubated beyond the attainment of maximal growth, particularly if the medium pH is altered. Many species can be maintained for weeks or months at 0–4°C, if the culture medium is first neutralised. Isolates of *Acholeplasma, Mycoplasma* and *Spiroplasma* spp. have been maintained viable for over three years at this laboratory, using an ordinary domestic freezer, but low temperature storage is to be recommended (−60 to −70°C, or in liquid nitrogen), and cycles of freeze-thawing will reduce viability drastically. Freeze-drying is preferred for long-term storage and transport of cultures, as described, for example, by Lapage *et al.* (1970) and Liao and Chen (this volume, Chapter 6).

F. Interpretation of Results

The history of claimed isolations of mycoplasmas from yellows diseases demonstrates the need for cautious evaluation of the relationship between a newly isolated organism and its presumed plant or insect host. Desirable steps for proving pathogenicity of an unknown isolate (after Davis and Whitcomb, 1971) are:

(i)   Consistent isolation from diseased, but not from healthy plant, and preferably insect hosts, by techniques that can be repeated at other laboratories. Replication and culture media controls must be adequate to exclude the possibility of contamination from such sources as animal sera or from the investigator. Where an organism is thought to be epiphytic or saprophytic, as with the acholeplasmas, isolations from hosts affected by other diseases with similar symptoms, but proven etiology, may help to clarify its origin.

(ii)   The organism must be passaged through sufficient subcultures to dilute out any nonmultiplying infectious agent in the original inoculum. Depending on the infectivity titre of the original inoculum (if known), this may demand a dilution factor greater than 10^{10}.

(iii)   Pure lines must be obtained by filter cloning or subculturing at limiting dilution. The significance of steps (ii) and (iii) is well illustrated by Faivre-Amiot *et al.* (1970), who obtained a mixed culture of mycoplasmal and bacterial forms from clover-phyllody-diseased *Vinca*. A low level of reinfection was produced on experimental inoculation, but only by cultures in up to the second or third passage, and no infective agent could be purified.

(iv)   The organism must be at least minimally characterised as a member of the Mollicutes. Wall-less L-phase variants of bacterial plant pathogens have been described (Rubio-Huertos and Beltra, 1962; Jones and Paton, 1973) and the similarities of colony morphology and ultrastructural features of L-phase bacteria to those of mycoplasmas are well documented (Anderson, 1969; Cole, 1971). The outer lipoprotein portion of the cell wall is retained in spheroplast or 'B-type' L forms of gram-negative bacteria, which may appear in ultrathin sections to be bound by two trilaminar membranes, but stable protoplast or 'A-type' L forms of gram-negative bacteria, and those of gram-positive bacteria, are limited by a single trilaminar membrane and are more easily confused with mycoplasmas.

(v)   Induction of the full disease syndrome in a representative range of natural hosts. This will usually require injection into a known or contrived vector, or acquisition by membrane feeding. As transmission characteristics, such as the efficiency of transmission by different vectors, may be specific properties of a given disease, this information may help establish relationships to, and possible confusion with, other cultured agents. Direct mechanical inoculations to plants, whilst unlikely to transmit MLO, may produce some symptoms of yellows disease (Alivizatos and Townsend, 1980).

(vi)   The agent must be reisolated from experimentally-infected plant and insect hosts, but not from suitable controls, and must be shown to resemble the original isolate.

In the absence of any means of transmitting the agent to its original host, transmission to an alternative host by an experimental vector may demonstrate plant pathogenicity, even where this cannot be ecologically related to the disease. Useful corroborative information on the specific association between a cultured organism and a plant disease might also be obtained by serological techniques, such as enzyme-linked immunosorbent assay (ELISA), to demonstrate mycoplasmal antigens in diseased plants or insects (Clark *et al.*, 1978; Bové *et al.*, 1979).

Finally, the possibility of natural dual infections should be considered: a disease associated with a noncultivable agent may be superinfected with a cultivable organism which may reproduce at least part of the original syndrome on experimental re-inoculation. Observations of dual infection of periwinkle by *S. citri* and a noncultivable MLO are cited by McCoy (1979) and Banttari and Zeyen (1979); the latter review other examples of dual infections, derived mainly from cross protection experiments involving symptomatologically distinct yellows diseases. In this connection, it is interesting to note the mounting evidence that the 'Rio Grande' and 'Mesa Centrale' strains of corn stunt are, in fact, associated with corn stunt spiroplasma and a non-helical MLO, respectively (Nault and Bradfute, 1979). These authors point out that plants and insects infected by 'Mesa Centrale' corn stunt, for which the name maize bushy stunt (MBS) has been proposed, can be superinfected with 'Rio Grande' corn stunt spiroplasma; plants showing MBS symptoms may thus contain spiroplasmas before 'Rio Grande' symptoms develop. The presence of a complex of mycoplasmal agents in clover-phyllody-diseased clover has recently been claimed by Giannotti *et al.* (1979) in explanation of earlier results.

4. Techniques for Handling Noncultivable Agents

Expectations that MLOs associated with yellows diseases could be cultured and manipulated by conventional microbiological techniques have tended to obscure earlier advances in handling these disease agents. It is ironic that a return to techniques that were under development when a viral etiology was suspected should now seem appropriate. With present knowledge of the likely *in vitro* behaviour of MLO, it is perhaps surprising that procedures for extraction, purification and bioassay of yellows agents, analogous to those developed for viruses, have not been more widely investigated. This section presents some suggestions for experimental work.

A. Bioassay and the Value of Model Systems

Many classical studies on plant virus diseases, including those now associated with prokaryotic agents, have centred on quantitative bio-assay of infectivity using plant indicator hosts infected via artificially-inoculated insect vectors. Studies on the extraction and purification of yellows 'viruses', such as those of Whitcomb *et al.* (1968), demonstrated properties which, had the work been pursued, would most probably have led to deduction of the real nature of the pathogens.

In the context of the present review, bioassays offer a means of monitoring the stages in attempted culture of a fastidious organism: extraction, purification and concentration of inoculum, and improvement of culture media to enhance survival and multiplication. Infectivity bioassay of yellows diseases requires a suitable vector (not necessarily a natural host) and many diseases are thus not amenable to study. Disease/vector combinations with the following features are favourable model systems: (i) plant host readily propagated, symptoms easily recognised and incubation period short; (ii) vector easily reared, large enough for injection, survives well, preferably on the experimental plant host, and transmits efficiently (i.e. a high proportion of experimentally-infected individuals transmit) after a short latent period. Additional factors such as the ease of obtaining infective extracts will influence the choice of starting material.

In practice, few disease/vector combinations fulfil these criteria, and the choice of experimental hosts will be based on material that is locally available. Model systems that have been used for monitoring attempted cultures by infectivity assay include aster yellows and vector *Macrosteles fascifrons* (R.E. Davis *et al.*, 1970; A.J. Smith, 1980); western X and vector *Colladonus montanus* (Whitcomb *et al.*, 1968; Nasu *et al.*, 1974a, b), and grapevine *Flavescence dorée* and vector *Euscelidius variegatus* (Caudwell *et al.*, 1973, 1974). A comprehensive review of practical and theoretical aspects has been presented by Whitcomb (1972) and statistical aspects have been described by Caudwell (1977).

B. Extraction and Purification of MLO

Extraction and maintenance of short-term viability of MLO will be influenced by mechanical factors affecting their release from host tissues and differences in physical factors, such as pH, hydrostatic and osmotic pressure, and redox potential, between the phloem or hemolymph environment and the extraction medium. Although incompletely defined, the many basic similarities between phloem sap and insect hemolymph (Saglio and Whitcomb, 1979) may serve as a basis for the design of media for extracting and culturing MLO.

Experimental studies on extraction and purification have been limited. Lee and Chiykowski (1963) showed that infective homogenates of aster yellows-infected *M. fascifrons* could be maintained for up to 48 hr at $5°C$ in phosphate-buffered saline both with and without 0.01M $MgCl_2$ + 0.1M glycine. Infectivity was sedimented at 40,000 rpm but only partially at 10,000 rpm. The sedimentation properties of the agent were confirmed by Whitcomb and Davis (1969), who with Steere (1967) described recovery of infectivity following filtration on agar and agarose gel columns eluted with 0.3M glycine in 0.03M $MgCl_2$ at neutral or slightly alkaline pH. These results, and ultra-filtration studies on extracts (Cohen *et al.*, 1969) were consistent with the known properties of mycoplasmas.

A more extensive investigation of the properties of extracts of the western X disease agent by Whitcomb *et al.* (1968) remains a valuable source of information on the extraction of plant MLO despite the fact that the investigators thought that they were working with a virus. The infectivity of insect extracts, estimated quantitatively by bioassay, was sedimented between 10,000–25,000 g and was concentrated after rate zonal density gradient centrifugation in the 30–40% w/v sucrose region of the gradient. Similar results were obtained by Nasu *et al.* (1974a, b), who claimed that slight differences in the concentration of 'large spherical electron transparent' and 'spherical electron dense' mycoplasmal forms could be detected in ultrathin sections prepared from different regions of the gradient and examined by electron microscopy. Differences in the infectivity of gradient fractions were not significant and comparative electron microscope examination of healthy plant and insect extracts, as controls, was not reported. Both leafhopper and celery plant extracts retained infectivity for up to two days in a leafhopper tissue culture medium (Chiu and Black, 1967) containing 0.9M sucrose. Interestingly, extracts from diseased celery plants were not infectious immediately after extraction, but infectivity increased to an apparent maximum after two days. The presence of a labile inhibitor in the fresh extracts was suggested to account for this and similar observations cited by the authors.

Sinha (1974) described the purification of the clover phyllody agent from aster plants. Diseased tissues were macerated in a glycine + $MgCl_2$ buffer, the extracts clarified by low-speed centrifugation followed by activated charcoal and Celite (diatomaceous earth) treat-ment, and fractionated on agarose columns. Fractions in which MLO could be detected by electron microscopy were pooled and centrifuged on 5–20% w/v sucrose gradients. A discrete fraction was reportedly recovered from diseased but not from healthy plants, which gave a low infectivity (5/50 plants) when assayed by injection into leafhoppers. The author (unpublished data) found that Celite irreversibly adsorbed a large proportion of *A. laidlawii* suspended in the same buffer, which suggests that this technique should, perhaps, be used with caution. Fractionated plant extracts examined by transmission electron microscopy (Sinha, 1976) showed numerous, mostly empty, membrane-bound bodies, but, whilst some of these resembled mycoplasmas (and the extracts were infective), the absence of an equivalent fraction from disease-free plant extracts precluded a comparative ultrastructural study of healthy controls. Similar structures were seen in ultrathin sections of extracts from both healthy and lethal yellowing-diseased coconut palms (Eden-Green, 1978). The interpretation of negatively-stained extracts examined by electron microscopy (Belli, 1969; Hirumi and Maramorosch, 1969) is particularly doubtful (Wolanski and Maramorosch, 1970; Wolanski, 1973).

C. Cell-free Media

Several authors have observed beneficial effects of mycoplasma or animal tissue culture media ingredients on the preservation of infectivity in diseased plant or insect extracts. Hirumi and Maramorosch (1969) maintained infectivity of aster yellows extracts for at least 6 hr at room temperature when these were mixed with an equal volume of leafhopper culture medium containing 20% w/v fetal bovine serum. R.E. Davis *et al.* (1970) prolonged survival of this agent from 3 to 48 hr in media containing amino acids, vitamins, inorganic salts, sucrose, cholesterol and 5% w/v horse serum, and incubated at 22°C under nitrogen or $CO_2 + N_2$. This approach was taken further in early attempts to culture corn stunt spiroplasma (Chen and Granados, 1970), where maintenance, and probably some multiplication of the agent, was achieved for up to 50 days in a complex partially-defined medium. Nasu *et al.* (1974c) maintained Western X infectivity from *C. montanus* for over two weeks in a leafhopper tissue culture medium containing sucrose and both with and without the addition of culture supernatant and cells from *C. montanus* cell cultures. An increase in infectivity, between one and two weeks after inoculation, was accompanied by the appearance of large pleomorphic electron transparent mycoplasma-like structures in sections from centrifuged cultures, and was considered to be evidence of primary culture of the western X agent in a cell-free medium.

A particularly methodical application of infectivity assay to the improvement of media for survival and culture of MLO is the study of Caudwell and co-workers on *Flavescence dorée* of grapevine (Caudwell *et al.*, 1973 to 1976; Caudwell, 1977, 1978). This agent survives only a few minutes in buffered saline or sucrose, but successive improvements in maintenance media, based on insect tissue culture and serum formulations, have prolonged infectivity for up to 44 hr (Caudwell *et al.*, 1975). A corresponding increase in titre has been reported, from 0.2 infection units (iu) per ml of medium to 10^5 iu/ml (Caudwell *et al.*, 1976) and most recently to 10^6 iu/ml (A. Caudwell, personal communication, 1979). These results strongly suggest that the agent is multiplying *in vitro*, although the titre is still well below that attained by most mycoplasma cultures grown under optimal conditions.

A novel approach, which mimics the *in vivo* environment of MLO in plants, is the use of media based on phloem sap. Phloem exudate can be collected in large quantities from certain species of monocotyledons (van Die and Tammes, 1975), and its suitability as a mycoplasma growth medium has been demonstrated. McCoy (1976, 1977) obtained vigorous growth of *A. laidlawii* and limited growth of *S. citri* and corn stunt spiroplasma in unsupplemented sap collected from healthy palm crowns. Addition of serum gave excellent growth of the two spiroplasmas and of *M. gallisepticum*. Eden-Green (1978) found that *A. laidlawii* and *A. axanthum* grew well in phloem sap from crowns of both healthy and lethal yellowing-diseased palms, and obtained excellent growth of *S. citri* and *M. fermentans* in sap containing combinations of 1% v/v serum fraction and 5% v/v yeast extract. Exudate collected from inflorescences of coconut palms, including varieties resistant to lethal yellowing, also supported growth of mycoplasmas (Eden-Green, unpublished data). Both authors have found that the pH of freshly collected sap increases rapidly to above 8.5 on exposure to air, and media must be incubated in sealed tubes or under liquid paraffin or nitrogen. No growth of the MLO associated with lethal yellowing disease was detected, but phloem sap media should be included in tests with a suitable model bioassay system. McCoy (1979) has called attention to the special hydraulic environment within phloem elements, and has suggested that cultures should be attempted under a continuous hydrostatic pressure in the region of ten atmospheres.

D. Tissue Cultures

An ingenious technique for transmitting aster yellows under aseptic conditions, using aseptically-reared plants and leafhopper vectors (*M. fascifrons*), enabled Mitsuhashi and Maramorosch (1964) to infect healthy carrot callus tissue *in vitro*. Disease-free leafhoppers re-acquired the agent from callus tissue 50 days after it had been inoculated, and transmitted it to aseptically-grown aster test seedlings. Infected calluses showed no visible symptoms but neither the degree of tissue differentiation nor the localisation of the agent within the tissues were ascertained. Several later reports described maintenance of MLO in tissue cultures established from diseased plants (Petrů *et al.*, 1971; Jacoli, 1974; Jacoli and Ronald, 1974; McCoy, 1979) and regeneration of both diseased and healthy plantlets from meristems and differentiated embryoids (Maia and Beck, 1976). Tobacco (*Nicotiana glauca*) callus and reconstituted plantlets, derived from plants infected with potato witches' broom and Crimean yellows, remained infective when grown in the presence of indole-3-acetic acid (IAA) and kinetin (Petrů and Ulrichová, 1975) but not when these hormones were substituted by 2, 4-dichlorophenoxy-acetic acid (2, 4-D). The authors attributed the loss of infectivity to the lack of vascular differentiation in tissues grown in the latter medium, in contrast to the presence of well differentiated xylem and phloem in the IAA + kinetin-grown explants. A later report (Petrů and Ulrychová, 1978) supported the suggestion that an important factor influencing the survival of MLO in callus was the rate of organogenesis, notably the differentiation of new phloem *in vitro*. Ultrastructural investigations of aster yellows-diseased carrot callus (Jacoli, 1974) and lethal yellowing diseased-coconut inflorescence tissue explants (McCoy, 1979) showed MLO persisting only in well-differentiated phloem, but subsequent reports by Jacoli (1978a, b) indicated that aster yellows MLO started to degenerate within 11–25 days in carrot callus grown in the presence of IAA + kinetin and did not spread to newly differentiated phloem elements.

In contrast, attempts to maintain MLO in insect tissue cultures have been less successful. Maramorosch (1956) maintained the aster yellows agent for ten days in excised vector (*M. fascifrons*) tissues incubated in hanging drops of a tissue culture medium. Infectivity was recovered only from tissue pieces, which derived from whole insects, and not from the suspending medium.

A later report (Hirumi and Maramorosch, 1963) suggested that the agent persisted only in Malpighian tubules, but the data were insufficient to confirm multiplication *in vitro*. Nasu *et al.* (1974c) detected slight western X infectivity in anterior lobes of salivary glands from infected *C. montanus* after one week incubation in tissue culture medium, and infectivity persisted for 28 days when dead salivary glands were maintained in a modified medium (Sugiura *et al.*, 1977). Infection of insect cell monolayers in a manner analogous to plant viruses (Chiu and Black, 1967) has not been reported (Maramorosch, 1979).

Although beyond the scope of this review, it would seem profitable to explore other *in vivo* systems that have been adapted to research on noncultivable groups of prokaryotes and viruses. Embryonated hens' eggs were utilised in classical studies on the agent of human primary atypical pneumonia (now recognised as *M. pneumoniae*) and other mycoplasmas, long before culture was achieved in cell-free media (Hayflick, 1969). This technique was recently employed to demonstrate multiplication and the spiroplasmal nature of the suckling mouse cararact agent (Tully *et al.*, 1976), prior to its axenic culture. Techniques for handling chicken eggs are described by Lennette (1969). An alternative model system, which appears more appropriate for plant and insect mycoplasmas, is suggested by recent work from McCoy *et al.* (1981) on wax moth larvae (*Galleria mellonella*). These insects are readily reared on artificial laboratory media, have a wide temperature range for growth, and are large enough to permit the sequential sampling of hemolymph. The authors found that several spiroplasma strains multiplied to high titres within 12 to 48 hr of injection into larvae, demonstrating the potential of this insect host for studying the multiplication and insect pathogenicity of yellows agents.

E. Characterisation and Preservation of MLO

Some attempts have been made to identify and characterise MLO *in vivo* by serological techniques. Gáborjányi and Bencsics (1968) reported preparation of an antiserum from stolbur-diseased tomato plants, which after absorption with healthy sap, gave a positive reaction with sap extracts from diseased tomato and potato, but not pepper and *Datura*, at dilutions of up to 1 in 64. This work was apparently repeated soon after MLO were associated with this disease (Marchoux *et al.*, 1979), but has not been substantiated since. Antisera prepared against relatively crude antigen preparations from corn stunt-diseased corn plants were used to demonstrate a serological relationship between the corn stunt agent and *S. citri*, before it was possible to culture the former (Tully *et al.*, 1973), and have since been shown to have a high titre against cultured corn stunt spiroplasma (Whitcomb, 1978). Charudattan and McCoy (1975) prepared antisera to phloem sap collected from lethal yellowing-diseased and healthy coconut palms and detected a distinct, disease-specific antigen in the former. Whether this derived from the pathogen or was due to a reaction by the host was not determined, but no cross reactions could be detected against antigen preparations from healthy and aster yellows-diseased periwinkle, *A. laidlawii* or *S. citri*. Reciprocal reactions between diseased coconut antigens and antisera to *S. citri* and *M. gallisepticum* gave similarly negative results, but the same antigen was detected in sap from declining *Veitchia* palms (McCoy and Charudattan, 1976).

In a recent report, Sinha (1979) described the preparation of antisera to purified mycoplasma extracts from aster yellows-diseased plants (see 4.B, above) which gave two disease-specific bands in agar double gel diffusion tests.

The absence of heterologous cross-reactions between antisera prepared against the aster yellows agent, *A. laidlawii* and *S. citri* and cultures of the latter two organisms was reported by McIntosh *et al.* (1974), although later reports from the same laboratories described the aster yellows as a spiroplasma (Kondo *et al.*, 1977) that was antigenically related to *S. citri* (McIntosh *et al.*, 1977). Recent preliminary reports have described both successful (Nomé *et al.*, 1980) and unsuccessful (Dollet *et al.*, 1980) detection of lethal yellowing disease in coconut tissues by ELISA, using respective antisera to spiroplasmas associated with aster yellows and pear decline, and to *S. citri*. The aster yellows spiroplasma was serologically closely related to *S. citri* (Raju *et al.*, 1980). The need for adequate controls and cautious interpretation in these and other serological tests on yellows-diseased plants (McCrum, 1974; de Leeuw, 1977) is underscored by the demonstration of a close serological relationship between glycolipids prepared from cultured *M. pneumoniae* and from chloroplasts of healthy plants (Kenny and Newton, 1973).

The long-term preservation of noncultivable agents poses special problems, particularly for the conservation and dissemination of standard reference strains. Subculturing from plant to plant, by grafting or via insect vectors, holds the risks that the former may result in loss of insect transmissibility, and the latter may lead to attenuation of pathogenicity (Chiykowski, 1977a). Musil (1964) demonstrated that the stolbur and clover phyllody agents remained infective after freezing in whole infected leafhoppers at $-20°C$, and preservation of viability after freezing has been demonstrated for both the western X agent in whole insects or saline extracts (Whitcomb *et al.*, 1968) and the aster yellows agent in cell culture medium (Davis and Whitcomb, 1970). A routine technique for preservation of yellows agents in whole frozen leafhoppers has been suggested only recently, however (Chiykowski,

1977b). If no vector is available, there seems no reason why the same techniques should not be applied to MLO in plant tissues, but the concentration of MLO may be lower and infectivity may be harder to recover in extracts. Presumably, infected host tissues could also be lyophilised to preserve the agents.

5. Isolation and Handling of Other Agents

A. *Rickettsia-like Organisms (RLO)*

Phloem-limited agents have not been cultured in cell-free media, although only a few attempts have been reported (Ghosh *et al.*, 1971). Similarities in habitat *in vivo* and transmission characteristics suggest that these agents can be handled by techniques found useful for MLO. Transovarial passage of the clover club leaf (Black, 1948) and rugose leaf curl (Grylls, 1954) agents provides an unusual opportunity for establishment of tissue cultures, infected from the egg stage, and could facilitate rearing of contamination-free infective insects.

Xylem-limited agents, in contrast, have been the subject of a number of additional techniques. In most diseases, xylem RLO can be identi- fied by light microscopy of sap extracted by the application of vacuum or positive pressure, or by squeezing with pliers. Immersion of cut stem tissues in 0.1M KOH enhanced the exudation of RLO from phony peach-diseased tissues and was suggested as a diagnostic aid (French, 1974). Sufficient bacteria were purified and concentrated from phony peach- (French *et al.*, 1978) and ratoon stunting- (Gillaspie, 1978) diseased plants for the preparation of specific antisera which have been used for diagnostic purposes, including demonstration of a relationship between the RLO associated with phony peach-disease and a similar organism in periwinkle (McCoy *et al.*, 1978). These should facilitate the verification of putative cultures of xylem RLO. The ratoon stunting disease agent differs from other RLO in several respects, including mechanical transmissibility from plant to plant (which may account for the apparent spread of disease via planting or harvesting operations; Steindl, 1961), but cultures of the Pierce's disease (= almond leaf scorch and alfalfa dwarf) bacterium were also successfully trans- mitted to grapevine (M.J. Davis *et al.*, 1978) and almond (M.J. Davis and Thompson, 1979) cuttings by vacuum infiltrations and to grape- vine, almond and alfalfa seedlings by needle injection (M.J. Davis and Thompson, 1979; Thompson *et al.*, 1979). This suggests that other xylem agents, in common with most plant pathogenic bacteria, will prove to be mechanically transmissible, but inoculum dose and viability and the method of inoculation may be critical. The non-cultivability of the phony peach group of RLO and the ratoon-stunting disease agent in conventional media, including those developed for the Pierce's disease bacterium, suggests that study of the survival and multiplication of these agents in media based on extracted xylem sap would be useful. A recent report by Nienhaus *et al.* (1979) suggests that infection of chicken embryos should also be attempted.

B. Phytomonas

Preliminary attempts to culture flagellates associated with coffee phloem necrosis (Vermeulen, 1963) and coconut Hartrot (Parthas-arathy and van Slobbe, 1978) have been unsuccessful, although the latter survived for several hours in media based on coconut milk (Dollet and Lopez, 1978). Phytomonads that inhabit laticiferous tissues are more widely distributed in nature, but successful axenic culture has been reliably reported only recently (McGhee and Postell, 1976). These authors were able to isolate *P. davidi* from a euphor-biaceous host, using various diphasic media with duck or outdated human blood in the agar phase. Pure cultures were established by allow-ing flagellates to swim clear of contaminants in migration tubes (Hanson and McGhee, 1961). Attempts to isolate *P. elmassiani* in these media were unsuccessful, however. McCoy (1978) subsequently reported excellent multiplication and serial passage of *P. davidi* in spiroplasma medium SP4 (Tully *et al.*, 1977), and the organism grew in conventional mycoplasma broth supplemented with yeast extract, and in coconut phloem sap. Mycoplasma media may thus facilitate the isolation of related organisms that are suspected pathogens in plant phloem and may, by a most circuitous route, come to find application in the wider field of medical and veterinary protozoology.

6. Conclusion: Areas for Future Work

If confirmed, the recent preliminary reports describing isolation of spiroplasmas from diseases previously associated with noncultivable MLO (Section 2.A) will suggest that the key to isolation of yellows agents lies in manipulation of the choice of host inocula, existing media and conditions of culture. Clearly, application of similar isolation techniques to other plant diseases will then be called for. At present, however, evidence for the separation of spiroplasmas from noncultivable polymorphic MLO, or virescence agents, rests on grounds of symptomatology, *in vivo* morphology, and the persistent failure of culture attempts by other workers.

Failure to culture yellows agents can be attributed to three factors: (i) failure in mechanical extraction of viable MLO from host tissues; (ii) inhibition of MLO in early passage by compounds derived from host tissue extracts; and (iii) inadequacy of present media and conditions of culture. Extraction of viable MLO from plant tissues may be strongly influenced by the effects of sudden release of hydrostatic pressure and rapid deposition of callose in ruptured sieve elements. Under these conditions, it is particularly difficult to envisage the release in intact and viable form of the complex, filamentous MLO recently observed ramifying between sieve elements of coconut palms affected by lethal yellowing disease (Waters and Hunt, 1980). But, whilst these factors may contribute to the low infectivity of plant extracts, the fact that such extracts are infective demonstrates that viable MLO are released from plant tissues. Further, these difficulties either do not arise, or are greatly reduced, in extractions from insects. Some support for the inhibition of MLO *in vitro* by factors released from damaged host plant tissues derives from early experiences with the corn stunt spiroplasma (Chen and Liao, 1975; Liao *et al.*, 1978) and the experimental studies reported by Teranaka *et al.* (1976). It seems less likely, however, that inhibitors from insect macerates could have had sufficient potency to affect the partially purified preparations obtained by Nasu *et al.* (1974c) and Caudwell *et al.* (1974); indeed, the most prolonged survival of the western X agent (28 days) was achieved in dead salivary glands incubated in culture medium (Sugiura *et al.*, 1977).

One is thus left with the conclusion that present media and conditions of culture are simply inadequate for the isolation of MLO. This may be due to some relatively simple deficiency and improvements in survival, multiplication and eventual subculture of these agents may come from chance combinations of culture conditions and reagents; however, the areas with the greatest logical potential lie in monitoring improvements in the survival of MLO *in vitro* by bioassay, as exemplified by the work of Caudwell and co-workers, and in the development of improved techniques for extraction and purification of these agents from their plant or insect hosts. The latter would facilitate study of the biochemical and serological properties of yellows agents, and could lead to elucidation of their relationships to known Mollicutes or to other groups of prokaryotes, as well as to the possible development of new diagnostic techniques.

Noncultivability may also reflect a truly obligate mode of parasitism,

involving a more intimate association with host metabolism such as is
exemplified by the Chlamydiales (R.E. Davis and Whitcomb, 1971;
Page, 1977). Several authors have commented that plant MLO are
intracellular parasites in their plant and insect hosts, whilst mycoplasma
infections of vertebrate tissues are extracellular, but this view holds
several contradictions. On the one hand, high concentrations of MLO
are frequently observed, and are presumed to multiply, in the lumen
of mature sieve elements of plants; a situation which is intracellular but
arguably is not intracytoplasmic. And on the other hand, it has become
widely accepted that MLO multiply extracellularly in the hemolymph
of insects. Ironically, the latter view seems to derive from earlier studies
on the development of yellows 'viruses' in their insect vectors (Whitcomb *et al.*, 1966; Sinha and Chiykowski, 1967), in which the authors
were careful to point out that the appearance of infective 'virus' in
hemolymph must have resulted from growth in, and subsequent release
from, intracellular sites such as haemocytes. Direct evidence for multiplication of MLO in insect hemolymph is limited to the high resolution
autoradiography study of Gouranton and Maillet (1973), in which
clover phyllody-infected *Euscelis lineolatus* were examined 1 to 24 hr
after injection with tritiated thymidine. Although groups of radio-
labelled MLO were detected in hemolymph attached to or trapped
between folds of salivary gland cells, it is difficult to exclude the
possibility that these organisms derived from an intracellular environment, prior to fixation. Whatever the significance of the distribution
of MLO *in vivo*, the development of either plant or insect cell cultures,
or other *in vivo* model systems, provides further possibilities for the
study of the properties of these organisms, and may prove central to
further progress in axenic culture.

Acknowledgements

Support from the Coconut Industry Board, Jamaica, and the United
Kingdom Overseas Development Administration is gratefully
acknowledged. I particularly wish to thank A. Caudwell, K. Maramorosch and R.E. McCoy for sending offprints and details of current
research.

Addendum

In the period between first drafting this review in December 1979 and its publication, several significant developments have been reported. At the third conference of the International Organisation for Mycoplasmology (Custer, S. Dakota, 3–9 September 1980) J.C. Vignault *et al.* described the isolation in SP4 medium of a novel *Mycoplasma* strain associated with apple proliferation disease, but the biological significance of this organism remains unclear. Details of natural dual infections in *C. roseus* by *S. citri* and a noncultivable MLO associated with virescence symptoms were reported by G. Oldfield at the same meeting, and there has been no confirmation of the association of spiroplasmas with aster yellows, western X and pear decline diseases during this period, now three years since the original reports. A more detailed account of the isolation, coidentity and etiological role of the RLB causing Pierce's disease and almond leaf scorch has been published by M.J. Davis *et al.* (*Phytopathology 70*, 472-5) and the isolation of the RLB causing ratoon-stunting disease was reported by M.J. Davis *et al.* and C.H. Liao and T.A. Chen, who also described the isolation of a similar organism associated with white leaf-diseased bermuda grass (abstracts of the American Phytopathological Society 1980 annual meeting, *Plant Disease*, in press). A xylem-limited RLB associated with Sumatra disease of cloves has also been cultured (P. Hunt and C.P.A. Bennett, personal communication) and it seems likely that the culture of other representatives of this group of agents will follow.

References

Alivizatos, A.S. and Townsend, R. (1980). Symptoms produced in plants in response to injection. In *Proceedings of the Fourth Meeting of the International Council on Lethal Yellowing, Fort Lauderdale, 1979*, p. 14. University of Florida Publication FL-80-1.

Anderson, D.R. (1969). Ultrastructural studies of mycoplasmas and the L-phase of bacteria. In *The Mycoplasmatales and the L-Phase of Bacteria*, pp. 365–402, L. Hayflick (ed). Amsterdam: North Holland Publishing Company.

Auger, J.G., Shalla, T.A. and Kado, C.I. (1974). Pierce's disease of grapevines: evidence for a bacterial etiology. *Science 184*, 1375-7.

Banttari, E.E. and Zeyen, R.J. (1979). Interactions of mycoplasmalike organisms and viruses in dually infected leafhoppers, planthoppers and plants. In *Leafhopper Vectors and Plant Disease Agents*, pp. 327-47, K. Maramorosch and K.F. Harris (eds). New York and London: Academic Press.

Barile, M.F. (1974). General principles of isolation and detection of mycoplasmas. *Les Mycoplasmes/Mycoplasmas. Les Colloques de l'Institut National de la Santé et de la Recherche Médicale 33*, 135-42.

Belli, G. (1969). Mycoplasma-like particles in clarified extracts of diseased rice plants. *Rivista di Patologia Vegetale 5*, 3-11.

Black, L.M. (1948). Transmission of clover club-leaf virus through the egg of its insect vector. *Phytopathology 38*, 2.

Bové, J.M., Moutous, G., Saillard, C., Fos, A., Bonfils, J., Vignault, J-C., Nhami, A., Abassi, M., Kabbage, K., Hafidi, B., Mouches, C. and Viennot-Bourgin, G. (1979). Mise en évidence de *Spiroplasma citri*, l'agent causal de la maladie du 'stubborn' des agrumes dans 7 cicadelles du Maroc. *Comptes Rendus Hebdomadaires des Séances de l'Académie des Sciences, Paris. Série D 288*, 335-8.

Caudwell, A. (1977). Aspects statistiques des épreuves d'infectivité chez les jaunisses (Yellows) des plantes et chez les viroses transmises selon le mode persistant. Intérêt de la Fève (*Vicia faba*) comme plante-test pour les jaunisses. *Annales de Phytopathologie 9*, 141-59.

— (1978). Étiologie des jaunisses des plantes. *Phytoma – Défense des Cultures 294*, 5-9.

Caudwell, A., Kuszala, C. and Larrue, J. (1973). Techniques utilisables pour l'étude de la flavescence dorée de la vigne. *Rivista di Patologia Vegetale 9*, 269-76.

— (1974). Sur la culture *in vitro* des agents infectieux responsables des jaunisses des plantes (MLO). *Annales de Phytopathologie 6*, 173-90.

— (1975). Conservation *in vitro* de l'agent pathogène de type mycoplasme (MLO) de la flavescence dorée de la vigne. *Comptes Rendus des Séances de la Société de Biologie 169*, 185-8.

— (1976). Progress in the culture of the etiologic agent, type mycoplasma, of the flavescence dorée of grapes. *Proceedings of the Society for General Microbiology 3*, 154.

Charbonneau, D.L., Hawthorne, J.D., Ghiorse, W.C. and VanDemark, P.J. (1979). Isolation of a spiroplasma-like organism from aster yellows infective leafhoppers. *Abstracts of the 79th Annual Meeting of the American Society for Microbiology, Los Angeles, California, 1979*, 86.

Charudattan, R. and McCoy, R.E. (1975). Antigenic difference in phloem exudates of healthy and lethal yellowing-diseased coconut palms. *Proceedings of the American Phytopathological Society 2*, 71.

Chen, T.A. and Granados, R.R. (1970). Plant pathogenic mycoplasma-like organism: maintenance *in vitro* and transmission to *Zea mays*. *Science 167*, 1633-6.

Chen, T.A. and Liao, C.H. (1975). Corn stunt spiroplasma: isolation, cultivation and proof of pathogenicity. *Science 188*, 1015-17.

Chiu, R.J. and Black, L.M. (1967). Monolayer cultures of insect cell lines and their inoculation with a plant virus. *Nature 215*, 1076-8.

Chiykowski, L.N. (1977a). Reduction in transmissibility of a greenhouse-maintained isolate of aster yellows agent. *Canadian Journal of Botany 55*, 1783-6.

— (1977b). Cryopreservation of aster yellows agent in whole leafhoppers. *Canadian Journal of Microbiology 23*, 1038-40.

Clark, M.F., Flegg, C.L., Bar-Joseph, M. and Rottem, S. (1978). The detection of *Spiroplasma citri* by enzyme-linked immunosorbent assay (ELISA). *Phytopathologische Zeitschrift 92*, 332-7.

Cohen, R., Purcell, R. and Steere, R.L. (1969). Ultrafiltration of the aster yellows agent. *Phytopathology 59*, 1555.

Cole, R.M. (1971). Some implications of the comparative ultrastructure of bacterial L forms. In *Mycoplasma and the L Forms of Bacteria*, pp. 49-83, S. Madoff (ed). London: Gordon & Breach.

Cousin, M-T., Perreau, P. and Kartha, K.K. (1974). Essais de caractérisation sur milieux artificiels d'agents pathogènes à partir de plantes atteintes de 'Jaunisse'. *Annales de Phytopathologie 6*, 277-84.

Daniels, M.J. and Meddins, B.M. (1972). Studies on plant mycoplasmas. In *63rd Annual Report, John Innes Institute, England, 1972*, 101.

Davis, M.J., Purcell, A.H. and Thomson, S.V. (1978). Pierce's disease of grapevines: isolation of the causal bacterium. *Science 199*, 75-7.

Davis, M.J. and Thompson, S.V. (1979). Pathological and serological relationship of the bacterium causing Pierce's disease of grapevines and almond leaf scorch disease. In *3rd International Congress of Plant Pathology, Abstracts of Papers*, 64. Berlin and Hamburg: Paul Parey.

Davis, R.E. (1979). Spiroplasmas: newly recognised arthropod-borne pathogens. In *Leafhopper Vectors and Plant Disease Agents*, pp. 451-84, K. Maramorosch and K.F. Harris (eds). New York and London: Academic Press.

Davis, R.E. and Whitcomb, R.F. (1971). Mycoplasmas, Rickettsiae and Chlamydiae: possible relation to yellows diseases and other disorders of plants and insects. *Annual Review of Phytopathology 9*, 119-54.

Davis, R.E., Whitcomb, R.F. and Purcell, R. (1970). Viability of the aster yellows agent in cell-free media. *Phytopathology 60*, 573-4.

Davis, R.E., Worley, J.F. and Basciano, L.K. (1977). Association of spiroplasma and mycoplasma-like organisms with flowers of tulip tree (*Liriodendron tulipifera* L.). *Proceedings of the American Phytopathological Society 4*, 185-6.

de Leeuw, G.T.N. (1977). Mycoplasmas in planten. *Natuur en Techniek 45*, 74-89.

Doi, Y., Teranaka, M., Yora, K. and Asuyama, H. (1967). Mycoplasma- or PLT-like microorganisms found in the phloem elements of plants infected with mulberry dwarf, potato witches' broom, aster yellows or *Paulownia* witches' broom. *Annals of the Phytopathological Society of Japan 33*, 259-66. English translation in *Review of Plant Protection Research 2*, 84-88 (1969).

Dollet, M., Saillard, C., Garcia-Jurado, O., Vignault, J.C., Gargani, D., Tully, J.G. and Bové, J.M. (1980). An approach to the serological study of the mycoplasmas of lethal yellowing in the coconuts in West Africa. In *Proceedings of the Fourth Meeting of the International Council on Lethal Yellowing, Fort Lauderdale, 1979*, p. 8. University of Florida Publication FL-80-1.

Dollet, M. and Lopez, G. (1978). Etude sur la association de protozoaires flagelles a la Marchitez sorpresiva du palmier à huile en Amerique du Sud. *Oleagineux 33*, 209-17.

Donovan, C. (1909). Kala Azar in Madras. *Lancet 177*, 1495.

Eden-Green, S.J. (1978). Attempts to extract and culture mycoplasmas from coconut palms. In *Proceedings of the Third Meeting of the International Council on Lethal Yellowing, West Palm Beach, 1977*, p. 20. University of Florida Publication FL-78-2.

Eden-Green, S.J., Markham, P.G. and Townsend, R. (1980). Acholeplasmas and lethal yellowing disease II. Transmission experiments. In *Proceedings of the Fourth Meeting of the International Council on Lethal Yellowing, Fort Lauderdale, 1979*, p. 10. University of Florida Publication FL-80-1.

Eden-Green, S.J. and Tully, J.G. (1979). Isolation of *Acholeplasma* spp. from coconut palms affected by lethal yellowing disease in Jamaica. *Current Microbiology 2*, 311-16.

Eden-Green, S.J. and Waters, H. (1981). Isolation of corn stunt spiroplasma in Jamaica, and probable dual infection with maize mosaic virus. *Annals of Applied Biology 99* (in press).

Faivre-Amiot, A., Moreau, J-P., Cousin, M-T. and Staron, T. (1970). Essai de mise en culture de l'agent de la phyllodie du trèfle. *Annales de Phytopathologie 2*, 251-8.

Fallon, R.J. and Whittlestone, P. (1969). Isolation, cultivation and maintenance of mycoplasmas. In *Methods in Microbiology*, Vol. 3B, pp. 211-67, J.R. Norris and D.W. Ribbons (eds). London & New York: Academic Press.

French, W.J. (1974). A method for observing rickettsialike bacteria associated with phony peach disease. *Phytopathology 64*, 260-1.

French, W.J. and Kitajima, E.W. (1978). Occurrence of plum leaf scald in Brazil and Paraguay. *Plant Disease Reporter 62*, 1035-8.

French, W.J., Stassi, D.L. and Schaad, N.W. (1978). The use of immunofluorescence for the identification of phony peach bacterium. *Phytopathology 68*, 1106-8.

Frey, M.L., Thomas, G.B. and Hale, P.A. (1973). Recovery and identification of mycoplasmas from animals. *Annals of the New York Academy of Sciences 225*, 334-6.

Gáborjányi, R. and Bencsics, M.Sz. (1968). Preparation of antiserum against stolbur virus. *Acta Phytopathologica Academiae Scientiarum Hungaricae 3*, 31-3.

Garnier, M. and Bové, J.M. (1978). The organism associated with citrus greening disease is probably a member of the Schizomycetes. *Zentralblatt für Bakteriologie, Parasitenkunde, Infektionskrankheiten und Hygiene. Erste Abteilung Originale 241*, 221-2.

Ghosh, S.K., Raychaudhuri, S.P., Varma, A. and Nariani, T.K. (1971). Isolation and culture of *Mycoplasma* associated with citrus greening disease. *Current Science 40*, 229-300.

Giannotti, J. and Vago, C. (1971). Rôle des mycoplasmes dans l'étiologie de la phyllodie du trèfle: culture et transmission expérimentale de la maladie. *Physiologie Végétale 9*, 541-53.

Giannotti, J., Vago, C. and Giannotti, D. (1979). Culture *in vitro* d'un mycoplasme agent étiologique de phyllodie chez le trèfle. *Comptes Rendus Hebdomadaires des Séances de l'Académie des Sciences. Paris. Série D 288*, 85-7.

Giannotti, J., Vago, C., Marchoux, C., Devauchelle, G. and Czarnecky, D. (1972). Caractérisation par la culture *in vitro* de souches de mycoplasmes correspondant à huit maladies différentes de plantes. *Comptes Rendus Hebdomadaires des Séances de l'Académie des Sciences. Paris. Série D 274*, 330-3.

Giannotti, J., Vago, C., Marchoux, G., Devauchelle, G. and Duthoit, J.L. (1970). Infection de plante par un type inhabituél de microorganisme intracellulaire. *Comptes Rendus Hebdomadaires des Séances de l'Académie des Sciences. Paris. Série D 271*, 2118-19.

Gillaspie, A.G. (1978). Ratoon-stunting disease of sugarcane: serology. *Phytopathology 68*, 529-32.

Goheen, A.C., Nyland, G. and Lowe, S.K. (1973). Association of a rickettsia-like organism with Pierce's disease of grapevines and alfalfa dwarf and heat therapy of the disease in grapevines. *Phytopathology 63*, 341-5.

Gouranton, J. and Maillet, P.L. (1973). High resolution autoradiography of mycoplasmalike organisms multiplying in some tissues of an insect vector for clover phyllody. *Journal of Invertebrate Pathology 21*, 158-63.

Grylls, N.E. (1954). Rugose leaf curl – a new virus disease transovarially transmitted by the leafhopper *Austroagallia torrida*. *Australian Journal of Biological Science 7*, 47-58.

Hampton, R.O., Stevens, J.O. and Allen, T.C. (1969). Mechanically transmissible *Mycoplasma* from naturally infected peas. *Plant Disease Reporter 53*, 499-503.

Hampton, R.O., Florance, E.R., Whitcomb, R.F. and Seidler, R.J. (1976). Evidence suggesting non-association of mycoplasma with pea disease. *Phytopathology 66*, 1163-8.

Hanson, W.L. and McGhee, R.B. (1961). The biology and morphology of *Crithidia acanthocephali* n. sp., *Leptomonas leptoglossi* n. sp. and *Blastocrithidia euschisti* n. sp. *Journal of Protozoology 8*, 200-4.

Hayflick, L. (1965). Tissue cultures and mycoplasmas. *Texas Reports on Biology and Medicine 23*, 285-303.

— (1969). Fundamental biology of the class Mollicutes, order Mycoplasmatales.

In *The Mycoplasmatales and the L-Phase of Bacteria*, pp. 15–17, L. Hayflick (ed). Amsterdam: North Holland Publishing Company.

Hayflick, L. and Arai, S. (1973). Failure to isolate mycoplasmas from aster yellows-diseased plants and leafhoppers. *Annals of the New York Academy of Sciences 225*, 494–502.

Hirumi, H. and Maramorosch, K. (1963). Recovery of aster yellows virus from various organs of the insect vector, *Macrosteles fascifrons. Contributions from the Boyce Thompson Institute 22*, 141–52.

— (1969). Further evidence for a mycoplasma etiology of aster yellows. *Phytopathology 59*, 1030–1.

Hopkins, D.L. (1977). Diseases caused by leafhopper-borne, rickettsia-like bacteria. *Annual Review of Phytopathology 17*, 277–94.

Hopkins, D.L., Mollenhauer, H.H. and French, W.J. (1973). Occurrence of a rickettsia-like bacterium in the xylem of peach trees with phony disease. *Phytopathology 63*, 1422–3.

International Committee on Systematic Bacteriology, Subcommittee on the Taxonomy of Mollicutes. (1979). Proposal of minimal standards for descriptions of new species of the class *Mollicutes. International Journal of Systematic Bacteriology 29*, 172–80.

Ishie, T., Doi, Y., Yora, K. and Asuyama, H. (1967). Suppressive effect of antibiotics of the tetracycline group on symptom development of mulberry dwarf disease. *Annals of the Phytopathological Society of Japan 33,* 267-75. English translation in *Review of Plant Protection Research 2*, 91–5 (1969).

Jacoli, G.G. (1974). Translocation of mycoplasma-like bodies through sieve pores in plant tissue cultures infected with aster yellows. *Canadian Journal of Botany 52*, 2085–8.

— (1978a). Sequential degeneration of mycoplasma-like bodies in plant tissue cultures infected with aster yellows. *Canadian Journal of Botany 56*, 133–40.

— (1978b). Early phases of degeneration of mycoplasma-like bodies in plant tissue cultures infected with aster yellows: morphological analogies with *Mycoplasma hominis. Canadian Journal of Microbiology 24*, 1053–7.

Jacoli, G.G. and Ronald, W.P. (1974). Electron microscope studies of plant tissue cultures infected with the aster yellows disease. *Journal of Ultrastructural Research 46*, 34–42.

Jones, S.M. and Paton, A.M. (1973). The L-phase of *Erwinia carotovora* var. *atroseptica* and its possible association with plant tissue. *Journal of Applied Bacteriology 36*, 729–37.

Kaloostian, G.H., Oldfield, G.N., Pierce, H.D. and Calavan, E.C. (1979). *Spiroplasma citri* and its transmission to citrus and other plants by leafhoppers. In *Leafhopper Vectors and Plant Disease Agents*, pp. 447–50, K. Maramorosch and K.F. Harris (eds). New York & London: Academic Press.

Kao, J. and Damann, K.E. (1978). Microcolonies of the bacterium associated with ratoon-stunting disease found in sugarcane xylem matrix. *Phytopathology 68*, 545–51.

Kenny, G.E. and Newton, R.M. (1973). Close serological relationship between glycolipids of *Mycoplasma pneumoniae* and glycolipids of spinach. *Annals of the New York Academy of Sciences 225*, 54–61.

Kleinhempel, H., Müller, H.M. and Spaar, D. (1972). Isolierung und Kultivierung von *Mycoplasmatales* aus Weissklee mit Blütenvergrünungssymptomen. *Archiv für Pflanzenschutz 8*, 361–70.

Kondo, F., Maramorosch, K., McIntosh, A.H. and Varney, E.H. (1977). Aster yellows spiroplasma: isolation and cultivation *in vitro. Proceedings of the American Phytopathological Society 4*, 190–1.

Laidlaw, P.P. and Elford, W.J. (1936). A new group of filterable organisms.

Proceedings of the Royal Society B 20, 292–303.

Lapage, S.P., Shelton, J.E., Mitchell, T.G. and Mackenzie, A.R. (1970). Culture collections and the preservation of bacteria. In *Methods in Microbiology*, Vol. 3A, pp. 135–228, J.R. Norris and D.W. Ribbons (eds). London & New York: Academic Press.

Lee, P.E. and Chiykowski, L.N. (1963). Infectivity of aster-yellows virus preparations after differential centrifugations of extracts from viruliferous leafhoppers. *Virology 21*, 667–9.

Lennette, E.H. (1969). General principles underlying laboratory diagnosis of viral and rickettsial infections. In *Diagnostic Procedures for Viral and Rickettsial Infections, 4th edition*, pp. 1–65, E.H. Lennette and N.J. Schmidt (eds). New York: American Public Health Association, Inc.

Liao, C.H., Chang, C.J. and Chen, T.A. (1978). Spiroplasmastatic action of plant tissue homogenates. *Proceedings of ROC-United States Cooperative Science Program, Joint Seminar on Mycoplasma Diseases in Plants, 27-31 March 1978*, p. 25. Taipei: National Science Council.

Lin, S.C., Lee, C.S. and Chiu, R.J. (1970). Isolation and cultivation of, and inoculation with, a mycoplasma causing white leaf disease of sugarcane. *Phytopathology 60*, 795–7.

Maia, E. and Beck, D. (1976). Culture d'organes *in vitro* et régénération de plantes infectées par des mycoplasmes. *Annales de Phytopathologie 8*, 303–6.

Maramorosch, K. (1956). Multiplication of aster yellows virus in *in vitro* preparations of insect tissues. *Virology 2*, 369–76.

— (1972). The enigma of mycoplasma in plants and insects. *Phytopathology 62*, 1230–1.

— (1978). New findings in the biology of plant yellows diseases. In *Proceedings of the third meeting of the International Council on Lethal Yellowing, West Palm Beach, 1977*, pp. 9–10. University of Florida Publication FL-78-2.

— (1979). Leafhopper tissue culture. In *Leafhopper Vectors and Plant Disease Agents*, pp. 485–511, K. Maramorosch and K.F. Harris (eds). New York & London: Academic Press.

Marchoux, G., Giannotti, J., Quiot, J.B., Marou, J. and Vago, C. (1969). Mise en évidence des propriétés antigéniques spécifiques des microorganismes de type mycoplasme isolés de tomate atteinte de Stolbur. *Comptes rendus de l'Académie d'Agriculture (1969)*, 191–6.

Markham, P.G. and Townsend, R. (1979). Experimental vectors of spiroplasmas. In *Leafhopper Vectors and Plant Disease Agents*, pp. 413–45, K. Maramorosch and K.F. Harris (eds). New York & London: Academic Press.

Markham, P.G., Townsend, R. and Plaskitt, K.A. (1975). A rickettsia-like organism associated with diseased white clover. *Annals of Applied Biology 81*, 91–3.

McCoy, R.E. (1976). Plant phloem sap: a potential mycoplasma growth medium. *Proceedings of the Society for General Microbiology 3*, 155.

— (1977). Growth of mycoplasmas in phloem sap from lethal yellowing resistant Malayan dwarf coconut palm. *Proceedings of the American Phytopathological Society 4*, 108.

— (1978). Growth of the plant parasitic protozoan *Phytomonas davidi* in mycoplasma media and in plant phloem sap. *Phytopathology News 12*, 217.

— (1979). Mycoplasmas and Yellows Diseases. In *The Mycoplasmas*, Vol. III, pp. 229–64, R.F. Whitcomb and J.G. Tully (eds). New York & London: Academic Press.

— (1980). Wall-free prokaryotes of plants and invertebrates. In *The Prokaryotes: a Handbook on Habitats, Isolation and Identification of Bacteria*. M.P. Starr, H. Stolp, H.G. Truper, A. Balows and H.G. Schlegel (eds). Berlin, Heidelberg & New York: Springer-Verlag, in press.

McCoy, R.E. and Basham, H.G. (1980). Isolation and characterisation of mycoplasmas from floral surfaces. In *Proceedings of the fourth meeting of the International Council on Lethal Yellowing, Fort Lauderdale, 1979*, p. 11. University of Florida Publication FL-80-1.

McCoy, R.E. and Charudattan, R. (1976). Progress towards the isolation and characterisation of the lethal yellowing pathogen. *Principes – Journal of the Palm Society 20*, 61.

McCoy, R.E., Davis, M.J. and Dowell, R.V. (1981). In vivo cultivation of spiroplasmas in larvae of greater wax moth. *Phytopathology 71*, 408-11.

McCoy, R.E., Thomas, D.L., Tsai, J.H. and French, W.J. (1978). Periwinkle wilt, a new disease associated with xylem delimited rickettsialike bacteria transmitted by a sharpshooter. *Plant Disease Reporter 62*, 1022-6.

McCrum, R.C. (1974). Antigens to *Mycoplasma orale* antisera in the sap of aster yellows infected plants. *Abstracts of the International Congress on Mycoplasmas of Man, Animals, Plants and Insects, Bordeaux*, 27.

McGhee, R.B. and Postell, F.J. (1976). Axenic cultivation of *Phytomonas davidi* Lafont (Trypanosomatidae), a symbiote of laticiferous plants (Euphorbiaceae). *Journal of Protozoology 23*, 238-41.

McIntosh, A.H. and Maramorosch, K. (1973). Mycoplasma and acholeplasma in plants. *Annals of the New York Academy of Sciences 225*, 330-3.

McIntosh, A.H., Maramorosch, K. and Kondo, F. (1977). Serological comparison of four plant spiroplasmas. *Proceedings of the American Phytopathological Society 4*, 193.

McIntosh, A.H., Skowronski, B.S. and Maramorosch, K. (1974). Rapid identification of *Spiroplasma citri* and its relation to other yellows agents. *Phytopathologische Zeitschrift 80*, 153-6.

Mircetich, S.M., Lowe, S.K., Moller, W.J. and Nyland, G. (1976). Etiology of almond leaf scorch disease and transmission of the causal agent. *Phytopathology 66*, 17-24.

Mitsuhashi, J. and Maramorosch, K. (1964). Inoculation of plant tissue cultures with aster yellows virus. *Virology 23*, 277-9.

Moll, J.N. and Martin, M.M. (1973). Electron microscope evidence that citrus psylla (*Trioza erytreae*) is a vector of greening disease in South Africa. *Phytophylactica 5*, 41-4.

— (1974). Comparison of the organism causing greening disease with several plant pathogenic gram-negative bacteria, rickettsia-like organisms and mycoplasma-like organisms. *Les Mycoplasmes/Mycoplasmas. Les Colloques de l'Institut National de la Santé et de la Recherche Médicale 33,* 89-96.

Mollenhauer, H.H. and Hopkins, D.L. (1974). Ultrastructural study of Pierce's disease bacterium in grape xylem tissue. *Journal of Bacteriology 119*, 612-18.

Musil, M. (1964). Persistence of infectivity of yellow-type viruses in frozen viruliferous leafhoppers. *Acta Virologia 8*, 92.

Nasu, S., Jensen, D.D. and Richardson, J. (1974a). Extraction of western X mycoplasma-like organism from leafhoppers and celery infected with peach western X disease. *Applied Entomology and Zoology 9*, 53-7.

— (1974b). Isolation of western X mycoplasma-like organism from infectious extracts of leafhoppers and celery. *Applied Entomology and Zoology 9*, 199-203.

— (1974c). Primary culturing of the western X mycoplasma-like organism from *Colladonus montanus* leafhopper vectors. *Applied Entomology and Zoology 9*, 115-26.

Nault, L.R. and Bradfute, E. (1979). Corn stunt: involvement of a complex of leafhopper-borne pathogens. In *Leafhopper Vectors and Plant Disease Agents*, pp. 561-86, K. Maramorosch and K.F. Harris (eds). New York & London:

Academic Press.

Nienhaus, F., Rumbos, I. and Green, S. (1979). Rickettsialike organisms isolated from plants cultivated in chick embryo. In *Third International Congress of Plant Pathology, abstracts of papers*, p. 62. Berlin & Hamburg: Paul Parey.

Nienhaus, F. and Sikora, R.A. (1979). Mycoplasmas, spiroplasmas, and rickettsialike organisms as plant pathogens. *Annual Review of Plant Pathology 17*, 37–58.

Nieschulz, O. (1931). Die parasitischen Protozoen der Pflanzen. In *Handbuch der Pathogenen Protozoen*, pp. 1799–813, S. von Prowarek and W. Noller (eds). Leipzig: J.A. Barth.

Nomé, S.F., Raju, B.C. and Nyland, G. (1980). ELISA for the detection of lethal yellowing agent in diseased coconuts. In *Proceedings of the Fourth Meeting of the International Council on Lethal Yellowing, Fort Lauderdale, 1979*, p. 11. University of Florida Publication FL-80-1.

Nyland, G., Goheen, A.C., Lowe, S.K. and Kirkpatrick, H.C. (1973). The ultrastructure of a rickettsialike organism from a peach tree affected with phony disease. *Phytopathology 63*, 1275–8.

Page, L.A. (1977). The Chlamydiae. In *CRC Handbook of Microbiology*, 2nd edn, pp. 397–404. A.I. Laskin and H.A. Lechevalier (eds). Cleveland: CRC Press Inc.

Parthasarathy, M.V. and van Slobbe, W.G. (1978). Hartrot or fatal wilt of palms I. Coconuts (*Cocos nucifera*). *Principes – Journal of the Palm Society 22*, 3–14.

Parthasarathy, M.V., van Slobbe, W.G. and Soudant, C. (1976). Trypanosomatid flagellate in the phloem of diseased coconut palms. *Science 192*, 1346–8.

Petrů, E., Limberk, J., Ulrychová, M. and Brčák, J. (1971). Growth and infectivity of callus cultures of tomato plants infected with a mycoplasma disease – potato witches' broom. *Biologia Plantarum 13*, 391–5.

Petrů, E. and Ulrychová, M. (1975). Persistence and spread of Mycoplasma in axenic callus tissue cultures of tobacco (*Nicotiana glauca* Grah.) in the presence of kinetin and IAA in the nutrient medium. *Biologia Plantarum 17*, 352–6.

— (1978). Behaviour of MLO evoking potato witches' broom in callus tissue culture of *Solanum laciniatum* Ait. and *Nicotiana tabacum* L. cv. Samsun. *Biologia Plantarum 20*, 383–6.

Poinar, G.O. and Thomas, G.M. (1978). *Diagnostic Manual for the Identification of Insect Pathogens*, p. 60. New York & London: Plenum Press.

Purcell, A.H., Latorre-Guzman, B.A., Kado, C.I., Goheen, A.C, and Shalla, T.A. (1977). Reinvestigation of the role of a lactobacillus associated with leafhopper vectors of Pierce's disease of grapevines. *Phytopathology 67*, 298–301.

Raju, B.C. and Nyland, G. (1978). Effects of different media on the growth and morphology of three newly isolated plant spiroplasmas. *Phytopathology News 12*, 216.

Raju, B.C., Purcell, A.H. and Nyland, G. (1980). Isolation of spiroplasmas from leafhoppers exposed to aster yellows and X-disease. In *Proceedings of the Fourth Meeting of the International Council on Lethal Yellowing, Fort Lauderdale, 1979*, p. 12. University of Florida Publication FL-80-1.

Rubio-Huertos, M. and Beltra, R. (1962). Fixed pathogenic L forms of *Agrobacterium tumefaciens. Nature 195*, 101.

Sabin, A.B. (1941). The filtrable microorganisms of the pleuropneumonia group. *Bacteriological Reviews 5*, 1–66 & 331–5.

Saglio, P.H.M. (1979). Motility and improvement in selective isolation of spiroplasmas. *Plant Disease Reporter 63*, 293–6.

Saglio, P.H.M., Daniels, M.J. and Pradet, A. (1979). ATP and energy charge as criteria of growth and metabolic activity of mollicutes: application to *Spiroplasma citri. Journal of General Microbiology 110*, 13–20.

Saglio, P., Laflèche, D., Bonissol, C. and Bové, M. (1971). Isolement, culture et observation au microscope électronique des structures de type mycoplasme associées à la maladie du Stubborn des agrumes et leur comparaison avec les structures observées dans le cas de la maladie du Greening des agrumes. *Physiologie Végétale 9*, 569–82.

Saglio, P.H.M. and Whitcomb, R.F. (1979). Diversity of wall-less prokaryotes in plant vascular tissue, fungi and invertebrate animals. In *The Mycoplasmas*, Vol. III, pp. 1–36, R.F. Whitcomb and J.G. Tully (eds). New York & London: Academic Press.

Schneider, E.L. (1975). Detection of mycoplasma contamination in cultured cells: comparison of biochemical, morphological and microbiological techniques. In *Methods in Cell Biology*, Vol. 10, pp. 261–75, D.M. Prescott (ed). New York & London: Academic Press.

Schneider, E.L. and Stanbridge, E.J. (1975). A simple biochemical technique for the detection of mycoplasma contamination in cultured cells. In *Methods in Cell Biology*, Vol. 10, pp. 277–90, D.M. Prescott (eds). New York & London: Academic Press.

Seiffert, G. (1937a) Über das Vorkommen filtrabler Mikroorganismen in der Natur und ihre Züchtbarkeit. *Zentralblatt für Bakteriologie, Parasitenkunde, Infectionskrankheiten und Hygiene, Erste Abteilung Originale 139*, 337–42.

— (1937b). Filtrabler Mikroorganismen in der freien Natur. *Zentralblatt für Bakteriologie, Parasitenkunde, Infectionskrankheiten und Hygiene, Erste Abteilung Originale 140*, 168–72.

Sethi, K.K. and Nienhaus, F. (1974). Attempts at reisolation of *Acholeplasma laidlawii* after experimental inoculation in plants. *Phytopathologische Zeitschrift 80*, 88–90.

Sinha, R.C. (1974). Purification of mycoplasma-like organisms from china aster plants affected with clover phyllody. *Phytopathology 64*, 1156–8.

— (1976). Ultrastructure of mycoplasma-like organisms purified from clover phyllody-affected plants. *Journal of Ultrastructural Research 54*, 183–9.

— (1979). Purification and serology of mycoplasma-like organisms from aster yellows-infected plants. *Canadian Journal of Plant Pathology 1*, 65–70.

Sinha, R.C. and Chiykowski, L.N. (1967). Initial and subsequent sites of aster yellows virus infection in a leafhopper vector. *Virology 33*, 702–8.

Smith, A.J. (1980). Factors affecting maintenance *in vitro* of aster yellows pathogenicity. In *Proceedings of the Fourth Meeting of the International Council on Lethal Yellowing, Fort Lauderdale, 1979*, p. 12. University of Florida Publication FL-80-1.

Smith, P.F. (1971). *The Biology of Mycoplasmas*. New York & London: Academic press.

Stahel, G. (1931). Zur Kenntnis der Siebrohrenkrankheit (Phloemnekrose) des Kaffeebaumes in Surinam I. Mikroskopische Untersuchungen und Infektionsversuche. *Phytopathologische Zeitschrift 4*, 65–82.

Steere, R.L. (1967). Gel filtration of aster yellows virus. *Phytopathology 57*, 832–3.

Steindl, D.R.L. (1961). Ratoon stunting disease. In *Sugarcane Diseases of the World*, Vol. 1, pp. 433–59, J.P. Martin, E.V. Abbott and C.G. Hughes (eds). Amsterdam: Elsevier.

Sugiura, M., Shiomi, T., Nasu, S. and Mizukami, T. (1977). Artificial culture of plant pathogenic mycoplasma-like organism (MLO). In *Tropical Agriculture Research Series 10: Symposium on Virus Diseases of Tropical Crops*, 85–91.

Teakle, D.S., Smith, P.M. and Steindl, D.R.L. (1973). Association of a small coryneform bacterium with the ratoon stunting disease of sugar-cane. *Australian Journal of Agricultural Research 24*, 869–74.

Teranaka, M., Okuda, S., Suzuki, I. and Wakaida, M. (1976). A trial to culture causal agent of plant mycoplasma disease and effect of plant macerating juice on growth of bovine mycoplasma (*Mycoplasma* sp.) and *Acholeplasma laidlawii*. *Bulletin of the College of Agriculture, Utsonomi University*, 1-9, (English summary and tables.)

Thompson, S.V., Davis, M.J. and Kloepper, J.W. (1979). Alfalfa dwarf: relationship to the bacterium causing Pierce's disease of grapevines and almond leaf scorch disease. In *Third International Congress of Plant Pathology, Abstracts of Papers*, p. 65. Berlin & Hamburg: Paul Parey.

Townsend, R., Eden-Green, S.J., Markham, P.G., Archer, D. and Clark, M.F. (1980). Acholeplasmas and lethal yellowing disease III: microbiological and serological studies. In *Proceedings of the Fourth Meeting of the International Council on Lethal Yellowing, Fort Lauderdale, 1979*, p. 11. University of Florida Publication FL-80-1.

Townsend, R., Markham, P.G. and Plaskitt, K.A. (1977). Multiplication and morphology of *Spiroplasma citri* in the leafhopper *Euscelis plebejus*. *Annals of Applied Biology 87*, 307-13.

Tully, J.G. (1979). Special features of the Acholeplasmas. In *The Mycoplasmas*, Vol. I, pp. 431-49, M. Barile and S. Razin (eds). New York & London: Academic Press.

Tully, J.G., Rose, D.L., Whitcomb, R.F. and Wenzel, R.P. (1979). Enhanced isolation of *Mycoplasma pneumoniae* from throat washings with a newly modified culture medium. *Journal of Infectious Diseases 139*, 478-82.

Tully, J.G., Whitcomb, R.F., Bové, J.M. and Saglio, P. (1973). Plant mycoplasmas: serological relation between agents associated with citrus stubborn and corn stunt diseases. *Science 182*, 827-9.

Tully, J.G., Whitcomb, R.F. and Clark, H.F. (1976). Suckling mouse cataract agent is a helical wall-free prokaryote (spiroplasma) pathogenic for vertebrates. *Nature 259*, 117-20.

Tully, J.G., Whitcomb, R.F., Clark, H.F. and Williamson, D.L. (1977). Pathogenic mycoplasmas: cultivation and vertebrate pathogenicity of a new spiroplasma. *Science 195*, 892-4.

Ulrychová, M. and Petrů, E. (1975). Elimination of mycoplasma in tobacco callus tissues. (*Nicotiana glauca* Grah.) cultured *in vitro* in the presence of 2, 4-D in nutrient medium. *Biologia Plantarum 17*, 103-8.

van Die, J. and Tammes, P.M.L. (1975). Phloem exudation from monocotyledonous axes. In *Transport in plants I: Phloem Transport (Encyclopedia of Plant Physiology, New Series, Vol. 1)*, pp. 196-222, M.H. Zimmermann and J.A. Milburn (eds). Berlin, Heidelberg & New York: Springer-Verlag.

Vermeulen, H. (1963). A wilt of *Coffea liberica* in Surinam and its association with a flagellate, *Phytomonas leptovasorum* Stahel. *Journal of Protozoology 10*, 216-22.

— (1968). Investigations into the cause of the phloem necrosis disease of *Coffea liberica* in Surinam, South America. *Netherlands Journal of Plant Pathology 74*, 202-18.

Waters, H. (1978). A wilt disease of coconuts from Trinidad associated with *Phytomonas* sp., a sieve tube-restricted protozoan flagellate. *Annals of Applied Biology 90*, 293-302.

Waters, H. and Hunt, P. (1980). The *in vivo* three-dimensional form of a plant mycoplasma-like organism by the analysis of serial ultrathin sections. *Journal of General Microbiology 116*, 111-31.

Whitcomb, R.F. (1972). Bioassay of clover wound tumor virus and the mycoplasma-like organisms of peach western X and aster yellows. *United States Department of Agriculture Technical Bulletin 1438*, 32 pp.

— (1978). Preparation of antisera from infected host antigen. In *Proceedings of the Third Meeting of the International Council on Lethal Yellowing, West Palm Beach, 1977*, p. 16. University of Florida Publication FL-78-2.

Whitcomb, R.F. and Davis, R.E. (1969). Properties of the aster yellows agent. *Phytopathology 59*, 1561.

Whitcomb, R.F., Jensen, D.D. and Richardson, J. (1966). The infection of leaf-hoppers by western X-disease virus II. Fluctuation of virus concentration in the hemolymph after injection. *Virology 28*, 454–8.

— (1968). The infection of leafhoppers by western X-disease virus V. Properties of the infectious agent. *Journal of Invertebrate Pathology 12*, 192-201.

Whitcomb, R.F., Tully, J.G., Bové, J.M. and Saglio, P. (1973). Spiroplasmas and acholeplasmas: multiplication in insects. *Science 182*, 1251-3.

Williamson, D.L. and Whitcomb, R.F. (1975). Plant mycoplasmas: a cultivable spiroplasma causes corn stunt disease. *Science 188*, 1018-20.

Windsor, I.M. and Black, L.M. (1972). Clover club-leaf: a possible rickettsial disease of plants. *Phytopathology 62*, 1112.

— (1973). Evidence that clover club leaf is caused by a rickettsia-like organism. *Phytopathology 63*, 1139-48.

Wolanski, B. (1973). Negative staining of plant agents. *Annals of the New York Academy of Sciences 225*, 223-35.

Wolanski, B. and Maramorosch, K. (1970). Negatively stained mycoplasmas: fact or artifact? *Virology 42*, 319-27.

8 SEROLOGICAL CHARACTERISATION OF SPIROPLASMAS AND OTHER MYCOPLASMAS

David L. Williamson

1. Introduction

Serological studies of mycoplasmas of plant and arthropod origin have been almost exclusively directed toward identification and classification. Except for *Acholeplasma* spp. isolated from phloem sap of coconut palms affected by lethal yellowing disease (Eden-Green, 1978; Eden-Green *et al.*, 1979) and from *Vinca rosea* (Spaar *et al.*, 1974) all mycoplasmas that have been cultivated from plants and insects and identified are *Spiroplasma* spp. Recently, however, other nonhelical mycoplasmas have been isolated from flowers, but have not been identified (Davis, 1978; Davis *et al.*, 1979) (see Chapter 1).

It is the purpose of this chapter to provide details of those serological procedures which have had or which should have great utility in the serological characterisation of plant and insect mycoplasmas. Most of the standard procedures such as growth inhibition, metabolism inhibition, complement fixation, interface precipitin ring and gel diffusion have been used in these studies and reference to their application will be cited as each procedure is considered. One new technique, the deformation (DF) test (Williamson *et al.*, 1978) has been

240

specifically devised for studies of spiroplasmas; more recently
(Williamson *et al.*, 1979) the DF test has been combined with the
classical metabolism inhibition test in single microtitre plates. The
epi-immunofluorescence test (Del Giudice *et al.*, 1967) and the enzyme-
linked immunosorbent assay (ELISA) (Engvall and Perlmann, 1971)
are highly useful serological procedures which are applicable to identification and classification of plant and insect mycoplasmas (Archer
and Best, 1980).

Other procedures, such as two-dimensional immunoelectrophoresis
(Wróblewski, 1975; Archer and Best, 1980), and immunoperoxidase
staining used to study specific cellular components (Williamson *et al.*,
1979) or the use of immunoperoxidase staining to identify mycoplasmas
in plant tissues (de Leeuw, 1977) are beyond the scope of this chapter.

2. Antigen Preparation and Antiserum Production

The availability of highly specific and potent antisera is absolutely
essential for meaningful serological studies. Some of the problems
which may be encountered in the preparation of these antisera and
approaches to dealing with them have been recently discussed in some
detail by Kenny (1979) and Tully (1979); they will be considered only
briefly here.

One of the most serious problems relates to the contamination of
pelleted mycoplasmas with substances from the medium. Because
serum proteins may be adsorbed on to the surface of mycoplasmas, it
is recommended (Kenny, 1979) that agamma serum or 1-5% bovine
serum fraction be used for supplementing media. Other approaches,
such as growth of the antigen in media supplemented with serum
homologous to the immunising animal, e.g. rabbit serum as a supplement
for antigens to be injected into rabbits (Bradbury and Jordan, 1972),
or growth of the immunising antigen and the test antigen in media
supplemented with sera from different sources (e.g. calf and horse)
have not been widely utilised in serological studies of plant and insect
mycoplasmas.

All culturable mycoplasmas to be used as antigens must be triply
cloned prior to immunisation to ensure that a single serotype is being
used. Plant and insect mycoplasmas refractory to *in vitro* cultivation
can be studied serologically by preparing antigens from diseased plants
(Tully *et al.*, 1973) or by pooling insect hemolymph (Williamson and
Whitcomb, 1974). Although it should be possible to use homogenates

of infected insects to prepare antigens for immunisation, this approach has received very little attention. The following procedures for the preparation of cultivatable mycoplasmas as immunising antigens and the schedule for the immunisation of rabbits are in routine use in the laboratory of Dr J.G. Tully, Mycoplasma Section, Laboratory of Infectious Diseases, National Institutes of Health, Bethesda, Maryland, USA. They are reproduced here with the permission of Dr Tully.

A. Antigen Preparation

(1) Antigens are grown in 500–1000 ml of broth culture medium and harvested before the pH of the medium becomes too acidic or too basic. Highly acidic conditions (pH 5–6) promote the precipitation of proteins on to the surface of mycoplasmas. This problem can be alleviated by the addition of 1.4% HEPES buffer to the medium (C. Mouches, personal communication).

(2) Mycoplasmas are harvested by centrifugation at 20,000–30,000 g for 30–45 minutes. The pellet is washed by resuspending it in 100–200 ml phosphate buffered saline, pH 7.3 (PBS) which is isotonic with the blood of the immunising animal. The resuspended pellet is recentrifuged at 20,000–30,000 g and the resulting pellet is washed a second time and centrifuged again. The pellet is then taken up in 4 ml PBS for each 500 ml of original broth culture and mixed by use of a vortex mixer to completely resuspend the cells.

(3) For immunisation, 4 ml of antigen suspension are mixed with 4 ml of Freund's complete adjuvant. This should be done just prior to injection. It is essential that the mycoplasma suspension and the adjuvant be completely emulsified. This can be done simply at room temperature by securely connecting two 10 ml syringes (plastic or glass) with a 1–2 inch piece of flexible plastic tubing. The mixture is poured into one syringe, or taken up prior to connecting the two syringes and then pushed back and forth until it is emulsified (a drop on the surface of clean water in a beaker should spread evenly). Remaining antigen suspension can be frozen at −70°C for later use (after mixing with adjuvant) in booster injections.

B. Immunisation Schedule

(1) Two rabbits, 1.5–2 kg, are immunised with the same antigen. The sex of the rabbits is not important, but males and females should be kept in separate cages. A pre-immunisation bleeding (10 ml) of each rabbit should be performed to provide approximately 5 ml of pre-immune serum from each animal. The following schedule has been

successful in providing high-titre antisera against many mycoplasmas
and spiroplasmas.

Day	Site	Inoculation Volume	Remarks
0	intramuscular	0.5 ml	Use high and low sites in right and left shoulder muscles (total volume 4 ml/2 rabbits)
	intradermal	0.8 ml	Divide among 4 sites in skin along centre of back after shaving hair (total volume 1.6 ml/2 rabbits)
21	–	–	Test bleeding (10 ml/rabbit)
	intramuscular	0.5 ml	Give booster shot in both right and left shoulders and in hip muscles (total volume 4 ml/2 rabbits)
28	–	–	Test bleeding (10 ml/rabbit)
35	–	–	Test bleeding (10 ml/rabbit)
42	–	–	Test bleeding. This usually proves to be an adequate time interval for development of good antiserum. However, if the titre is still increasing, continue test bleeding at 1 week intervals until it stabilises.

(2) At the end of the immunisation schedule the rabbits are anaesthetised and ex-sanguinated by heart puncture. Removal of food 18 hours
prior to this procedure will greatly decrease the lipid content of the
blood; lipids can cause problems in the precipitin ring and spiroplasma
deformation tests. Collected blood is dispensed gently into centrifuge
tubes to avoid hemolysis, allowed to clot and then centrifuged ($1000\,g$).
Antiserum is kept at $-70°C$ for long-term storage and at $-20°C$ for
current usage.
(3) The potencies of the antisera are usually tested by growth inhibition
(see below).

3. Serological Procedures

The serological procedures presented here are those having widest
application in the identification and classification of plant and insect
mycoplasmas. The test chosen should be determined by the level of

classification desired. Most of the tests recognise inter- and intra-species relationships based on membrane-derived antigens, but at varying levels of sensitivity. However, the complement fixation, precipitin ring and immunodiffusion tests involve soluble, presumably cytoplasmic, antigens as well as membrane antigens and the antisera used in such tests may therefore show considerable cross-reactivity.

A. Growth Inhibition

The growth inhibition (GI) test is presented first because it is the most useful test for evaluating the quality of an antiserum produced against a cultivable mycoplasma and because it has widest application in separating mycoplasma species (Subcommittee on the Taxonomy of Mollicutes, 1979). The test is based upon the observation that mycoplasma growth on solid media is inhibited by antiserum. A complete discussion of the method, including pertinent references, is provided by World Health Organisation Working Document VPH/MIC/76.7. Three basic variations have been described for the application of antiserum: (1) agar-well, (2) serum-drop, and (3) filter paper disc. Only the paper disc method introduced by Huijsmans-Evers and Ruys (1956) and refined by Clyde (1964), has received wide acceptance. The disc growth inhibition method currently in use is as follows:

(1)   Preparation of Paper Discs.
(a)   Filter paper discs 5.5–7 mm in diameter are autoclaved in Petri dishes and allowed to dry thoroughly.
(b)   Using sterile technique, a single disc is saturated with 25 μl of undiluted antiserum or preimmune serum previously sterilised by membrane filtration (450 nm).
(c)   Discs are allowed to become thoroughly dry at 37°C. Dried discs can be stored in sterile vials at 4°C for short-term and −20°C for long-term storage.

(2)   Preparation of Agar Plates.
(a)   Agar plates are poured (60 x 15 mm) to a depth of 3.5–4 mm.
(b)   Plates should be dried at 37°C for one or more hours to free them of condensed water.

(3)   Antigen Titration and Plate Inoculation.
(a)   Antigens to be tested are grown in broth medium and a sample from each is removed for titration of the culture by colony forming units (cfu). The cultures are frozen at −70°C for later use in GI tests.
(b)   Following determination of the titre of each antigen to be tested, frozen cultures are removed from the freezer, thawed at 37°C, and

three 1 ml volume dilutions made to contain 10^4, 10^5 and 10^6 cfu/ml.

(c) The agar plate is inoculated by placing 0.1 ml of each broth culture dilution on the agar surface at the centre of each plate. The plate is tipped to spread the inoculum and set aside until the inoculum has been absorbed (approximately 30 minutes).

(4) Antiserum Application.

(a) Using sterile forceps, a paper disc saturated with homologous or heterologous antiserum and a saturated disc with pre-immune serum are placed on the surface of each test plate.

(b) The disc is pressed gently, without deforming the agar surface, to assure adherence of the disc. The bottom surface of the plate is marked to identify each disc.

(5) Incubation and Evaluation of Plates.

(a) Each plate is inverted and incubated at the temperature and atmosphere which are optimal for growth of the colonies.

(b) Plates are observed daily with the use of a dissecting microscope or low-power objectives of a compound microscope. The zone of inhibition is measured from the edge of the paper disc to the edge of the area of colonies. Zones of inhibition may not always be well-defined; partial inhibition, in which there is a marked reduction in the size and/or number of colonies around the disc, may occur with weak antisera. Total inhibition has been defined by Ernϕ and Jurmanova (1973) as inhibition associated with the occurrence of less than ten breakthrough colonies. Zones of inhibition which are less than 1–2 mm are equivocal.

(c) After utilisation of the immunisation schedule outlined above, inhibition zones should be 5–15 mm around discs soaked with undiluted antiserum. Zones smaller than 5 mm indicate weak antisera and the immunisation period may be extended for 3–4 weeks in an attempt to improve the quality of the antiserum. After this period, any rabbit that fails to produce a 5–7 mm zone should be bled out and the immunisation repeated with new animals.

B. Immunofluorescence

Fluorescent antibody (FA) staining of mycoplasmas is *direct* if the fluorescing compound (fluorescein isothiocyanate) is conjugated with the antibody made against the mycoplasma. It is *indirect* if the conjugated antibody is directed against the IgG of the species of animal immunised against the mycoplasma and secondarily coupled to specific antibody bound to mycoplasmal antigen. Although it is a sensitive and useful technique, the indirect FA procedure has had little application in the study of plant and insect mycoplasmas and no further consideration will be given to it. However, the direct FA technique has proved to be a highly useful serological procedure for the identification of all mycoplasmas. Its application to the study of plant and insect mycoplasmas will now be considered.

The direct FA test on agar colonies compares favourably to the GI test in its specificity, but is much more sensitive because conjugation with fluorescein permits detection of small amounts of antigen-antibody complexes. Furthermore, the FA test can be used to determine the presence of mixtures of serotypes on the culture plate. The original FA technique (Clark *et al.*, 1961; Carski and Shepard, 1961) in which stained agar colony impressions on glass slides or coverslips were observed microscopically with transmitted ultra-violet light has now been largely replaced by the *epi-fluorescent antibody* technique in which the stained colonies are observed under incident UV illumination (Del Giudice *et al.*, 1967). Further refinements of the epi-FA procedure have been made which lessen the amount of conjugated antibody needed for the test (Al-Aubaidi and Fabricant, 1971; Rosendal and Black, 1972).

The procedure described here is based on that currently used by David L. Rose in the laboratory of Dr Joseph G. Tully, National Institutes of Health, Bethesda, Maryland, USA.

(1) Antiserum. Antisera should be selected on the basis of their growth-inhibiting activity. A proper experimental set consists of an antiserum and a similar volume of pre-immunisation serum. Those antisera producing GI zones of 5–10 mm will usually be suitable for fluorescein conjugation.

(2) Immunoglobulin Fractionation from Whole Serum.

(a) Using a flask or beaker, add 10 ml of the antiserum to be conjugated to 10 ml saturated ammonium sulfate (80–90 g/100 ml distilled water) to precipitate the globulin. Stopper or cover and place at 4°C overnight.

(b) The following day centrifuge the suspension at 15,000 g for 20 minutes. Resuspend the pellet in 2 ml sterile distilled water.

(c) Transfer dissolved globulin to dialysis tube and dialyse against 1 litre PBS (0.15M sodium chloride, 0.01M sodium phosphate buffer, pH 7.5) at 4°C with stirring. Change PBS 3 or 4 times during the day and before leaving at night. Continue dialysis overnight.

(3) Conjugation of Globulin with Fluorescein.

(a) Prepare carbonate buffer:
    (1) Add 420 mg sodium bicarbonate to 10 ml distilled water.
    (2) Add 530 mg sodium carbonate to 10 ml distilled water.
    (3) Mix 10 ml solution (1) with 1.9 ml solution (2) (pH 9.0).

(b) Transfer globulin fraction from dialysis tube to 50 ml graduated flask or cylinder and bring volume to 20 ml with PBS.

(c) Add 3 ml of carbonate buffer (3) to 20 ml globulin solution.

(d) Add 15 mg fluorescein isothiocyanate (FITC) to the carbonate buffered globulin solution and stir on a magnetic stirrer overnight at 4°C.

(4) Purification of Conjugate.

(a) Following conjugation, free FITC is removed from the crude conjugate by dialysis for 6–8 hours against one-litre volumes of PBS (pH 7.5) at 4°C. The PBS is changed every two hours.

(b) The crude conjugate is purified further by passing it through a 1 cm x 40 cm Sephadex G-25 (course) column at 4°C. PBS is used for equilibration and elution of the column.

(c) Aliquots of 0.5–2 ml of FITC-labelled globulin are frozen at −70°C.

(d) Twofold dilutions of the conjugate in PBS (1:2–1:2048) are tested against homologous mycoplasma colonies. Fluorescence of dilution is judged at 0, +, ++, +++, ++++ for none, weak, moderate, strong and very strong fluorescence. Dilutions giving 3+ or 4+ fluorescence are used for future tests involving the conjugate.

(5) Procedure for Staining of Agar Colonies.

(a) Agar plate procedure:
    (1) Flood plate with 5 ml PBS. Decant PBS and repeat once or twice. Decant last wash after 10–15 minutes' incubation.
    (2) Cover the surface of the agar with 1–2 ml of the working dilution of the conjugate. Cover the plate. Incubate at room temperature for 30 minutes with periodic (5-minute intervals) gentle swirling of the conjugate over the agar surface.
    (3) Decant conjugate. Wash surface 3 times with 3–5 ml PBS. Allow the last wash to incubate at room temperature for 10–15 minutes. Last wash can incubate overnight if PBS contains 1:2000 parts thallium acetate and 1000 units of penicillin/ml.
    (4) Decant PBS. Rinse once with distilled water. Dry agar surface (lid off) by placing in 37°C incubator for 30–60 minutes.
    (5) One agar plate should be stained with FITC-labelled pre-immunisation globulin.

(b) Agar block procedure:
  (1) Wash plate with PBS as described in 5(a)(1) above.
  (2) Cut agar into blocks (5 mm x 5 mm) each containing at least one colony.
  (3) Place 4-6 blocks on a single microscope slide, colony side up. Blocks can be secured to slide by ringing each block with a warm mixture of 65% paraffin wax and 35% vaseline.
  (4) One drop (approx. 25 μl) of the working dilution of the conjugate is placed on each agar block. One or more blocks should be stained with FITC-labelled pre-immunisation globulin.
  (5) Place slide in a dish or tray with moistened paper or towel in the bottom, cover and incubate at room temperature for 30 minutes.
  (6) Remove conjugate by flooding tray with PBS. Repeat once or twice, allowing last wash to incubate at room temperature for 10-15 minutes.
  (7) Pour off PBS. Rinse once with distilled water. Dry agar surface in 37°C incubator.
(c) Microscopic examination of stained colonies with incident illumination:
  (1) First locate colonies with visible light and then switch to ultra-violet light.
  (2) The following equipment provides high-quality FITC epifluorescence. It is presented here as a guide for those laboratories not already equipped for epifluorescence. All items mentioned are obtainable from Carl Zeiss, Oberkochen, West Germany.
      (i) Quartz halogen light source (Halogen Illuminator for Zeiss Standard or WL Microscopes). High light emission in the blue range (up to 490 nm) for FITC (peak excitation wavelength for fluorescein is 492 nm).
      (ii) Vertical illuminator III RS (Zeiss Number 46 62 49 9904) containing exciter-barrier filter and reflector combination for FITC fluorescence (Zeiss Number 48 77 09).

C. The Spiroplasma Deformation (DF) Test

The deformation test (tube method) (Williamson *et al.*, 1978) was devised specifically for spiroplasmas. It is a simple and highly sensitive technique capable of demonstrating significant antigenic differences among spiroplasmas. The test is based on the fact that helical spiroplasmas when exposed to specific antibody are completely or partially deformed. Partially deformed spiroplasmas are affected at only one point, usually at an end. Such helices are freely moving at the unaffected end. The DF test utilises small amounts of antiserum and results can be obtained 30 minutes after antiserum and antigen are mixed. It requires the use of a high-quality dark-field microscope for evaluation and determination of titres. The details of the DF procedure are given in the report by Williamson *et al.* (1978). It can be performed either in small culture tubes or in microtitre plates. The tube method is described here.

(1) Antigens. Broth cultures of spiroplasmas are diluted (1:2, 1:4 or greater if necessary) in medium used for their cultivation and in volumes sufficient to perform the test. A dilution providing a mean number of 40–60 spiroplasmas per 1,250x field should be used for performing the test. The uninoculated culture medium should be free of small particulate material which may be confused with deformed helices; it should be filtered through a 450 nm membrane filter.

(2) Antiserum Dilutions.

(a) Antisera are heat-inactivated (56°C for 30 minutes) and filtered through 450 nm membrane filters prior to use. Pre-immunisation sera are included as controls for each antiserum used.

(b) Twofold or threefold dilutions are made in tubes in the medium used to grow the spiroplasmas. For high-quality antisera, 10–12 dilution tubes will be required for the test.

(c) Dilutions of a pre-immunisation serum should also be made. Twofold dilutions to 1:64 or threefold to 1:81 are normally sufficient for this control series.

(d) Twofold and/or threefold dilutions of both antisera and pre-immunisation sera can be prepared as stock dilutions in 200–400 μl aliquots in 400–500 μl volume stoppered plastic tubes and frozen at −70°C for future serological tests.

(3) Test Procedure.

(a) Glass culture tubes (6 x 50 mm) are placed in a rack and marked for identification.

(b) Transfer 0.025 ml (25 μl) from each serum dilution to its appropriate culture tube. One culture tube should receive only 25 μl of medium and serves as an antigen control.

(c) Add 0.025 ml (25 μl) of the appropriate spiroplasma suspension to each dilution tube plus the antigen control tube. Cover tubes with plastic wrap or parafilm and incubate at room temperature.

(d) DF endpoint determination can be made after 30 minutes incubation.

    (1) Remove 5–7 μl from the antigen control tube, place on a clean

microscopic slide, cover with a No. 1 coverglass and examine the preparation by dark-field microscopy. Note the density of the spiroplasmas (there should be 20–30/1250x field) and their condition – they should be helical, motile, and free of distortion in size and shape.

(2) Read the pre-immunisation serum dilution series next. Begin with the highest dilution and examine progressively lower dilutions, sampling as described above. Each tube should be examined for completely free and motile spiroplasmas, as well as for evidence of deformed helices.

(3) Read the antiserum dilution series. Again, start at the highest dilution and examine progressively lower dilutions. Assuming that the spiroplasmas are free and not deformed at the highest dilution, a dilution will be found in which all organisms are completely or partially deformed.

(4) The tube in which approximately one-half the spiroplasmas are completely free and motile and one-half either completely or partially deformed, is called the DF endpoint. The reciprocal of the total antiserum dilution (taking into account the two-fold dilution by the antigen suspension) is the DF titre.

(5) If the endpoint is determined to be between two tubes, the lower antiserum dilution is used for the DF endpoint.

D. The Metabolism Inhibition (MI) Test

The metabolism inhibition test (Taylor-Robinson *et al.*, 1966) is a very specific and highly sensitive test for identification and characterisation of mycoplasmas at the species or intraspecies levels. The test is similar to the growth inhibition test except that it measures inhibition of growth in a liquid medium. Mycoplasma growth is evaluated by a change in colour of a pH indicator. Specific antibody inhibits the growth of the organism and thus production of the metabolic products that cause the colour change. The MI endpoint is determined by titrating the antiserum against a previously determined fixed number of colour changing units (CCU) of the organism being tested. Utilisation of such substrates as glucose (Taylor-Robinson *et al.*, 1966), arginine (Purcell *et al.*, 1966a), urea (Purcell *et al*, 1966b) or tetrazolium (Senterfit and Jensen, 1966) has been used to measure inhibition.

Chen and Liao (1975) used the MI test (Taylor-Robinson *et al.*, 1966) to study relationships between spiroplasmas. A more complete study of spiroplasma interrelationships was done by Williamson *et al.* (1979) using a combined deformation-metabolism inhibition test (see below).

A detailed discussion of the MI test procedure is provided by World Health Organisation Working Document VPH/MIC/75.6; additional information can be obtained from the review by Purcell *et al.* (1969).

(1) Antigen Titration.

(a) In the MI procedure, antiserum is titrated against a fixed number of organisms. It is therefore necessary to standardise the amount of antigen (in colour changing units/ml) in a preliminary titration. At the same time the antigen is being titrated, the need for complement can be assessed in the test system. Mycoplasmas for titration are grown in broth medium in 100 ml volumes, monitored to obtain organisms from logarithmic phase cultures, and the culture is then distributed into 2-3 ml vials which are frozen at $-70°C$.

(b) Antigen dilutions.

(1) Vials of frozen stock antigen are removed from the freezer and allowed to thaw at room temperature.

(2) A tenfold dilution series $(10^{-1}-10^{-8})$ in 1 ml volumes is made in broth medium that contains a pH indicator, such as phenol red.

(i) Place 0.9 ml broth medium in each of 8 small sterile vials or tubes and mark the tubes 10^{-1} through 10^{-8}.

(ii) Transfer 0.1 ml of a frozen-thawed antigen stock to the 10^{-1} tube, mix thoroughly, and using a clean pipette, transfer 0.1 ml of the 10^{-1} dilution to the 10^{-2} tube. Continue the dilutions in the same manner through the 10^{-8} tube. Some antigens may require higher dilutions to obtain an endpoint, making it necessary to use an additional microtitre plate.

(c) Preparation of microtitre plates (e.g. Cooke Laboratory Products, Alexandria, Virginia, USA) (each plate contains eight rows (A-H) of twelve wells). Sterile procedures should be used in setting up the plate. The use of sterile, rigid, plastic lids (Linbro Scientific, Incorporated, Hamden, Connecticut, USA) is recommended.

(1) Place 0.025 ml (25 μl) sterile broth medium (containing phenol red) in wells 1-9 and antigen control wells 11 and 12, rows A-H.

(2) Place 0.075 ml (75 μl) sterile broth medium in well 10, rows A-H. These wells serve as medium controls.

(3) Add 0.025 ml (25 μl) of heat-inactivated, membrane-filtered (450 nm) homologous antiserum to well 1, rows A-H.

(4) Using 25 μl microdiluters (flamed and cooled), make twofold dilutions in all rows by mixing the antiserum in well 1 and

transferring 25 μl serially through well 9.

(5) Add 0.050 ml (50 μl) of the 10^{-1} antigen dilution to wells 1–9 and 11, 12 of row A. Add 50 μl of the 10^{-2} antigen dilution to wells 1–9 and 11, 12, row B. Continue for each of the other rows: row C (10^{-3}), row D (10^{-4}), row E (10^{-5}), row F (10^{-6}), row G (10^{-7}), row H (10^{-8}). Volume of antigen dilution used for each row is 0.55 ml (550 μl).

(6) Add 0.125 ml (125 μl) of broth medium to each well, all rows. The final volume in each well should be 200 μl. The final dilution of serum in well 1 is 1:16, 1:32 in well 2, 1:64 in well 3, etc.

(7) The rigid plastic lid is removed and the plate is sealed with pre-cut Pressure Sensitive Film (Falcon Plastics, Los Angeles, California, USA) and incubated at the optimal temperature for the growth of the organism.

(8) The need for complement in the MI test is assessed by setting up a second plate identical to the first except that an 8–10% solution of complement in broth medium is added to each well.

 (i) For this purpose, commercially available lyophilised guinea pig complement (e.g. Cappel Laboratories, Downingtown, Pennsylvania, USA) is resuspended in phosphate buffered saline, distributed in vials (1–3 ml/vial) and frozen at $-70°C$.

 (ii) For use in the MI test, an 8–10% solution of complement in broth medium is prepared: 0.8 ml frozen-thawed complement stock plus 9.2 ml cold broth medium for an 8% solution; 1 ml complement stock plus 9 ml cold broth medium for a 10% solution. The solution is membrane filtered (450 nm) and kept at 4°C until added to the plate.

 (iii) The solution is added (125 μl/well) to all wells at step (6) above (rather than broth medium without complement), thus giving a final concentration of 5–6% complement.

 (iv) The two plates are compared for evidence of enhancement, suppression, or stabilisation of the MI titre by the presence of complement (Taylor-Robinson and Berry, 1969).

(9) The plates are read over diffuse light at one- or two-day intervals. Colour changes in the antigen control wells (11 and 12), indicating a pH drop of about 0.5 unit, are interpreted as evidence of metabolism. The endpoint can be determined when the number of wells showing change has stabilised (3–10 days).

(10) The antigen titration endpoint is the highest dilution of antigen which has changed colour in the control wells (11 and 12) at a specified time (time elapsed since setting up the plate). This dilution becomes one colour changing unit (CCU), and each *decreasing* tenfold dilution from that point provides a factor of 10 CCUs. For example, if 10^{-6} is the highest dilution of antigen providing a colour change, that dilution contains 1 CCU; the 10^{-5} dilution contains 10 CCUs, etc. Antigen concentrations for use in the MI test should be 10–1,000 CCUs.

(2) Homologous Antiserum Titration.

(a) The homologous antiserum MI endpoint can be obtained from these plates by recording the highest dilution of antiserum that has inhibited colour change in wells 1–9 for each antigen dilution. The MI titre for each antigen dilution is the reciprocal of the highest antiserum dilution that prevented colour change.

(b) For subsequent MI tests employing any of the frozen antigens, the antigen dilution to be used is that which provides 10–1,000 CCUs/0.05 ml and which also has the highest MI titre.

(3) Heterologous MI Tests.

(a) One antiserum can be tested in heterologous combinations against seven different antigens in a single microtitre plate. The eighth row of the plate is reserved for the homologous control test.

(b) It is also possible to test a single antigen in heterologous combinations against seven different antisera, with the eighth being reserved for the homologous control test.

(c) Prior to setting up the test, a chart of the tests to be performed should be prepared. Antigens and antisera should be placed in a rack in the sequence to be used.

(d) Procedure:

(1) Antigen stocks are removed from the freezer and diluted as previously determined. The volume of antigen dilution required for the test should be computed, allowing an excess of 50–100%.

(2) Compute and prepare volume of membrane filtered (450 nm) complement solution (8–10%) in cold broth medium required to perform tests (12 ml/full plate). Store at 4°C.

(3) Preparation of the microtitre plate.

(i) Place 25 μl broth medium in wells 1–9 and 11, 12, rows A–H.

(ii) Place 75 μl broth medium in well 10, rows A–H.

(iii) Add 25 μl heat-inactivated, membrane-filtered (450 nm) antiserum to well 1, rows A–H. If a single antigen is to be tested against several different antisera, add 25 μl homologous antisera to well 1, row A and 25 μl of each of the heterologous antisera to well 1 in each of the remaining rows.

(iv) Using 25 μl microdiluters, make twofold dilutions through well 9, rows A–H.

(v) Add 50 μl of the homologous antigen dilution to wells 1–9 and 11, 12, row A. Add 50 μl of the other antigen dilutions to wells 1–9 and 11, 12 in their respective rows. If a single antigen is to be tested against several antisera, the same antigen dilution is added to wells 1–9 and 11, 12 in *all* rows.

(vi) Add 125 μl complement solution to all wells.

(vii) Seal plate and place in incubator.

(viii) Readings of the plate are made in accordance with the previously determined time for observation of colour change for each antigen being tested. The antigen control wells (11 and 12) in each row should show colour change at the time of MI endpoint determination.

E. Combined Deformation and Metabolism Inhibition Test for Spiroplasmas

The deformation (DF) and metabolism inhibition (MI) tests are very sensitive serological tests: both tests are capable of demonstrating spiroplasma relationships at the intraspecific level, and groupings obtained are usually closely correlated. Performing the DF test in microtitre plates rather than tubes has simplified the test. The incorporation of a standardised spiroplasma MI test with the DF procedure permits the collection of data from two serological tests in a single test run. For the combined DF/MI test the volumes of materials used in the standard DF and MI procedures were modified to permit the use of threefold antiserum dilutions which provide a greater range of dilutions in a single row of the microtitre plate. Details of the procedure have been published (Williamson *et al.*, 1979).

(1) Antigens. Antigens (spiroplasmas) are grown in 100 ml broth medium. Their morphological adequacy for the DF test is monitored by dark-field microscopy. They are then frozen at −70°C in 3 ml aliquots.

(2) Antisera. Antisera are heat-inactivated (56°C for 30 minutes). Stock dilutions (1:3) are made in broth medium, filtered through

450 nm membrane filters and frozen at $-20°C$ in 200-400 μl aliquots in polyethylene micro-tubes.

(3) Titrations. Preliminary titrations of each frozen antigen are performed in microtitre plates to determine the titre of the antigen suspension in CCUs and to determine the appropriate antigen dilution for carrying out the DF and MI tests.

(a) Frozen spiroplasma suspensions and antisera are allowed to thaw at room temperature.

(b) Spiroplasma antigens are prepared (in 3 ml vials) in volumes sufficient to carry out the test (2-3 ml) to the following dilutions: undiluted, 1:2, 1:4, 10^{-1}, 10^{-2}, 10^{-3}, 10^{-4}, 10^{-5}.

(c) For homologous tests, the 1:3 stock dilution of antiserum is further diluted to 1:27 or 1:81 and used as a base dilution for preparation of the antiserum dilutions in microtitre plates. The 1:3 stock dilutions are used to make the antiserum dilutions in heterologous tests.

(d) Preparation of plates for test:

    (1) Place 100 μl of growth medium in wells 1-9 and 11, 12 (antigen titration wells), and 150 μl in well 10 (medium control well).

    (2) Add 50 μl of 1:81 antiserum dilution in well 1, rows A-H, producing a 1:243 initial antiserum dilution in well 1.

    (3) Using 50 μl microdiluters, threefold dilutions are made by mixing the antiserum in the first well and transferring 50 μl serially through well 9.

    (4) Add 50 μl of each antigen suspension, one dilution for each row, beginning with row A, to wells 1-9, 11 and 12.

    (5) Add 50 μl 8-10% guinea pig complement solution in growth medium to each well in all rows. See standard MI procedure outlined above for the handling of complement.

    (6) The plate is covered with a rigid plastic lid and allowed to incubate at room temperature for 30 minutes before beginning DF titre determinations:

        Antigen control wells containing undiluted, 1:2, 1:4, and, if necessary, 1:10 dilutions are examined to find the dilution which provides the appropriate number of spiroplasmas (20-30 per 1250x microscope field). This dilution of this frozen spiroplasma stock is then used in all future DF tests.

    (7) After DF titres have been determined, the plate is sealed with Pressure Sensitive Film and incubated at the optimal

temperature for spiroplasma growth.

(e) The plate is read daily over a test mirror and the pH shift from red to yellow (1–1.5 pH units) is observed in wells 11 and 12, rows A–H. At the highest dilution of antigen giving a colour change, the number of colour changing units (CCU) is one per 50 μl.

(f) When the number of antigen control wells showing change has stabilised (4–9 days), the pH change in wells 1–9, rows A–H is recorded.

    (i) The MI titre of the antiserum for each antigen dilution is defined as the reciprocal of the highest antiserum dilution that prevented colour change.

    (ii) For subsequent MI tests employing this frozen spiroplasma, the dilution to be used should provide 10–1,000 colour changing units (CCU) per 50 μl and which also has the highest MI titre. The appropriate DF and MI dilutions and the time for reading the MI test are recorded and kept with vials of each frozen spiroplasma antigen.

(4) Homologous and Heterologous Test Procedures. DF/MI tests are performed in which single spiroplasmas are tested in homologous combination against their specific antisera and in heterologous combinations against other spiroplasma antisera. The antigen dilutions used for the DF and MI tests are those previously determined by antigen titration. Heterologous DF/MI tests for each spiroplasma strain are completed in a single run if possible. Fresh vials of frozen spiroplasma suspensions are used in subsequent tests, but the use of frozen suspensions permits the elimination of homologous tests in continued testing of each spiroplasma strain.

(a) Two rows of wells are used to test the spiroplasmas against each antiserum; the first row is used for the DF test and the second for the MI test.

(b) For each antiserum, 100 μl of growth medium are added to wells 1–9, 11 and 12, and 150 μl to well 10.

(c) For homologous tests, 50 μl of a 1:81 antiserum dilution are added to the 100 μl of medium in well 1 in both the DF and MI test rows. Threefold dilutions are then made in well 1–9, using 50 μl microdiluters.

(d) For heterologous tests, 50 μl of a 1:3 stock dilution of each antiserum are added to the 100 μl of medium in well 1 in both the DF and MI test rows. Threefold dilutions are then made in wells 1–9 using 50 μl microdiluters.

(e) 50 μl of spiroplasma suspension at the previously determined dilution are added in the appropriate rows to wells 1-9, 11 and 12.

(f) 50 μl of 8-10% guinea pig complement solution are added to each well in all rows.

(g) The plate is covered with a rigid plastic lid and incubated for 30 minutes at room temperature.

(h) Deformation titres are determined as previously described.

(i) The plate is sealed with Pressure Sensitive Film and incubated at the temperature optimal for growth.

(j) If MI titres have stabilised, they are read on the day previously determined as optimal for the spiroplasma being tested.

F. The Enzyme-linked Immunosorbent Assay (ELISA)

Enzyme-labelled antibodies were first used by Nakane and Pierce (1966) to detect the presence of virus antigens in tissue sections. A quantitative enzyme immunoassay, with a sensitivity comparable with that of radio-immunoassay was developed by Engvall and Perlmann (1971, 1972). It is now most commonly known by the acronym ELISA (enzyme-linked immunosorbent assay).

ELISA has been used by Saillard *et al.* (1978) to detect *S. citri* in extracts of leaves of sweet orange and periwinkle, in which *Spiroplasma* antigens were detectable at concentrations of 5-10 ng. Recently, Dollet *et al.* (1979) used the ELISA technique to search for *Acholeplasma* in the tissues of coconut palms suffering from lethal yellowing disease. Archer *et al.* (1979) used ELISA to study the distribution of *S. citri* in various tissues of periwinkle during the course of infection by grafting, and Archer and Best (1980) studied the serological relatedness of various spiroplasmas by ELISA. At the time of this writing, there are no reported studies of the application of ELISA to insect-derived mycoplasmas. An important caveat in the use of ELISA for studying plant infections is that certain plants possess the enzyme phenol oxidase which is capable of reacting with the ELISA substrate to produce a colour change similar to that produced by enzyme-linked immunoglobulin.

A collection of articles edited by Engvall and Pesce (1978) provides an excellent description of ELISA procedures and their application, and is recommended reading for anyone interested in using this technique. The ELISA procedure to be presented below was adapted from Clark and Adams (1977) by Saillard *et al.* (1978) for their studies on *S. citri* in extracts of leaves of sweet orange and periwinkle. It was presented in the Mycoplasma Techniques Course given at Bordeaux, France, 3-21 September 1979. Permission to reproduce it here was kindly provided by Dr Colette Saillard, Institut National de la Recherche Agronomique (INRA), Laboratoire de Biologie Cellulaire et Moléculaire, Pont-de-la-Maye, France. Modifications of the procedure may be required for some mycoplasma-antisera systems.

(1) Antigens. Antigens for immunisation are prepared and inoculated into rabbits as described above (2.A).

(2) Antisera. IgG from hyperimmune serum and pre-immunisation serum is prepared as follows (one-step chromatographic procedure, Fahey, 1967):

(a) Dialyse at 4°C 1 ml antiserum (or pre-immunisation serum) against 500 ml 0.05M Tris-HCl buffer (pH 8.0). Change the buffer during the day and before leaving at night. Continue dialysis overnight.

(b) The following day, remove the serum from the dialysis tube and centrifuge at 10,000 g for 15 minutes.

(c) Remove supernatant and pass through 20 ml DEAE cellulose (Whatman DE52, Whatman Ltd., Maidstone, Kent, England) pre-equilibrated with 0.05M Tris-HCl (pH 8.0).

(d) Elute IgG with 0.05M Tris-HCl (pH 8.0). Collect two bed volumes. IgG is the first protein fraction to come off the column. Monitor effluent at 280 nm and pool the fractions containing IgG.

(e) Precipitate IgG with an equal volume of saturated ammonium sulfate solution (80–90 g/100 ml glass distilled water).

(f) Mix thoroughly and leave at 4°C with stirring for 30–60 minutes.

(g) Centrifuge at 15,000 g for 20 minutes.

(h) Dissolve precipitate in 2 ml PBS (0.02M sodium-potassium phosphate buffer, pH 7.4, plus 0.15M sodium chloride and 0.02% sodium azide).

(i) Transfer to dialysis tube and dialyse 48 hours against PBS at 4°C with stirring. Change PBS twice during the day and before leaving at night. The absence of ammonium ions, which can interfere with glutaraldehyde conjugation of the alkaline phosphatase with IgG, can be confirmed with Nessler reagent.

(j) Remove the IgG from the dialysis tube. Determine the concentration of IgG at OD_{280} and adjust with PBS to read 1.4 OD units (equals approximately 1 mg IgG/ml). Store at −20°C in 1 ml aliquots.

(3) Conjugation of the Enzyme Alkaline Phosphatase with IgG (One-step Glutaraldehyde Coupling Procedure).

(a) Centrifuge 2 ml (2 mg) alkaline phosphatase suspension (calf intestine, Type VII, suspension in 3.2M $(NH_4)_2$ SO_4 solution; Sigma Chemical Company, St Louis, Missouri, USA) at 12,000 g

at 4°C for 20 minutes. Discard the supernatant and dissolve the pellet in 0.8 ml IgG (= 0.8 mg IgG) solution.

(b) Dialyse the mixture for 48 hours against 1 litre PBS (use 1 litre for each 1 ml of enzyme–IgG solution) at 4°C. Change PBS at least 3 times.

(c) Remove from dialysis tube and, while mixing, add fresh glutaraldehyde (electron microscope grade) solution to 0.06% final concentration.

(d) Leave mixture at room temperature for 3–4 hours. A yellow-brown colour should develop.

(e) Remove glutaraldehyde by dialysing the mixture against PBS as for step (b) above.

(f) Add bovine serum albumin (BSA) (RIA grade; Sigma Chemical Co., St Louis, Missouri, USA) (5 mg BSA per ml conjugate) and store at 4°C.

(4) Preparation of Cultured Mycoplasmas for Antigen Titration.

(a) Mycoplasmas are grown in broth medium and harvested by centrifugation. The pellet of organisms is resuspended in sample buffer (osmotically suitable PBS, pH 7.4). The pellets are washed and recentrifuged three times.

(b) Protein concentrations of each antigen are determined and the concentration of each is adjusted to 0.5 mg/ml sample buffer. For the assay make 0.5 ml volume dilutions of 10^{-2}, 10^{-3}, 10^{-4}, 10^{-5}.

(5) Preparation of Plant Homogenates. (Procedures for preparation of insect homogenates for ELISA have not yet been reported.)

(a) One gram of plant tissue is homogenised with a mortar and pestle in 1 ml of buffer osmotically compatible with survival of the organisms.

(b) Filter homogenate through four layers of cheese cloth. Hold filtrate at 4°C until used. For the assay use undiluted filtrate and a 10^{-1} dilution.

(6) ELISA Test Procedure.

(a) The assay is performed in microtitre plates. Nonspecific reactions sometimes occur in the outer rows of the plate and, for this reason, they are not used.

(b) Make dilution of purified IgG (1 mg/ml) in coating buffer (0.05M sodium carbonate buffer, pH 9.6, plus 0.02% sodium azide) to provide 1–10 μg IgG/ml. Low-titre antisera may require higher concentration of IgG for maximum coating efficiency (see Clark and Adams, 1977).

(c) Coat microtitre wells by adding 250 μl purified IgG dilution to each well to be used in the test. Tests are run in duplicate or triplicate. Cover plate and place at 37°C for 2-6 hours.

(d) Wash by flooding wells with PBS-Tween 20 (PBS plus 0.05% Tween 20). Allow PBS-Tween to stand in wells for 3 minutes. Repeat 3 times. Empty plate.

(e) Add 250 μl of each antigen dilution to duplicate or triplicate wells. For example, row B: homologous antigen dilutions 10^{-2} (wells 2 and 3); 10^{-3} (wells 4 and 5); 10^{-4} (wells 6 and 7); 10^{-5} (wells 8 and 9). Rows C–F: heterologous antigen dilutions may be added in duplicate to the appropriate wells. Row G is used for control wells.

(f) If plant homogenates are to be tested, 250 μl each of undiluted filtrate and 10^{-1} dilution are added to wells 10 and 11, rows B–F. Filtrates of homogenates of healthy plants are tested in row G.

(g) The plate is covered and left at 4-6°C overnight or at 37°C for 4-6 hours.

(h) Wash plate with PBS-Tween as in (d) above.

(i) Add to each well 250 μl of enzyme-labelled IgG in enzyme IgG buffer (PBS-Tween containing 2% polyvinyl-pyrrolidone (PVP) and 0.2% ovalbumin). Cover plate and incubate at 37°C for 3-6 hours.

(j) Wash plate with PBS-Tween as in (d) above.

(k) Add to each well 250 μl freshly prepared substrate (p-nitrophenyl-phosphate) in substrate buffer (10% diethanolamine adjusted to pH 9.8 with HCl; 0.02% sodium azide). Cover and incubate at room temperature for 30 minutes.

(l) Stop reaction by adding 50 μl of 3MNaOH to each well.

(m) Evaluate results: a yellow colour in the well indicates a positive reaction. Quantitative data may be obtained by transferring the contents of duplicate wells to a spectrophotometer cuvette and measuring absorbance at 405 nm. The results of the optical density readings at 405 nm are translated as follows (Tully *et al.*, 1980):

0.0-0.1 (−)	0.5-1.0 (3+)
0.1-0.5 (1+)	1.0-1.5 (4+)
0.2-0.5 (2+)	1.5-2.0 (5+)

G. Precipitin Ring, Gel Diffusion and Complement-fixation Tests

In the serological procedures outlined thus far the reactions involve antibodies directed primarily against membrane antigens. Most of the tests, except growth inhibition, can detect intraspecific antigenic differences. The precipitin ring, gel diffusion and diagnostic complement-fixation tests are less sensitive because they involve soluble antigens in addition to membrane antigens and the antisera produced against such antigen preparations may show considerable cross-reactivity, especially if the immunisation schedule is prolonged (Lemcke, 1973). It may be that this lack of sensitivity would permit the use of one or all of these tests to establish or recognise intraspecific cross-reactivities between spiroplasmas, a test which is currently missing from the repertoire of spiroplasma serology. However, as yet, none of these three procedures has been used on a sufficiently broad scale to determine its utility as a group test.

The gel diffusion and complement fixation tests have been used only rarely and no detailed procedures for their application to plant and insect mycoplasmas have been published; therefore, only references to the standard procedures, and not the procedures themselves, will be provided. Some details of the precipitin ring test procedure as applied to spiroplasmas are available and these will be presented next.

(1) Precipitin Ring Test. This test, adapted from studies of viral soluble antigens (Whitcomb and Black, 1961), has had very limited use in serological studies of plant and insect mycoplasmas. Tully *et al.* (1973) used the precipitin ring test to compare the antigens of *S. citri*, the only spiroplasma cultivable at that time, with extracts of corn plants affected by the corn stunt spiroplasma. Later, Tully *et al.* (1976, 1977) used the precipitin ring test to study the serological relationships between two isolates of the tick-derived spiroplasma, the suckling mouse cataract agent (SMCA), *S. citri*, the corn stunt spiroplasma (CCS), and the sex ratio organism (SRO) of certain *Drosophila* species. More recently, Davis *et al.* (1979) used the precipitin ring test to study serological relationships among spiroplasmas from several sources. The following procedure is based on the precipitin ring test of Whitcomb and Black (1961) and follows recommended procedures of R.F. Whitcomb.

(a) Antigens.

(1) Mycoplasmas grown in broth culture are harvested by centrifugation.

(2) Resuspend pellets in a sufficient volume of osmotically appropriate PBS to provide a 10–50-fold concentration of original culture.

(3) Subject suspension to ten cycles of rapid freezing and thawing at $-70°C$ and $37°C$. Ultrasound is also useful for disruption of organisms.

(4) Centrifuge suspension at 85,000 g for 1 hour at $4°C$.

    (5) Remove supernatants and prepare antigen dilutions for use in the precipitin ring test. Make an initial 1:10 dilution in PBS and then twofold dilutions (1:20, 1:40, 1:80, 1:160, 1:320, 1:640). Keep dilutions at 4°C.

(b) Antiserum.

    (1) Follow previously outlined procedure for antiserum production, with special emphasis on starvation of rabbits before bleeding to minimise lipoproteins in the serum.

    (2) Centrifuge at 85,000 g for 1 hour. Antiserum must be free of particulate material or lipoproteins which could result in a misinterpretation of the results.

    (3) Beginning with an initial dilution of 1:10, prepare twofold dilutions of antisera in 1 ml volumes in a solution of 10% glycerol in PBS. Carry dilution to 1:320 or 1:640.

(c) Test procedure.

    (1) Transfer 50-100 μl of each serum dilution to the bottom of a small glass tube (inside diameter of 4 mm) in a rack.

    (2) Overlay 50-100 μl of each antigen dilution on to each antiserum dilution.

    (3) Incubate at room temperature for 1 hour.

    (4) Read results in a darkened room by focusing a narrow beam of light on the interface. A heat filter should be used to avoid the production of convection currents which can cause the diffusion of an existing ring. A positive reaction is one in which a ring of precipitation is observed at the antigen-antiserum interface.

    (5) Tubes which fail to react positively within 1 hour are considered to be negative.

    (6) The endpoint for any antigen dilution is the highest antiserum dilution which gives a precipitate; the antiserum titre is the reciprocal of that dilution.

    (7) The initial tenfold antigen dilution should be tested against pre-immune serum dilutions.

    (8) The antigen dilution providing the highest antiserum titre should be used in heterologous tests. Alternatively, the protein concentration of each antigen preparation can be determined and the concentration adjusted to 1-0.5 mg/ml; all heterologous tests can be run with the same antigen concentration.

(2) Gel Diffusion. Although double immunodiffusion (Ouchterlony) has had wide usage in serological studies of animal and human mycoplasmas, it has only rarely been used for plant and insect mycoplasmas.

McBeath and Chen (1973) used this technique in serological studies involving extracts from healthy corn plants and corn stunt infected plants; it was also used by McCoy and Basham (1979) as a procedure in their studies of mycoplasma isolates from floral surfaces. Both reports are abstracts and details of the procedure were not presented. No attempt will be made here to devise a procedure for gel diffusion as applied to plant and insect mycoplasmas. Investigators desiring to use this technique are referred to the procedure as outlined by Taylor-Robinson *et al.* (1963), Lemcke (1964, 1965) and by Kenny (1971a, 1971b).

Immunoelectrophoretic separation of antigens prior to application of antiserum increases the resolving power of the gel procedure but has the disadvantage of requiring relatively large amounts of antiserum for each test. There are no published reports of the use of this method in the serological characterisation of plant and insect mycoplasmas, although Wróblewski (1975, 1979) and Wróblewski *et al.* (1978) used the two-dimensional (crossed) immunoelectrophoresis method to study proteins in the membranes of *Spiroplasma citri*.

(3) Complement Fixation. The complement fixation test of Taylor-Robinson *et al.* (1963) was one of the tests used by Tully *et al.* (1977) to show that the SMCA spiroplasma was only distantly related to *S. citri* and corn stunt spiroplasmas. There are no recent published reports of the further use of the complement fixation test with plant and insect mycoplasmas.

The microtitre plate method is a convenient modification of the standard diagnostic complement fixation test and interested investigators are referred to the technique of Lennette and Schmidt (1979) for the detailed procedure.

Acknowledgements

I am grateful to Dr C. Saillard, Dr J.G. Tully and Dr R.F. Whitcomb for thoughtful and critical reading of the manuscript.

References

Al-Aubaidi, J.M. and Fabricant, J. (1971). The practical application of immuno-fluorescence (agar block technique) for the identification of Mycoplasma. *Cornell Veterinarian 61*, 519–42.
Archer, D.B. and Best, J. (1980). Serological relatedness of Spiroplasmas

estimated by enzyme-linked immunosorbent assay and crossed immunoelectrophoresis. *Journal of General Microbiology 119*, 413–22.

Archer, D.B., Best, J. and Plaskitt, K.A. (1979). The distribution of spiroplasmas within infected plants varies during the course of infection. *Proceedings of the Fourth Meeting of the International Council on Lethal Yellowing. Fort Lauderdale, 1979*, p. 9. University of Florida Publication FL-80-1.

Bradbury, J.M. and Jordan, F.T.W. (1972). Studies on the absorption of certain medium proteins to *Mycoplasma gallisepticum* and their influence on agglutination and haemagglutination reactions. *Journal of Hygiene, Cambridge 70*, 267–78.

Carski, T.R. and Shepard, C.C. (1961). Pleuropneumonia-like (mycoplasma) infections of tissue culture. *Journal of Bacteriology 81*, 626–35.

Chen, T.A. and Liao, C.H. (1975). Corn stunt spiroplasma: Isolation, cultivation, and proof of pathogenicity. *Science 188*, 1015–17.

Clark, H.W., Fowler, R.C. and McP. Brown, T. (1961). Preparation of pleuropneumonia-like organisms for microscope study. *Journal of Bacteriology 81*, 500–2.

Clark, M.F. and Adams, A.N. (1977). Characteristics of the microplate method of enzyme-linked immunosorbent assay for the detection of plant viruses. *Journal of General Virology 34*, 475–83.

Clyde, W.A., Jr. (1964). Mycoplasma species identification based upon growth inhibition by specific antisera. *Journal of Immunology 92*, 958–65.

Davis, R.E. (1978). Spiroplasma associated with flowers of the tulip tree (*Liriodendron tulipifera* L.). *Canadian Journal of Microbiology 24*, 954–9.

Davis, R.E., Lee, I.-M. and Basciano, L.K. (1979). Spiroplasmas: serological grouping of strains associated with plants and insects. *Canadian Journal of Microbiology 25*, 861–6.

de Leeuw, G.T.N. (1977). Mycoplasmas in planten. *Natur en techniek 45*, 74–89.

Del Giudice, R.A., Robillard, N.F. and Carski, T.R. (1967). Immunofluorescence identification of *Mycoplasma* on agar by use of incident illumination. *Journal of Bacteriology 93*, 1205–9.

Dollet, M., Saillard, C., Garcia-Jurado, O., Vignault, J.C., Gargani, D., Tully, J.G. and Bové, J.M. (1979). An approach to the serological study of the Mycoplasmas of lethal yellowing in the coconuts in West Africa. *Proceedings of the Fourth Meeting of the International Council of Lethal Yellowing. Fort Lauderdale, 1979*, p. 8. University of Florida Publication FL-80-1.

Eden-Green, S.J. (1978). Isolation of Acholeplasmas from coconut palms affected by lethal yellowing disease in Jamaica. *Zentralblatt für Bakteriologie, Parasitenkunde, Infektionskrankheiten und Hygiene. Erste Abteilung Originale 241*, 226.

Eden-Green, S.J., Tully, J.G. and Townsend, R. (1979). Acholeplasmas and lethal yellowing disease. I. Present status. *Proceedings of the Fourth Meeting of the International Council on Lethal Yellowing. Fort Lauderdale, 1979*. p. 10. University of Florida Publication FL-80-1.

Engvall, E. and Perlmann, P. (1971). Enzyme-linked immunosorbent assay (ELISA). Quantitative assay of immunoglobulin G. *Immunochemistry 8*, 871–4.

— (1972). Enzyme-linked immunosorbent assay, ELISA. III. Quantitation of specific antibodies by enzyme-labelled antiimmunoglobulin in antigen-coated tubes. *Journal of Immunology 109*, 129–35.

Engvall, E. and Pesce, A.J. (eds) (1978). *Quantitative Enzyme Immunoassay. Scandinavian Journal of Immunology Supplement*, no. 7, vol. 8. Oxford: Blackwell Scientific Publications Ltd.

Ernø, H. and Jurmanova, K. (1973). Bovine mycoplasmas: serological studies by double immunodiffusion, growth precipitation and growth inhibition. *Acta Veterinaria Scandinavica 14*, 524-37.

Fahey, J.L. (1967). Chromatographic separation of immunoglobulins. In *Methods in Immunology and Immunochemistry*, Vol. I. pp. 321-32, C.A. Williams and M.W. Chase (eds). New York: Academic Press.

Huijsman-Evers, A.G.M. and Ruys, A.C. (1956). Microorganisms of the pleuropneumonia group (family of Mycoplasmataceae) in man. II. Serological identification and discussion of pathogenicity. *Antonie van Leeuwenhoek 22*, 377-84.

Kenny, G.E. (1969). Serological comparison of the glycolytic *Mycoplasma* species. *Journal of Bacteriology 98*, 1044-55.

— (1971a). Immunogenicity of *Mycoplasma pneumoniae*. *Infection and Immunity 3*, 510-15.

— (1971b). Serological cross-reactions between lipids of *Mycoplasma pneumoniae* and *Mycoplasma neurolyticum*. *Infection and Immunity 4*, 149-53.

— (1979). Antigenic determinants. In *The Mycoplasmas*, Vol. I, pp. 351-84, M.F. Barile and S. Razin (eds). New York: Academic Press.

Lemcke, R.M. (1973). Serological reactions of Mycoplasmas. *Annals of the New York Academy of Sciences 225*, 46-53.

— (1964). The serological differentiation of Mycoplasma strains (pleuropneumonia-like organisms) from various sources. *The Journal of Hygiene, Cambridge 62*, 199-219.

— (1965). A serological comparison of various species of mycoplasma by an agar gel double-diffusion technique. *Journal of General Microbiology 38*, 91-100.

Lennette, E.H. and Schmidt, N.J. (1979). General principles underlying laboratory diagnosis of viral infections. In *Diagnostic Procedures for Viral, Rickettsial and Chlamydial Infections*, 5th edn, pp. 35-42. Washington, DC: American Public Health Association.

McBeath, J.H. and Chen, T.A. (1973). Serological studies of corn stunt diseases. Abstracts: *Phytopathology 63*, 803.

McCoy, R.E. and Basham, H.G. (1979). Isolation and characterization of Mycoplasmas from floral surfaces. *Abstracts: Fourth Meeting of the International Council on Lethal Yellowing*. Fort Lauderdale, Florida, USA, 13-17 August 1979.

Nakane, P.K. and Pierce, G.B. (1966). Enzyme-labelled antibodies: preparation and application for the localisation of antigens. *The Journal of Histochemistry and Cytochemistry 14*, 929-31.

Purcell, R.H., Chanock, R.M. and Taylor-Robinson, D. (1969). Serology of the mycoplasmas of man. In *The Mycoplasmatales and the L-phase of Bacteria*, pp. 221-64, L. Hayflick (ed). New York: Appleton-Century-Crofts.

Purcell, R.H., Taylor-Robinson, D., Wong, D.C. and Chanock, R.M. (1966a). A color test for the measurement of antibody to the non-acid-forming human mycoplasma species. *American Journal of Epidemiology 84*, 51-66.

— (1966b). Color test for the measurement of antibody to T-strain mycoplasmas. *Journal of Bacteriology 92*, 6-12.

Rosendal, S. and Black, F.T. (1972). Direct and indirect immunofluorescence of unfixed and fixed mycoplasma colonies. *Acta Pathologica et Microbiologica Scandinavica, Section B 80*, 615-22.

Saillard, C., Dunez, J., Garcia-Jurado, O., Nhomi, A. and Bové, J.M. (1978). Detection de *Spiroplasma citri* dans les agrumes et les pervenches par la technique immuno-enzymatique 'ELISA'. *Comptes Rendus Hebdomadaires des Séances de l'Academie des Sciences, Paris, Série D 286*, 1245-8.

Senterfit, L.B. and Jensen, K.E. (1966). Antimetabolic antibodies to *Mycoplasma pneumoniae* measured by tetrazolium reduction inhibition. *Proceedings of the*

Society for Experimental Biology and Medicine 122, 786-90.

Spaar, D., Kleinhempel, H., Muller, H.M., Stanarius, A. and Schimmel, D. (1974). Culturing mycoplasmas from plants. *Les Mycoplasmes/Mycoplasmas. Les Colloques de l'Institut National de la Santé et de la Recherche Médicale 33,* 207-14.

Subcommittee on the Taxonomy of *Mollicutes* (1979). Proposal of minimal standards for descriptions of new species of the class *Mollicutes. International Journal of Systematic Bacteriology 29,* 172-80.

Taylor-Robinson, D. and Berry, D.M. (1969). The evaluation of the metabolic-inhibition technique for the study of *Mycoplasma gallisepticum. The Journal of General Microbiology 55,* 127-37.

Taylor-Robinson, D., Purcell, R.H., Wong, D.C. and Chanock, R.M. (1966). A colour test for the measurement of antibody to certain mycoplasma species based upon the inhibition of acid production. *Journal of Hygiene, Cambridge 64,* 91-104.

Taylor-Robinson, D., Somerson, N.L., Turner, H.C. and Chanock, R.M. (1963). Serological relationships among human mycoplasmas as shown by complement-fixation and gel diffusion. *Journal of Bacteriology 85,* 1261-73.

Tully, J.G. (1973). Biological and serological characteristics of the acholeplasmas. *Annals of the New York Academy of Sciences 225,* 74-93.

— (1979). Special features of the acholeplasmas. In *The Mycoplasmas,* Vol. I, pp. 431-49, M.F. Barile and S. Razin (eds). New York: Academic Press.

Tully, J.G., Rose, D.L., Garcia-Jurado, O., Vignault, J.C., Saillard, C., Bové, J.M., McCoy, R.E. and Williamson, D.L. (1980). Serological analysis of a new group of spiroplasmas. *Current Microbiology 3,* 369-72.

Tully, J.G., Whitcomb, R.F., Bové, J.M. and Saglio, P. (1973). Plant mycoplasmas: Serological relation between agents associated with citrus stubborn and corn stunt disease. *Science 182,* 827-9.

Tully, J.G., Whitcomb, R.F., Clark, H.F. and Williamson, D.L. (1977). Pathogenic mycoplasmas: Cultivation and vertebrate pathogenicity of a new spiroplasma. *Science 195,* 892-4.

Tully, J.G., Whitcomb, R.F., Williamson, D.L. and Clark, H.F. (1976). Suckling mouse cataract agent is a helical wall-free prokaryote (spiroplasma) pathogenic for vertebrates. *Nature 259,* 117-20.

Whitcomb, R.F. and Black, L.M. (1961). A precipitin ring test for estimation of relative soluble-antigen concentrations. *Virology 15,* 507-8.

Williamson, D.L., Blaustein, D.I., Levine, R.J.C. and Elfvin, M.J. (1979). Anti-actin-peroxidase staining of the helical wall-free prokaryote, *Spiroplasma citri. Current Microbiology 2,* 143-5.

Williamson, D.L., Tully, J.G. and Whitcomb, R.F. (1979). Serological relationships of spiroplasmas as shown by combined deformation and metabolism inhibition tests. *International Journal of Systematic Bacteriology 29,* 345-51.

Williamson, D.L. and Whitcomb, R.F. (1974). Helical, wall-free prokaryotes in *Drosophila,* leafhoppers and plants. In *Les Mycoplasmes/Mycoplasmas. Les Colloques de l'Institut National de la Santé et de la Recherche Médicale 33,* 283-90.

Williamson, D.L., Whitcomb, R.F. and Tully, J.G. (1978). The spiroplasma deformation test, a new serological method. *Current Microbiology 1,* 203-7.

Working Group of the FAO/WHO Programme on Comparative Mycoplasmology (1975). The metabolic-inhibition test. World Health Organisation Working Document, VPH/MIC/75.6. (WHO unpublished document).

— (1976). The growth inhibition test. World Health Organisation Working Document, VPH/MIC/76.7 (WHO unpublished document).

Wróblewski, H. (1975). Dissolution sélective de protéines de la membrane de

Spiroplasma citri par le désoxycholate de sodium. *Biochimie 57*, 1095–8.
— (1979). Amphiphilic nature of spiralin, the major protein of the *Spiroplasma citri* cell membrane. *Journal of Bacteriology 140*, 738–41.
Wróblewski, H., Burlot, R. and Johansson, K.-E. (1978). Solubilisation of *Spiroplasma citri* cell membrane proteins with the anionic detergent sodium lauroyl-sarcosinate (sarkosyl). *Biochimie 60*, 389–98.
Wróblewski, H., Johansson, K.-E. and Burlot, R. (1977). Crossed immunoelectrophoresis of membrane proteins from *Acholeplasma laidlawii* and *Spiroplasma citri*. *International Journal of Systematic Bacteriology 27*, 97–103.

9 PHYSICOCHEMICAL CHARACTERISATION OF PLANT AND INSECT MYCOPLASMAS

R. Townsend and M.J. Daniels

1. Biochemical Tests
   - A. Sterol Dependence
   - B. Glucose Fermentation
   - C. Arginine Hydrolysis
   - D. Carotenoid Production
   - E. Other Tests
2. Electrophoretic Analysis of Mycoplasma Proteins in Gels
   - A. Growth of Cells
   - B. Solubilisation
   - C. Polyacrylamide Gel Electrophoresis
   - D. Isoelectric Focusing
   - E. Two-dimensional Gel Electrophoresis
   - F. Crossed Immunoelectrophoresis
   - G. Staining and Recording
   - H. Autoradiography and Fluorography
3. Genome Properties
   - A. DNA Preparation
   - B. Determination of Base Composition
   - C. Genome Size
   - D. Analysis by Restriction Endonucleases
   - E. Nucleic Acid Hybridisation for Investigating Relatedness

The diminutive size of mycoplasma cells invited speculation that such tiny organisms might have developed unique biochemical pathways designed to make the most efficient use of the restricted coding capacity afforded by their small genomes. It has transpired that their physiology and metabolism generally resemble that of bacteria although they have complex nutritional requirements, reflecting a limited biosynthetic capacity and very restricted metabolic capabilities. As a consequence the diversity of biochemical properties available to the bacterial tax-onomist is denied to the mycoplasmologist. A few biochemical and physiological tests have been developed to aid identification but taxonomic classification depends to a large extent on serological techniques and genome properties (ICSB Subcommittee on the Taxonomy of Mollicutes, 1979). Electrophoretic analysis of cell proteins has also been found of great value, particularly in the classification of spiroplasmas (Davis *et al.*, 1969; Mouches *et al.*, 1979; Daniels *et al.*, 1980).

1. Biochemical Tests

A. Sterol Dependence

Two mechanisms operate within the Mycoplasmatales to ensure maintenance of membrane fluidity over a limited temperature range. Members of the essentially saprophytic family *Acholeplasmataceae* are capable of *de novo* fatty acid synthesis and are therefore able to vary the lipid composition, and hence the fluidity of the cytoplasmic membrane. Organisms belonging to the families *Mycoplasmataceae* and *Spiroplasmataceae*, which are parasites of animals, insects and plants, have very limited or no capacity for lipid biosynthesis, instead they maintain the cytoplasmic membrane in an intermediate fluid state by incorporation of large quantities of sterols. The absolute requirement for a sterol source capable of sustaining cell growth therefore represents a fundamental division in the classification of mycoplasmas.

In culture media sterol is usually provided in the form of bound cholesterol present in animal sera; however, the absence of growth in a serum-free medium does not constitute a reliable test for sterol dependence. Some mycoplasmas require only very small quantities of sterols and repeated passages in serum-free media are required to eliminate all traces of cholesterol from the inoculum Two tests, one direct and one indirect, are recognised to determine sterol dependence.

The digitonin inhibition test (Freundt *et al.*, 1973) is based on the ability of digitonin to bind to cholesterol preventing its incorporation into the cell membrane. An ethanolic solution of digitonin (1.5% w/v) is applied to sterile filter paper discs which are placed on freshly inoculated and dried lawns or streaks of the test organism and appropriate controls. After inoculation, sterol-requiring organisms exhibit inhibition zones (3–11 mm) around the impregnated discs. An important feature of this method is that the medium should contain 20% (v/v) of horse serum since it has been found that the use of serum fraction can lead to false positive results with *Acholeplasmas*.

The direct method (Razin and Tully, 1970; Edward, 1971) measures the actual growth occurring in the presence of varying concentrations of cholesterol. Test organisms are inoculated into equal volumes of medium containing bovine serum albumin (0.5%) (BSA) and palmitic acid (10 µg/ml) and increasing concentrations of cholesterol from 0–20 µg/ml with Tween 80 (0.02%). Controls should include media supplemented with serum fraction (1%) or horse serum (2% v/v) and serum-free medium with and without BSA and palmitic acid.

After incubation the cells are harvested from each culture by centrifugation, washed and the total protein determined by a calorimetric method (Lowry *et al.*, 1951). Alternatively a radioactive nucleic acid precursor such as [^{32}P] phosphate or [^{14}C] thymidine may be incorporated in the medium and the amount of cell growth determined by scintillation counting (Saglio *et al.*, 1973). Sterol-requiring organisms show an increasing cell yield with increasing cholesterol concentration, whereas nonsterol-requiring organisms will grow irrespective of sterol concentration.

B. Glucose Fermentation

A second fundamental division of the Mollicutes is based on their ability to ferment glucose. The simple method of detecting glucose utilisation is to observe a pH shift due to the acid products of fermentation (Aluotto *et al.*, 1970). A basic growth medium is supplemented with 1% (w/v) glucose and 0.05% phenol red and the pH adjusted to pH 7.5. A log phase culture is used to inoculate aliquots of this medium and controls from which glucose is omitted. During subsequent incubation glucose fermenters will produce a colour change in the medium from red to orange to yellow. A fall of pH may also be apparent in cultures of some nonfermenters, presumably because they are able partially to degrade substrates in complex components, such as yeast extract, to yield acid metabolites. However, a similar fall in pH should be apparent in the control culture (Edward and Moore, 1973). The extent of pH fall can be judged by comparison with a sample of uninoculated supplemented medium.

Direct measurement of glucose disappearance by the glucose oxidase reaction (Huggett and Nixon, 1957) has been used to detect mycoplasmas capable of metabolising that sugar (Edward and Moore, 1973) but the method requires a large number of cells. Much more sensitive techniques are available using radioactively-labelled glucose. The method of Cirillo and Razin (1973) combines a fermentation assay based on detection of labelled acid products with determination of hexokinase activity by measuring sugar phosphorylation. Cells from a 500 ml culture are washed and divided into two fractions. One fraction (at two concentrations 1 mg and 10 mg cell protein/ml) is inoculated in a reaction mixture containing 5×10^{-4} or 10^{-2} M [^{14}C] glucose. After cessation of the reaction the mixture is passed down a Dowex 1-X2 column (Cl⁻ form). Unutilised sugar passes straight down the column but acid products are bound and can be subsequently released with 1M lithium chloride. For glucose fermenters much of the activity will be stuck to the column; with nonfermenters all the activity will be in the column eluant. The remaining volume of washed cells is lysed by freezing and thawing and reacted with $[^{14}C]$ glucose in the presence of ATP, magnesium chloride and sodium fluoride. The amount of phosphorylated sugar is also determined by binding to Dowex 1-X2. If results are expressed as nanomoles of glucose phosphorylated per mg of cell protein then nonfermenters phosphorylate less than 0.001 nmoles/mg of cell protein/min.

C. Arginine Hydrolysis

Most nonfermentative mycoplasmas can derive energy from the hydrolysis of arginine by the arginine dihydrolase pathway (Schimke and Barile, 1963). The ammonia released by the degradation of arginine causes an alkaline pH shift in the medium. A test similar to that for glucose fermentation can be used to detect a change in phenol red indicator from orange to red in media supplemented with 1% arginine hydrochloride. Similar controls should be employed (Aluotto *et al.*, 1970). Because some organisms are inhibited by higher concentrations of arginine or its metabolites, lesser amounts of amino acid should also be tested (Leach, 1976). Some organisms, notably *S. citri*, are capable of metabolising both glucose and arginine in which case the acid from glucose fermentation may neutralise the ammonia released by hydrolysis of arginine (Townsend, 1976). For some reason which is not clear, this organism can only degrade arginine when actively growing and to maintain its growth a source of fermentable sugar such as glucose or fructose is essential. It is therefore necessary to include in the test a culture containing both arginine (0.5%) and glucose (0.1%) which has been adjusted to a pH of 7.5. Organisms which degrade both the amino acid and the carbohydrate will show an initial drop in pH which will then be reversed so that the culture finally returns to the same or a slightly higher pH. Organisms unable to break down arginine will show a steady fall in pH. Confirmation of arginine degradation can be obtained by demonstrating an increase in accumulation of the breakdown product citrulline (Weickmann *et al.*, 1978).

D. Carotenoid Production

All members of the genus *Acholeplasma* so far examined produce carotenoid pigments which in nearly all instances impart a yellow colour to cell pellets. Carotenoids are synthesised from acetate or mevalonate as demonstrated by incorporation of [^{14}C] acetate or [^{14}C] mevalonate into the neutral lipid fraction, which contains carotenoids (Rottem and Razin, 1967; Smith, 1979). Carotenoids (with the exception of *Acholeplasma axanthum* (Tully and Razin, 1969)) can be extracted with boiling ethanol and give an absorption spectrum with three maxima at around 418, 442 and 472 nm, the highest of which is at 442 nm (Razin and Cleverdon, 1965). The carotenoid pigments of *A. axanthum* have recently been shown to have different spectral characteristics with absorption maxima mostly in the range 270–295 nm. A full discussion of the detection of carotenoids in this species and the implication of these findings on established carotenoid detection methods can be found in the paper by Smith and Langworthy (1979).

E. Other Tests

(i)   Urea hydrolysis: breakdown of urea to carbon dioxide and
       and ammonia is the fundamental property of the genus *Ureaplasma*. This property is unlikely to be encountered in isolates
       from plant or insect sources but could be associated with
       contaminants of human origin. Tests for the hydrolysis of urea
       are described by Shepard and Howard (1970) and Masover *et al.*
       (1976, 1977).

(ii)   Aesculin and arbutin hydrolysis: degradation of aesculin (6,
       7-dihydrocoumarin-6 glucoside) by the β-D-glucosidase pathway
       (Williams and Wittler, 1971) and arbutin (hydroquinone β-D-
       glucopyranoside) (Ernø and Stipkovits, 1973) can be diagnostic
       for some species of acholeplasmas (Tully, 1979).

(iii) Phosphatase activity (Williams and Wittler, 1971).

(iv)   Proteolytic activity (Aluotto *et al.*, 1970).

(v)   Tetrazolium reduction – anaerobic and aerobic (Aluotto *et al.*,
       1970).

(vi)   Production of films and spots (Fabricant and Freundt, 1967).

2. Electrophoretic Analysis of Mycoplasma Proteins in Gels

An extensive range of electrophoretic techniques is available for the separation of constituent cell proteins and polypeptides in gels. The resulting pattern of proteins can be regarded as 'fingerprints' of the mycoplasmas (Razin and Rottem, 1967) and provide a basis for assessing the similarity of the organisms which is a reflection of genetic homology.

A. *Growth of Cells*

Sufficient cell protein for a single analysis can be obtained from as little as 1 ml of culture but, unless radioisotopes are used, it is more convenient to harvest cells from 100–200 ml and have enough material to perform a number of separations. The electrophoretic pattern can be affected by components of the medium, usually those derived from whole serum supplements and which may be precipitated by fast-growing acid-producing strains. Since this material is not removed by washing it may be preferable to grow such organisms in a serum-free medium containing 1–2% (v/v) PPLO serum fraction. For the more nutritionally fastidious organisms, fetal calf serum, extensively dialysed against 0.1M potassium chloride, may be used as a compromise since it supports good growth with the minimum of preciptitation. The problem can be entirely avoided by *in vivo* labelling with radioisotopes and autoradiographic detection of radioactive cell-synthesised proteins (Mouches *et al.*, 1979).

Harvested cells are resuspended in a buffer of appropriate osmotic pressure (5% w/v sorbitol in 0.1M phosphate pH 7.5) and the protein content determined by the method of Lowry *et al.* (1951). An approximate estimate can be obtained turbidimetrically (Daniels and Meddins, 1973).

B. *Solubilisation*

Only a small percentage of mycoplasma proteins are normally soluble in aqueous media so the cells must be broken down and the proteins dissociated. A mixture of phenol, acetic acid and water (2:1:0.5) (Razin and Rottem, 1967) will solubilise a large number of mycoplasma proteins in 10–30 minutes at 37°C (Rhoades *et al.*, 1974). However, solubilisation is incomplete, even after extended incubation. Some insoluble material can be removed by centrifugation but appreciable amounts of protein fail to enter the gel during electrophoresis. Although it was stated that this represents nonspecific aggregation (Razin *et al.*, 1969) a large proportion of the remaining protein migrates as a single fast-moving component (Daniels and Meddins, 1973).

A very effective solubilising agent is the anionic detergent sodium dodecyl sulphate (SDS) which binds in a 1:1 ratio with almost all proteins, conferring on them an overall negative charge. The resulting complex is a straight particle whose length is directly proportional to the molecular weight of the polypeptide (Reynolds and Tanford, 1970). During electrophoresis the mobilities of these complexes are related solely to the molecular weights of their polypeptide chains so that the molecular weights of individual protein subunits can be determined by reference to the electrophoretic mobilities of standards of known molecular weight (Shapiro *et al.*, 1967; Weber and Osborn, 1969). Whole cells can be solubilised in 1–2% (w/v) SDS containing β-mercaptoethanol or dithiothreitol to reduce disulphide bonds. It is usual to boil the cells in this solution for 3 minutes to inactivate proteolytic enzymes.

In methods such as isoelectric focusing where proteins are separated according to their natural charge, solubilisation must be accomplished with nonionic detergents. Tween-20 or Triton X-100 are reasonably efficient at solubilising mycoplasma cells (Sayed and Kenny, 1980) and their efficiency can be enhanced by the addition of urea to 8M and β-mercaptoethanol (Archer *et al.*, 1978); however some proteins remain insoluble (Townsend *et al.*, 1980). For some applications it is possible to render them soluble by first treating with SDS which is subsequently displaced by addition of excess nonionic detergent (Ames and Nikaido, 1976). In immunoelectrophoretic techniques, where the conformation of proteins must be extensively conserved, solubilisation is normally achieved with nonionic detergents alone (Thirkill and Kenny, 1974). In order to prevent aggregation or reassociation of solubilised proteins during any electrophoretic separation, it is essential that the gels should also contain the same solubilising agent present in the sample.

Cell lysis is accompanied by release of DNA which makes the material difficult to handle and may block the gel pores and distort the gel surface. To prevent this the nucleic acid strands can be sheared by sonication or repeated passage through a fine bore needle (Daniels and Meddins, 1973) or digestion with DNAase I (O'Farrell, 1975).

C. Polyacrylamide Gel Electrophoresis

If an electrical current is passed through a solution buffered at constant pH and ionic strength and containing a mixture of proteins, the proteins will move towards the anode or cathode according to their overall charge. In practice the separation is carried out in a porous support medium and the proteins are applied in a thin layer. During electrophoresis they are resolved into a number of bands containing proteins of similar charge properties. Analysis of constituent proteins by electrophoresis has been extensively applied to mycoplasmas. Except where very large molecules or supramolecular complexes are of interest, the starch gel support systems employed in early studies (Fowler *et al.*, 1963) have been superseded by polyacrylamide gels which offer much greater resolution and, because of the ease with which the pore size of the gel matrix can be varied, introduce an element of separation according to molecular size. It is beyond the scope of this chapter to review the principles and systems available for polyacrylamide gel electrophoresis (PAGE) or the factors which govern the choice of pore size, degree of cross linking, choice of buffer, etc. Extensive discussions of these topics can be found elsewhere (Davis, 1964; Ornstein, 1964; Gordon, 1969; Maurer, 1971; Allen and Maurer, 1974). Instead we will limit ourselves to a discussion of two systems of proven use in analysing mycoplasma proteins.

The continuous buffer system used by Daniels and Meddins (1973), which is based on the method described by Hull (1971) is very simple and particularly suited for use in cylinder gels. Acrylamide (5% w/v) containing 0.1% SDS is polymerised in 75 x 5 mm int. diam. chromic acid-cleaned glass tubes sealed at one end. Care should be exercised when handling acrylamide since it is poisonous in the unpolymerised state. The most critical part of the operation is overlaying the unpoly-merised gel with buffer to produce a sharp flat interface. Gelling time should be adjusted by varying catalyst concentration so that the acrylamide does not set while there is still turbulence at the interface or excessive heat generation produces an uneven top to the gel and consequently deformed protein bands, or so slowly that considerable diffusion and resulting dilution of the upper part of the gel occurs – about 15-20 min is optimum. After polymerisation the seal is removed and the tubes suspended between the anode and cathode reservoirs which contain 0.0125M phosphate buffer pH 7.1 with 0.1% SDS. The samples of SDS solubilised protein are layered from a capillary tube under the buffer on to the surface of the gel, a procedure which is facilitated by including 10% (w/v) sucrose or glycerol in the sample. The sample volume should be kept as small as possible (10-25 μl) to reduce broadening of the bands and the amount of protein should not exceed 150 μg/gel. Separation is effected by passing a constant current of 3 mA/gel for 1 hr, after which time the lowest molecular weight components will have migrated about 5 cm into the gel. If a marker dye such as bromophenol blue (0.01%) is incorporated in the sample, it will run just ahead of the fastest moving proteins, allowing progress of the separation to be visualised. Increased separation of the protein bands can be achieved by using longer gel tubes. After electrophoresis the gels should be removed from the tubes by 'ringing' with a long hypodermic needle and fixed and stained as soon as possible to minimise diffusion of the smaller components.

Although cylinder gels can achieve a very rapid separation they suffer from a number of drawbacks, the most important of which is lack of comparability. It is almost impossible to produce two identical cylinder gels and run them under exactly similar conditions, which is a source of error in critical comparisons of gel patterns or molecular weight determinations. By using thin slabs of acrylamide to which the samples are applied from slots formed in the slab during polymerisation, up to 25 individual samples may be run under identical conditions (Wreghitt *et al.*, 1974). The best separations have been achieved using the discontinuous SDS system of Laemmli (1970) as modified for slab gels (Laemmli and Favre, 1973). The system consists of a short nonsieving stacking gel of low acrylamide concentration and containing a tris/HCl buffer of low ionic strength and pH (0.125M, pH 6.8) and a longer separating gel of higher acrylamide concentration containing a tris/HCl buffer of higher ionic strength and pH (0.375M, pH 8.8). The electrode vessels contain a tris/glycine buffer (0.025M tris, 0.192M glycine, pH 8.3). The low pH of the stacking gel causes the sample to concentrate into a thin band, sandwiched between the leading (Cl^-) and trailing (Gly^-) ions, in which individual proteins are sequentially stacked (Davis, 1964; Ornstein, 1964; Williams and Reisfeld, 1964). This effect ceases when the migrating protein zone enters the higher pH gel where normal separation occurs according to molecular weight. Because of the concentrating effect of the stacking gel, this system is capable of handling larger volumes of sample without loss of resolution by band broadening.

The apparatus for running slab gels is similar to that described by Reid and Bieleski (1968) except that the slot in the upper reservoir is extended upwards to form a deep notch corresponding to a similar notch cut in the back gel supporting plate so that the buffer flows over the gel surface but is retained by the square front supporting plate (Studier, 1973). The separating gel is poured to a depth of 10–15 cm between the two glass plates which are held apart by plastic spacers 1.5 mm thick which are coated in petroleum jelly to make a water-tight seal. The solution is overlayed, carefully, with water and allowed to polymerise; then the stacking gel is poured on top to a depth of 5 cm. The sample slots are formed by introducing a 'comb', which is very slightly thinner than the spacers, into the unpolymerised stacking gel. A typical comb has rectangular teeth 2.5 cm long and 5 mm wide spaced 2.5 mm apart which leaves a series of flat-bottomed sample wells of the same dimensions in the polymerised gel when the comb is removed. Good separations of spiroplasma proteins have been achieved using a 4% stacking gel and a 12 or 15% separating gel (Archer and Best, 1980; Townsend *et al.*, 1980), but the resolution can be increased by the formation of a linear gradient of acrylamide concentration in the separation gel, e.g. 15-20% (w/v) (Mouches *et al.*, 1979). Linear gradients can be formed using a normal two-chambered gradient mixer. The catalyst concentration must be adjusted so that the complete gel can be poured and overlayed before polymerisation occurs. An exponential acrylamide gradient can be made by plugging the front chamber of the mixer with an air-tight stopper so that the volume of the chamber remains constant (O'Farrell, 1975). The amount of whole cell protein loaded should be in the order of 2.5-5 μg/sq mm of slot surface. A typical 1.5 mm thick gel is run at a current of 2 mA/cm during sample concentration in the stacking gel which is increased to 2.5 mA/cm when the sample enters the separating gel. A complete 15 cm long separation will take about 3-4 hours. If increased currents are applied to achieve faster separations then some form of cooling system will be required to prevent band distortion.

D. *Isoelectric Focusing*

At its isoelectric pH (pI) a protein has no net electrical charge and will not move in an electrical field. Consequently, if a mixture of proteins is placed in a stabilised pH gradient and a potential difference is applied across the gradient, each protein will migrate until it reaches the pH corresponding to its pI where it will stop or 'focus'. Since the pI is a reflection of amino acid composition, isoelectric focusing represents a powerful tool capable of separating proteins having only minor differences in amino acid sequence (Garrels and Gibson, 1976). Unlike separations by electrophoresis where protein bands become more diffuse as the separation continues, isoelectric focusing causes the bands to concentrate allowing larger amounts of protein to be analysed.

The pH gradient is established by carrier ampholytes which are mixtures of aliphatic polyamino-polycarboxylic acids. When subjected to an electrical field each component ampholyte will migrate to a position defined by its pI and, because they have a high buffering capacity, produce in the surrounding medium a pH corresponding to that pI. The range and profile of the resulting pH gradient can be varied according to the ampholytes chosen.

For analytical purposes the pH gradient is stabilised in a nonsieving polyacrylamide gel (4-5% w/v). Ampholines should be present at a concentration of 2-3% (v/v). The polyacrylamide can be cast in tubes but the same lack of comparability referred to in association with PAGE in tubes means that slab gels are the system of choice. Gels are normally pre-run to establish the pH gradient before application of the sample. Since much higher voltages are applied to isoelectric focusing gels, some method of cooling is required. After completion of a run the pH gradient may be measured directly with a microelectrode or by cutting a strip of the gel into slices which are soaked in water for 30 minutes and then measuring the pH of the solution.

General references to the theory and practice of isoelectric focusing can be found in Arbuthnot and Beeley (1975) and Righetti and Drysdale (1976) and details of its application to the analysis of mycoplasma proteins in papers by Sayed and Hatten (1976) and Sayed and Kenny (1980). For taxonomic studies SDS-PAGE is simpler, cheaper and achieves better solubilisation of membrane proteins than is possible with nonionic detergents but, in certain instances, such as the analysis of cytoplasmic proteins, isoelectric focusing may yield more information (Sayed and Kenny, 1980).

E. Two-dimensional Gel Electrophoresis

Analysis of whole spiroplasma cells by SDS-PAGE seldom resolves more than 40 separate protein bands (Figure 9.1a) while the genome molecular weight (1×10^9) represents a coding capacity of between 1×10^3 and 1.4×10^3 average polypeptides. Obviously some may not be expressed while others are transient or simply in such small quantities that they are below the detection threshold of the system, but many proteins will have the same or very similar molecular weights or pIs and will be superimposed on each other. However, only a fraction of these proteins will share the same molecular weight and pI, so by combining the two separation techniques into a two-dimensional method it is possible to increase hugely the resolution of constituent polypeptides.

An excellent two-dimensionsl method is described in great detail by O'Farrell (1975), which, with a few minor modifications (Archer *et al.*, 1978), can be applied to mycoplasmas. The basis of the system is a first dimension separation of urea/nonionic detergent-solubilised protein in a thin cylindrical isoelectric focusing gel containing urea and having a pH gradient from pH 4.5 to pH 10, and a second dimension separation in an SDS-PAGE slab gel with an exponential acrylamide gradient from 5–22.5% (w/v) and a stacking gel of 4.75% (w/v) acrylamide. Because of the instability of the basic end of the pH gradient this method is unsuitable for resolving basic proteins in urea. A modified non-

Figure 9.1: Comparison of the Separation of Proteins of a Strain of *S. citri* by (a) One-dimensional SDS/PAGE which Resolves about 40 Components after Staining and (b) Two-dimensional Electrophoresis which Shows more than 300 Components by Fluorography.

(a)   (b)

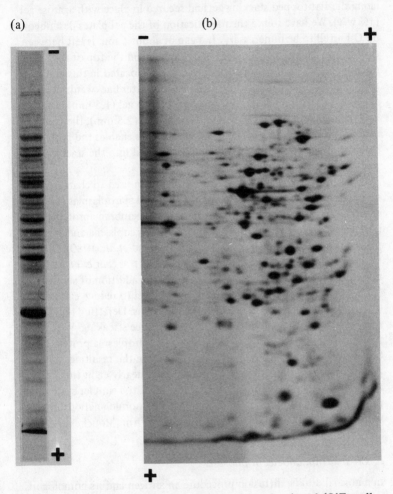

equilibrium pH gradient electrophoresis has been developed (O'Farrell *et al.*, 1977) as an alternative first dimension which gives high resolution of both basic and acidic proteins. This method uses a shorter time of electrophoresis which takes place towards the cathode. In this rapidly formed pH gradient separation appears to be achieved by a combination of isoelectric focusing of acidic proteins and nonequilibrium electrophoresis of basic proteins. The nonequilibrium system extends the analysis to include 15–30% of the proteins excluded from normal isoelectric focusing gels. After the first dimension isoelectric focusing has been completed, the gels are equilibrated in SDS for 1–2 hr, laid along the flat-topped stacking gel and secured in place with agarose gel (1% w/v). We have found the modification of the gel plates described by O'Farrell to be unnecessary. If a gap of about 1 mm is left between the bottom of the notch in the back gel plate and the top of the stacking gel, the isoelectric focusing gel can be located in this groove and embedded in agarose while inclining the plates backwards at an angle of 45°. Although the thickness of the slab gel (1.5 mm) is about half the diameter of the isoelectric focusing gel (2.5 mm), the continuity of the agarose between the two gel surfaces enables the protein bands to move out of the first dimension gel and into the stacking gel without mixing.

Two-dimensional gel electrophoresis has been used to characterise mycoplasmas (Rodwell and Rodwell, 1978) and spiroplasmas (Mouches *et al.*, 1979), to determine the distribution of membrane proteins (Archer *et al.*, 1978) and to identify specific mycoplasma and spiroplasma proteins (Rodwell *et al.*, 1979; Townsend *et al.*, 1980). In all cases the basic method of O'Farrell was used but Archer *et al.* (1978) recommend certain modifications including the addition of sucrose (12% w/v) to the samples and first dimension gel to reduce cathodic drift and limit aggregation of solubilised proteins. Defatting the membranes prior to solubilisation helps to reduce streaking. With these modifications 25 μg of [^{35}S] labelled whole spiroplasma protein can be resolved into about 300 polypeptide spots on the resulting fluorograph (Figure 9.1b). Although the method has nearly eight times the resolving power of one-dimensional SDS-PAGE, the simpler system may provide sufficient information to establish taxonomic relationships which two-dimensional separations merely confirm (Mouches *et al.*, 1979; Daniels *et al.*, 1980).

F. Crossed Immunoelectrophoresis

In a normal double diffusion procedure an antigen and its homologous antibody are allowed to diffuse freely through an agarose gel matrix. At the point where they are present in optimal proportions a visible immunoprecipitate is formed (Crowle, 1961). In immunoelectrophoresis the antigen is separated into its constituent protein components by one-dimensional electrophoresis in agarose, and the proteins are then located by allowing antiserum to diffuse into the gel from a slot cut alongside the length of the electrophoresis path (Grabar and Williams, 1953). The resulting pattern of immunoprecipitates reflects reactions of identity between individual components and the antigen mixture and their homologous antibodies in the whole antiserum but, although this represents good qualitative information, it is not quantitative. In the crossed immunoelectrophoresis method of Laurell (1965) as modified by Clark and Freeman (1967), a second dimension electrophoresis is introduced causing the separated antigens to migrate into a small slab of antiserum-containing agarose which is buffered at pH 8.6, which represents the pI of gamma globulins. Reactions of homology give rise to immunoprecipitin peaks whose area is directly proportional to the antigen concentration and inversely proportional to the antibody concentration; thus the method combines identification with quantification.

In the first dimension the sample is applied to a well cut in the agar and electrophoresed over a distance of about 8 cm towards the anode. Progress of the separation, which usually takes 2–3 hr, can be observed if bromophenol blue bound to a strongly anionic protein such as bovine serum albumin is added to the sample. The electrophoresis track is then cut out and placed along the bottom edge of a 10 x 5 cm glass plate, the remainder of which is filled with molten agarose containing antiserum. In order to achieve complete immobilisation of gamma globulins agarose should be of the low electroendosmosis type. When it has set the second dimension separation is performed overnight. Apparatus for running these gels is commercially available but perfectly good results can be achieved using a water-cooled plate, two buffer reservoirs and an ordinary electrophoresis power supply.

Crossed immunoelectrophoresis has been used to study serological relationships between mycoplasmas (Wróblewski and Ratanasavanh, 1976; Wróblewski *et al.*, 1977) to examine the nature and distribution of membrane proteins (Johansson and Hjertén, 1974; Thirkill and Kenny, 1974; Johansson *et al.*, 1975; Alexander and Kenny, 1977) and to identify specific proteins (Wróblewski *et al.*, 1977; Johansson and Wróblewski, 1978). In all cases the method used was essentially that of Clark and Freeman (1967) using material solubilised in Tween 20 or Triton X-100 or the anionic detergent sodium deoxycholate (SDOC) which is relatively non-denaturing (Ne'eman *et al.*, 1972) but alters the first dimension separation because it imparts a negative charge to the proteins. Recently a different buffer system has been described which gives improved resolution of spiroplasma antigens (Archer and Best, 1980). About 20 μg of cell protein is separated in the first dimension in a 1% agarose gel containing 50mM tris buffered to pH 8.6 with citric acid and either 2% (v/v) Triton X-100 or 5% (w/v) SDOC. A similar buffer is used in the second dimension gel which also contains 2-10% (v/v) antiserum. Using this system a spiroplasma reacted against its homologous antiserum produces between 20 and 30 precipitin peaks (Figure 9.2), although the number will depend on whether the antiserum was raised against fixed whole cells, lysed cells or membranes.

Figure 9.2: Crossed Immunoelectrophoresis of Solubilised Whole Cells of a Strain of *S. citri* with Antiserum Prepared against Lysed Whole Cells of that Strain. More than 25 individual peaks representing different antigens are apparent.

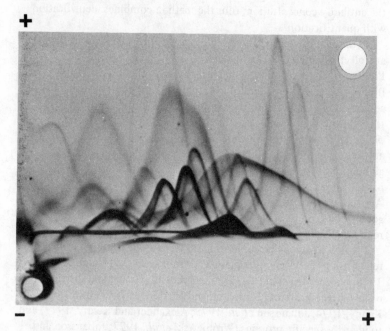

If two different organisms produce similar peaks in a gel containing antiserum to only one of them then it is an indication that they share antigens. This can be confirmed by tandem-crossed immunoelectrophoresis (Bjerrum and Bøg-Hansen, 1976). The antigen preparations are applied as two separate samples in adjacent wells about 2.5 mm apart along the electrophoresis path and the first and second dimension separations performed as usual. In the resulting gel, antigens having similar electrophoretic properties will form tandem peaks and if the

Figure 9.3: Tandem-crossed Immunoelectrophoresis of Solubilised Whole Cells of the BC3 (i) and SP-4 (ii) Strains of *S. citri* with Antiserum Prepared against Lysed Whole Cells of the SP-4 Strain. Continuity of the precipitin line between peaks (examples arrowed) indicates antigenic identity and shows that about 15 antigens are common to both strains.

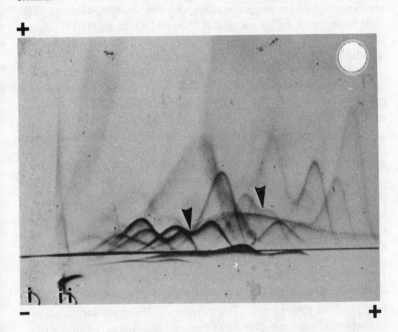

antigens are homologous the tandem peak will be fused (Figure 9.3); if they are heterologous the peaks will cross over each other. By using this method it was possible to show common antigens between *S. citri* and several other spiroplasmas (Archer and Best, 1980; Archer and Townsend, 1981).

Individual antigenic components in complex mixtures can be identified by the use of intermediate gels (Bjerrum and Bøg-Hansen, 1976). The intermediate gel containing monospecific antibody to the antigen is placed between the first dimension electrophoresis and the second dimension slab containing antibodies against the complete mixture. During the second dimension electrophoresis the single antigen will be precipitated as a peak in the intermediate gel while the remaining components of the mixture will pass through to the main slab, where they will be precipitated. This approach has been used by

Archer and Best (1980) and Archer and Townsend (1981) to
investigate the occurrence of spiralin (Wróblewski *et al.*, 1977) and a
closely related protein in different spiroplasmas.

In some circumstances it may be more appropriate to use SDS-PAGE
to achieve the first dimension separation since precipitin rockets can be
identified by their approximate molecular weights. In order to prevent
interference with the antigen/antibody binding reaction, unbound SDS
must be removed. In the method of Chau and Blomberg (1979) this is
accomplished by the presence of an SDOC containing gel at the cathode,
an intermediate gel containing the nonionic detergent, Lubrol and an
anodal gel also with Lubrol. Unbound SDS complexes with the SDOC
and is moved out of the antibody containing gel during the second
dimension separation. The SDOC also serves to enhance the mobility
of the proteins and helps move them out of the SDS gel into the
second dimension gel. The apparent function of the Lubrol intermediate
gel is to remove any traces of unbound SDS. However it may also
displace SDS from the protein complex resulting in precipitation of
proteins not soluble in nonionic detergent. Archer and Townsend
(1981) have described a modification to this method which is simpler
and gives improved resolution. The SDS gel strips are equilibrated overnight in buffer containing 0.5% (w/v) SDOC and the anodal gel is
eliminated. The cathodal, intermediate and antibody gels are retained
but Lubrol is omitted and instead all the gels contain 0.5% (w/v) SDOC.
Using this method the band corresponding to spiralin was identified in
the pattern of proteins resolved by SDS-PAGE (Archer and Townsend,
1981) and the fibril protein (Townsend *et al.*, 1980) was identified
in twelve different spiroplasmas (Townsend and Archer, unpublished)
(Figure 9.4).

Although some mycoplasma proteins do retain a degree of anti-
genicity (Kahane and Razin, 1969) many will be denatured by the
binding of SDS (Tanford and Reynolds, 1976) so that the antisera
raised against native proteins may not react with SDS-solubilised
components. Even when an antiserum raised against SDS-solubilised
spiroplasmas was used few peaks were observed (Archer and Townsend,
1981) indicating that the method is probably much less sensitive than
normal crossed immunoelectrophoresis.

Individual peaks formed in crossed immunoelectrophoresis represent
a single species of antibody/antigen complex and as such are a source
of purified cell components. Consequently individual peaks may be
excised, emulsified and used as immunogens to prepare monospecific
antisera against cell components. Alexander and Kenny (1977)

employed this technique to raise monospecific antibodies against the major membrane component of *Mycoplasma arginini.*

Figure 9.4: Crossed Immunoelectrophoresis of (a) 5 μg of SDS Solubilised Fibril Protein (Molecular Weight 55,000) from the BC3 Strain of *S. citri* and (b) Whole SDS Solubilised BC3 Cells Both Separated by SDS/PAGE in the First Dimension and Electrophoresed into Monospecific Antiserum against SDS Solubilised Fibril Protein in the Second Dimension. Stained first dimension gels are included as a reference. The similar dimensions and positions of the two peaks show that the whole cell preparation contains approximately the same amount of fibril protein which has a similar molecular weight to the purified material.

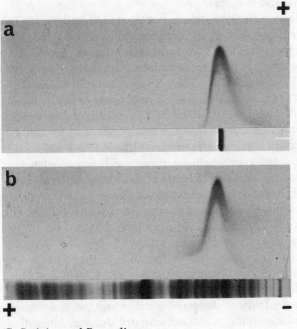

G. Staining and Recording

Immediately after electrophoresis is completed, gels should be fixed and stained to locate protein bands. In most cases the two processes can be carried out simultaneously, except that the ampholines must be removed from isoelectric focusing gels because they have a strong affinity for most protein stains. There are a variety of methods available for the fixation, removal of ampholines and staining of electrofocusing gels but we have found the most reliable is that described in LKB Application Note 75 (LKB-Produkter, Bromma, Sweden) which uses a fixing solution of 5% (w/v) 5-sulphosalicyclic acid in 10% (v/v) methanol (60°C for 30 min) and a staining solution of Coomassie Brilliant Blue R250 in 25% (v/v) ethanol and 8% (v/v) acetic acid in water.

Excess antiserum must also be removed from crossed immunoelectrophoresis gels since it will produce a heavily stained background. Gels, still attached to the glass plate, are pressed between several sheets of filter paper, soaked in 0.1M sodium chloride for 15 min, then pressed again and dried with a warm air blower. Plates are stained for 5 min in 0.5% Coomassie Brilliant Blue R250 in 45% (v/v) ethanol and 10% (v/v) acetic acid in water.

The use of amido black for staining gels (Razin and Rottem, 1967) has been superseded by the use of Coomassie Brilliant Blue R250 which has ten times the affinity for proteins (Groth *et al.*, 1963) facilitating the detection of minor components and allowing less protein to be loaded. Coomassie Brilliant Blue also exists as G250 which is marginally better for some applications since it produces less background staining (Diezel *et al.*, 1972). Optimal staining, capable of detecting 0.5 μg or less of protein in a single band, can be achieved using the method of Fairbanks *et al.* (1971), which combines high sensitivity with minimum loss of low molecular weight components and extremely low background staining. However, the method uses several different solutions and gels take at least 48 hours to destain completely. A more rapid method which gives almost as good results is to stain for 1 hr with 0.1% Coomassie Brilliant Blue G250 in 45% (v/v) methanol and 10% (v/v) acetic acid in water. Destaining is achieved with several changes of the same solution without the dye but, if swelling of the gel can be tolerated, then the methanol can be reduced to 15% (v/v) or lower and the acetic acid to 7% (v/v). Destaining can be accelerated by constant agitation and more frequent changes of destain which can be decolourised and re-used after filtration through activated charcoal. Alternatively, anion-exchange resin beads can be suspended in the destaining solution to accelerate dye removal.

Various electrolytic destaining devices are commercially available but in our experience the results obtained are highly variable — destaining is often uneven and some bands appear to be lost altogether.

For most purposes photography offers the best method of recording gels; if necessary filters can be used to enhance the contrast of the stained bands (Daniels and Meddins, 1973). In our experience visual analysis also offers the most convenient method of comparing gel patterns for taxonomic purposes (Daniels *et al.*, 1980). For comparing two-dimensional gels it is often easier to have the prints made into transparent overlays allowing common spots to be marked (Rodwell and Rodwell, 1978). The staining pattern of gels themselves or of photographic negatives can be recorded by scanning densitometry. The resulting profiles are not easy to compare visually but can form the basis for a computer based storage and retrieval system and pro-grammes exist for computerised analysis and comparison of one-dimensional (Daniels and Johnson, 1978) and two-dimensional (Garrels, 1979) gels.

It should be remembered that the intensity of staining does not necessarily reflect the true concentration of different proteins since stain binding is determined by the number of binding sites present. Coomassie Brilliant Blue binds to NH_3^+ groups, so protein low in these groups will bind less dye than the same quantity of a different protein having more such groups (Groth *et al.*, 1963).

The gels themselves may be stored in destain for some considerable time but it is more convenient to store them dried flat. Slab gels, or thin strips of cylinder gels, are placed flat on Whatman 3MM filter paper and covered with clear cellophane sheet. The area below the gel is supported on a porous polythene sheet in a holder through which a vacuum can be applied to the gel. The speed of drying is increased by placing the gel surface over a boiling water bath (Bonner and Laskey, 1974).

H. Autoradiography and Fluorography

Proteins labelled with [^{14}C, ^{35}S, ^{135}I or ^{32}P] can be located on dried gels by autoradiography (Fairbanks *et al.*, 1965). The gel is held in intimate contact with X-ray film for sufficient time to achieve exposure. Sensitivity of detection can be increased by exposing at $-70°$C. It has been shown that under these conditions a single protein spot on a two-dimensional gel emitting 1 cpm can be detected on a film of optical density 0.01 after 20 days exposure (O'Farrell, 1975).

The range of detectable isotopes can be extended to include [^{3}H] and the sensitivity of [^{14}C] etc., correspondingly increased tenfold by fluorography (Bonner and Laskey, 1974). The scintillator 2,5-diphenyl-oxazole (PPO) (20% w/w) dissolved in dimethyl sulphoxide (DMSO) is introduced into gels by diffusion after they have been fixed and dehydrated in DMSO. Care should be exercised since DMSO can penetrate the skin. The gel is then hydrated and dried under vacuum before being placed in contact with X-ray film and exposed at $-70°C$. About 3,000 [^{3}H] disintegrations (dis)/min or 130 [^{14}C] dis/min located in a single band can be detected on film after 24 hr. This sensitivity can be increased still further by pre-exposing the film before exposure to the gel (Laskey and Mills, 1975). Using pre-exposed film, 300 [^{3}H] dis/min or 30 [^{14}C] dis/min can be detected in 24 hr. The use of DMSO has several drawbacks; not only is it unpleasant to handle but it is expensive and complete dehydration of the gel takes several hours. An alternative method using the water-soluble fluor, sodium salicylate, is available (Chamberlain, 1979) — however the spots tend to be a little more diffuse than when DMSO/PPO is used.

Because of its extreme sensitivity fluorography has been used to locate mycoplasma proteins separated by two-dimensional electrophoresis (Rodwell and Rodwell, 1978; Archer *et al.*, 1978; Mouches *et al.*, 1979). Fluorography in combination with staining has been used to demonstrate the cellular origin of specific mycoplasma proteins (Neimark, 1979a) and to compare the electrophoretic properties of unlabelled muscle actin with proteins synthesised by mycoplasmas (Rodwell *et al.*, 1979).

3. Genome Properties

The mycoplasma genome consists of a circular DNA molecule (Bode and Morowitz, 1967) packaged in the cell as a 'folded chromosome' (Teplitz, 1977). Two features of the genome serve to set mycoplasmas apart from bacteria. The first is the base composition: all mycoplasmas have DNA of low guanine + cytosine content, in the range 24 to 40 moles % (guanine + cytosine), whereas bacteria span the full theoretically possible range of 24 to 72%. The second is the genome size, that is the molecular weight of the nonreplicating chromosome. Mycoplasmas have genomes weighing either about 5×10^8 or 1×10^9 daltons, whereas bacteria range from 8×10^8 to about 15×10^9. These properties are summarised in Table 9.1. Fuller information together with a discussion of its significance is given by Stanbridge and Reff (1979).

Since the genome contains all the information specifying the structure and activities of the mycoplasma, its characterisation is an important goal. If it were possible fully to characterise the genome, that is to determine the total base sequence, then all other properties of the cell could in principle be deduced and other characterisation techniques

Table 9.1: Properties of Mycoplasma Genomes

Genus	Guanine + Cytosine Content (moles %)	Genome Size (daltons x 10^{-8})
Mycoplasma	23–35	5
except *M. pneumoniae*	41	5
Ureaplasma	27–30	5
Acholeplasma	30–33	10
Anaeroplasma	30–33, 40	?
Spiroplasma	26–29	10
Thermoplasma	46	9

would theoretically be redundant. In practice, however, base sequences have not yet been established for DNA molecules larger than plasmids or those of small viruses and, moreover, even if the process could be extended to a cell we are still lacking the means to deduce the structure and function of proteins from their primary amino acid sequences, which are equivalent to DNA base sequences. Nevertheless characterisation of the mycoplasma genome at lower levels yields valuable information on taxonomy and offers a method for investigating relationships with other organisms. Determination of the base composition of the DNA is now mandatory when new mycoplasmas are described (ICSB Subcommittee on Taxonomy of Mycoplasmatales, 1979).

A. DNA Preparation

With the exception of base composition determination from buoyant density measurements in caesium chloride gradients, all genome characterisation techniques require highly purified DNA, free of RNA, protein and polysaccharide. Many procedures have been published for preparing DNA, but almost all involve similar basic steps. The cells are lysed with detergents, the lysate is deproteinised with phenol or organic solvents, and nucleic acids are precipitated with alcohols. Further purification depends on ribonuclease treatment to destroy RNA, additional deproteinising treatments and further selective precipitation steps to remove polysaccharides and oligonucleotides. Mycoplasmas seem in general to present few problems. The lack of a cell wall renders them easily lysed by detergents and polysaccharide contamination is not usually encountered. Against this must be set the disadvantage that mycoplasma yields in culture are low compared with bacteria, so that larger volumes of expensive culture medium must be used. In the authors' experience 500 ml of a typical culture yields ample material for DNA preparation. At many steps of the purification it is essential to avoid exposure of the sample to deoxyribonucleases whether originating from the mycoplasmas or from external sources such as fingers or contaminated glassware. In addition, for some purposes (e.g. restriction enzyme analysis) shearing of the DNA must be minimised by avoiding shaking of solutions or passage through narrow bore pipettes.

Cultures should be chilled and the cells harvested by centrifugation in a refrigerated centrifuge. A spin for 15 minutes at $10,000\,g$ is adequate to recover most of the cells. It is advisable not to wash the cells by resuspension in buffer and recentrifugation because some mycoplasmas, notably spiroplasmas, lyse in the process and premature lysis means that much DNA is lost.

The pellet is suspended in a suitable solution which minimises DNAase action, for example saline-EDTA in the method of Marmur (1961). Lysis is effected with detergents such as sodium dodecyl-sulphate, sodium lauroylsarcosinate or with the triisopropyl naphthalene sulphonate-4 aminosalicylate mixture of Kirby (1965). Lysis is usually immediate and complete. Deproteinisation is then begun, if necessary, after adjusting the ionic strength of the solution. The deproteinising agent is usually either chloroform/isoamylalcohol (24/1) (Marmur, 1961) or a phenol mixture. Good results are obtained with a mixture of phenol (redistilled), *m*-cresol, 8-hydroxyquinoline, but a variety of solutions have been used (Kirby, 1968). The mixture is vigorously shaken in a stoppered tube for several minutes, but if shearing must be minimised, the tube should be gently rocked instead. Centrifugation yields two phases separated by a mat of denatured protein. Nucleic acids are found in the upper, aqueous phase, which is removed and subjected to several further cycles of deproteinisation. It is prudent not to discard the organic layers and the protein interface material at this stage because significant quantities of DNA may be trapped therein, particularly if the cell suspension was too dense when lysed.

After the deproteinisation cycles the amount of protein precipitated at the interface should be markedly less than before, and it is usual at this stage to precipitate nucleic acids by gently mixing the separated aqueous layer with two volumes of cold ethanol. DNA may either be 'spooled' on to a clean glass rod or recovered by centrifugation. The pellet or spool is rinsed with alcohol to remove much of the denaturing agent, and the process is completed by dissolving the crude DNA in a suitable aqueous solution (e.g. dilute saline-citrate in the method of

Marmur, 1961) and reprecipitating with alcohol.

It is now possible to treat the preparation with ribonuclease (e.g. 50 μg/ml at 37°C for 1 hour) after suitable adjustments to the buffer. If there is reason to doubt the purity of the enzyme preparation available, contaminating deoxyribonuclease can be destroyed by heating the enzyme solution at 80° for 20 min. The ribonuclease and remaining cellular protein which is released following hydrolysis of RNA is now removed by a further series of deproteinisation steps, and many workers precede the phenol or chloroform extractions with a proteolytic digestion using enzymes such as pronase or proteinase K. When, finally, no denatured protein remains at the interface, the DNA is precipitated with ethanol then redissolved and dialysed. If the DNA is required for hybridisation experiments it may be advantageous to add one final purification step, namely centrifugation in caesium chloride. The high salt concentration removes any residual protein, and RNA is precipitated. The DNA band is removed from the centrifuge tube with a wide-bore pipette and dialysed to remove the caesium chloride.

DNA solutions are stored at 4°C with a preservative to discourage microbial growth (e.g. a few drops of chloroform) or at −20°C, but repeated freezing and thawing of solutions of high molecular weight DNA may cause appreciable shearing.

B. Determination of Base Composition

Two indirect methods are commonly used to measure the proportion of guanine + cytosine residues in double-stranded DNA: (1) determination of 'melting temperature', i.e. the midpoint of the thermal transition from double- to single-stranded structures; and (2) determination of the buoyant density in caesium chloride solution. Both of these quantities are related in a simple manner to the base composition.

It is also possible to measure base composition directly, i.e. by chromatographic analysis of hydrolysates, but the indirect methods are much more convenient. Razin and Razin (1980) in the course of a study of methylated bases in mycoplasma DNA separated bases in acid hydrolysates by high performance liquid chromatography, and found that the base composition calculated from their data agreed well with determinations by indirect methods. If highly purified DNA is available, some information about the base composition can be deduced from the ultra-violet absorption spectrum because the four bases have somewhat different spectral characteristics (Ulitzur, 1972), but this method is highly sensitive to contaminating impurities and is rarely used.

(1)   Melting Temperature. A sensitive spectrophotometer with a
temperature-controlled cell holder is required, equipped with a thermo-
couple or electronic thermometer for measuring the temperature of the
cell contents. All solutions must be degassed with a vacuum pump to
prevent air bubbles forming and giving spurious absorbance readings.
Stoppered quartz cuvettes are used to prevent evaporation of the
solvent. One cuvette contains the unknown DNA, another contains a
reference DNA solution of known base composition (e.g *Escherichia
coli* DNA), a third cell contains solvent only and a fourth may contain
the temperature-measuring probe. The experiment is started at 25°C,
and readings are taken as the temperature is raised at about 1°C per
minute. When the absorbance begins to increase the temperature may
be increased more slowly, a few minutes being allowed for equilibrium
at each temperature before taking a reading. The total increase in
absorbance (hyperchromicity) should be about 40% of the initial
reading, and the heating should be continued for several degrees after
the absorbance has ceased to increase. Before the data can be plotted it
is necessary to correct the absorbance values to take account of the
thermal expansion of the solution, which has the effect of diluting the
DNA. Tables for performing this correction are given by Mandel and
Marmur (1968). The corrected absorbance values A_T are plotted against
temperature T, usually as the ratio $A_T/A_{25°}$ and the melting temperature, T_m, at which the value attains half its maximum value is read
from the graph. The relationship between T_m and base composition
depends on the ionic composition of the solvent, but in the commonly-
used solution SSC (0.15M sodium chloride and 0.015M sodium citrate)
the equation is

$$T_m = 69.3 + 0.41 \ (G + C)$$

where (G + C) is the guanine + cytosine content of the DNA in moles
per cent (Marmur and Doty, 1962).

(2)   Buoyant Density. An analytical ultracentrifuge such as the
Beckman Model E or MSE Centriscan is required. Using ultra-violet
optical systems, samples containing 1–5 μg DNA give excellent results.
Our standard procedure is to prepare samples containing 2 μg each of
mycoplasma and *E. coli* DNA in a total volume of 0.6 ml, usually in
0.1 x SSC buffer; 0.8 g solid caesium chloride (optical grade) is added,
and the refractive index of the solution is measured to check that the
density is approximately 1.700 g cm^{-3}. The relationship between
refractive index (η) and density (ρ) of caesium chloride may be found

from tables, or the relationship

$$\rho_{25}° = 10.8601\eta_{25}° - 13.4974$$

may be used (Ifft *et al.*, 1961). Portions of 0.6 ml of the solution are introduced into the ultracentrifuge cells, and centrifuged for 20–24 hours at about 45,000 rpm, at 20°C. The operation of the centrifuge is outside the scope of this discussion and reference should be made to the instruction manuals. Ultra-violet absorption photographs are scanned with a densitometer and from the tracing the actual position of the DNA bands in the centrifuge cell can be calculated, knowing the dimensions of the rotor and the position of the marker slots (which are given by the manufacturer). The density of the mycoplasma DNA, ρ_M, can then be calculated knowing ρ_E (the density of *E. coli* marker DNA, 1.709 gcm^{-3}), τ_M and τ_E, the distances from the rotor axis of the mycoplasma and marker DNA bands, respectively, and W, the angular velocity, using the equation of Schildkraut *et al.* (1962):

$$\rho_M = \rho_E + \frac{W^2}{2\beta} (\tau_M{}^2 - \tau_E{}^2)$$

The quantity β depends on the density of the solution and its value may be found from the paper of Ifft *et al.* (1961). Using our standard conditions described above, centrifuging at 44,770 rpm in the Beckman Model E machine, the coefficient $\frac{W^2}{2\beta}$ has a value of 0.0092 gcm^{-5}.

Finally, from the density the base composition (moles per cent G + C) is calculated using the relationship

$$\rho - 1.660 = \frac{0.098 (G + C)}{100}$$

(Schildkraut *et al.*, 1962). This method is very accurate, the standard error on a series of determinations being less than 1% (G + C).

C. Genome Size

Determination of genome size is important for characterisation of mycoplasmas because all genera so far studied seem to fall into two classes, with genome size either 5×10^8 or 1×10^9 (Table 9.1), and therefore the parameter has taxonomic significance. It is possible to measure the size of mycoplasma chromosomes directly, by careful lysis and electron microscopy to determine contour lengths of circular

DNA molecules, as was done by Bode and Morowitz (1967) for *M. hominis*, but the procedures are excessively tedious, and an indirect method is normally used instead. The principle is to measure the rate of renaturation of single-stranded fragments of DNA, for as Wetmur and Davidson (1968) showed, the rate depends not only on the size of the fragments (which can be measured), but upon the size of the genome from which the fragments were prepared. The experiment, strictly speaking, yields the 'kinetic complexity' of the DNA, which for prokaryotes is the same as the genome size.

The requirements for the experiments are purified DNA from the mycoplasma and from a bacterium of known complexity (e.g. *E. coli* or *M. hominis*), an analytical ultracentrifuge for measuring the size of the DNA fragments and a recording spectrophotometer with thermostatted cells.

The DNA solution is first sheared by sonication to give double-stranded fragments of a fairly uniform length. The size of the single-stranded fragments resulting from denaturation of the sheared double-stranded DNA is found by sedimentation in the analytical ultracentrifuge using a solvent of 0.9M NaCl containing 0.1M NaOH (Studier, 1965). The sedimentation constant, S, is obtained in the usual way, and is corrected for solvent density and viscosity effects by multiplying

by a factor 1.16, i.e. $S_{20°,W}^{pH13}$ = 1.16 S.

A sample dissolved in 0.1 x SSC is then degassed and heated in the spectrophotometer to determine the hyperchromicity and the melting temperature, T_m. This part of the experiment may conveniently be combined with measurements of % (G + C) by melting temperature. The temperature is then rapidly lowered to a value of $T_m - 25°C$ (at which temperature the renaturation is performed) and the absorbance again measured. It will be found to have decreased by about 3% because of some secondary structures formed by the single-stranded DNA. The corrected value is taken as A_o, the initial absorbance of the denatured DNA.

A further sample of sonicated DNA is now prepared and denatured by boiling for 15 min in a stoppered tube and then rapidly cooled in ice and 5M NaCl is added to give a final concentration of 1M. It is loaded into the spectrophotometer maintained at a temperature 25°C less than the T_m in this solvent (which can be calculated from the previously determined value using an equation given by Mandel *et al.*, 1970). The absorbance values decrease as the DNA renatures, and the data are plotted against time as the fraction $(A_o - A_\infty) \div (A_t - A_\infty)$

where A_o is the initial value for the denatured DNA deduced from the melting experiment, A_∞ is the absorbance of the fully renatured material, obtained by dividing A_o by the hyperchromicity factor, and A_t is the value at time t. A straight line is obtained of slope k_2, which is related to the genome size N_D and the sedimentation coefficient $S_{20, W}^{pH13}$ by the equation given by Wetmur and Davidson (1968):

$$N_D = \frac{5.5 \times 10^8 \ (S_{20^\circ,W}^{pH13})^{1.25}}{k_2}$$

Examples of the application of this technique to spiroplasmas and other mycoplasmas are given by Saglio *et al.* (1973) and Bak *et al.*, (1969).

D. Analysis by Restriction Endonucleases

Restriction endonucleases are enzymes produced by bacteria which cleave DNA at certain sites defined by specific sequences of 4–6 nucleotides. It is believed that the enzymes function *in vivo* to protect cells against 'foreign' DNA, while host DNA is protected against cleavage by selective base modification, usually methylation. Assuming that nucleotide sequences are approximately random in DNA, a specific hexanucleotide sequence would be expected to occur once in 4^6 (= 4096) such groups, or once in 25,000 bases, which corresponds to about 30 typical genes. It is clear that an enzyme recognising such a sequence would produce a limited number of fragments from a mycoplasma genome. Harris-Warrick *et al.* (1975) introduced the technique of enzyme cleavage followed by electrophoretic separation to fractionate the bacterial genome.

Bové and Saillard (1979) have exploited restriction enzymes to compare spiroplasma strains and have found that it is possible to detect differences between *S. citri* strains which are otherwise indistinguishable. Needless to say, since the technique depends upon specific cleavage of DNA molecules, nonspecific breaks must be avoided and so methods for DNA preparation must be chosen which minimise shearing. The procedure of Gross-Bellard *et al.* (1973) has been found satisfactory. DNA samples (about 1 μg) are cleaved with commercially-available enzymes such as *Eco*RI or *Hind*III and the digestion products are analysed by electrophoresis in slabs of polyacrylamide and agarose, which effects a separation according to molecular weight. The gels are stained with ethidium bromide, a fluorescent intercalating agent, and examined under a UV light. The bands on the gel fluoresce red and can be photographed. The band pattern is used as a 'fingerprint' of the strain in the same way that polyacrylamide gel electrophoresis patterns of cell proteins can be used (see Section 2.C). At present it is not known what the basis of strain differences in DNA fragment patterns may be, but obvious possibilities include the presence of extrachromosomal DNA molecules (e.g. plasmids or virus DNA), or point mutations, base modifications or deletions in the chromosome. Only limited experience has so far been gained with this technique for characterising the myco-plasma genome but it may well develop into a standard comparative procedure. A similar procedure has also been reported by Kieser *et al.* (1981) for comparing *Streptomyces* genomes.

E. Nucleic Acid Hybridisation for Investigating Relatedness

The determination of genome size described in Section C (above) depends on the property of the two strands of native DNA to dissociate and reassociate *in vitro*, first described by Marmur and Lane (1960) and Doty *et al.* (1960). It was soon realised that the phenomenon made possible an approach to analysing genetic relatedness essentially by mixing dissociated DNA strands from two organisms and, after sub-sequently allowing reassociation to proceed, looking for 'hybrid' double-stranded molecules composed of one strand from each parent organism. An extensive literature exists recording experiments along these lines, and early work with mycoplasmas in the late 1960s, largely aimed at seeking relatedness with bacteria, is summarised by Stanbridge and Reff (1979) and Neimark (1979b).

Hybridisation reactions have great inherent specificity and can dis-tinguish components of complex mixtures of polynucleotides, but the limits of the specificity and the interpretation of experiments depend critically on details of the methodology to an extent which is not always realised. McCarthy and Church (1970) reviewed the factors governing specificity in hybridisation reactions, and their paper should be consulted by all who intend to undertake hybridisation work.

DNA strands from different organisms, whether they are members of different species or independent isolates of the same species, will have base sequences which are more or less different, and the ability of hybridisation experiments to distinguish the two organisms depends on the answers to two related questions: (1) What is the degree of base sequence complementarity in the two strands necessary to give a stable duplex? and (2) What is the minimum proportion of non-complemen-tary base pairs in a hybrid duplex which can be detected by virtue of an effect on the properties of the duplex? The answers to these questions depend on the conditions under which the reaction takes place, particularly the temperature, cation concentration, length of the interacting strands, base composition and the nature of any un-paired regions. A useful measure of the quality of hybrids is the thermal dissociation temperature, T_m, which we have mentioned in Section B above in connection with determinations of base composition. Under standard conditions the T_m can give valuable information about the proportion of noncomplementary (unpaired) bases in hybrid duplex molecules, for experiments with synthetic and natural polynucleotides have shown that 1% of unpaired bases lower the T_m of the duplex by $0.7°C$, and this relationship holds up to 20–25% unpaired bases. Thus in an experiment to study hybridisation between two related strains the difference in T_m between homologous and heterologous hybrids can be used as a measure of sequence divergence. Formation of stable hybrids probably requires sequences of not less than 10–15 bases, and stability increases with chain length up to about 50 bases. If hybrid-isation is carried out at low temperatures nonspecific duplex structures are formed, and as the temperature is raised specificity increases. It is customary to work at temperatures about $25°C$ below the T_m of the DNA in the chosen solvent to give maximum rate of hybridisation (cf. Section C), and to use salt concentrations around 1M. Prolonged exposure of DNA to such temperatures may cause damage such as chain scission and depurination, so it is customary to incorporate an organic solvent which reduces the T_m, usually formamide, in buffers so that reactions can be performed at lower temperatures (McConaughy *et al.*, 1969).

Many methods differing mostly in detail have been used for DNA hybridisation. Two techniques are described below, one using filter-immobilised DNA and one using DNA free in solution. Both methods have been used for mycoplasmas: Davis *et al.* (1974) applied filter hybridisation to compare *S. citri* with the corn stunt spiroplasma, whereas the liquid system was used by Aulakh *et al.* (1979) for achol-eplasmas and by Junca *et al.* (1980) for spiroplasmas.

The filter technique depends on the observation by Nygaard and Hall (1963) that single-stranded DNA binds strongly to membrane filters, and Gillespie and Spiegelman (1965) found that bound DNA could still participate in hybridisation reactions with RNA free in the bathing solution. Application to DNA-DNA hybridisation was at first ruled out because of adsorption of DNA from the solution to the filter, obscuring binding caused by hybridisation to strands originally bound.

However Denhardt (1966) found that if filters to which DNA was bound were incubated in a mixture of bovine serum albumin, polyvinylpyrrolidone and Ficoll, further binding was suppressed whereas hybridisation was unimpaired, and a very convenient system thereby became available for studying genetic relatedness.

The DNA to be fixed to the filter is first denatured either by boiling for 15 min and then rapidly cooling in ice, or by treatment with alkali followed by neutralisation. The solution is passed slowly through a cellulose nitrate membrane filter, and the filter is then washed, usually on both sides, with buffer to remove unbound DNA, and dried at room temperature for several hours and then at 80°C in a vacuum oven. Filters can be stored in a desiccator for periods of several weeks. The capacity of the filters for binding DNA is about 10 μg cm^{-2}. It is often convenient to load DNA on to large filters which, after drying, can be cut into small pieces to give suitable amounts of bound DNA for particular experiments. The amount of DNA bound can be easily found by hydrolysing samples of the filter with acid and measuring the ultraviolet absorbance of the released nucleotides and nucleosides.

Before performing the hybridisation the filter pieces are incubated in the polymer mixture of Denhardt (1966). Radioactive DNA for hybridisation is prepared in two ways: mycoplasmas may be grown in the presence of a radioactive precursor of DNA such as [^{3}H] or [^{14}C] thymidine or [^{32}P]-phosphate, or alternatively nonradioactive DNA may be labelled *in vitro* by the so-called 'nick translation' procedure using limited nuclease digestion followed by DNA polymerase action with radioactive substrates (Maniatis *et al.*, 1975). Radioactive DNA is sheared by sonication, denatured, and incubated in the chosen buffer at the appropriate temperature. Incubation is continued until the reaction approaches completeness, which with DNA of the complexity of mycoplasmas is achieved overnight. The kinetics of the reaction have been studied by Flavell *et al.* (1974), and their paper indicates factors which should be taken into account when performing the experiment. At the end of the incubation period the filters are removed from the hybridisation mixture and washed several times to remove unhybridised material, dried, and the radioactivity measured. The 'quality' of the hybrids can be tested by immersing the filters for 15 min in a series of tubes of buffer solution, each maintained at a higher temperature than its predecessor. The DNA eluted from the filter at each temperature is found by precipitating with 5% trichloroacetic acid, collecting the precipitate on a filter by suction, and counting the radioactivity on the filter. If the cumulative radioactivity eluted from the hybrid-bearing filter is plotted against temperature a 'melting curve' is generated from which the T_m may be read, and comparison of the T_m of the hybrid with similar preparations of homologous DNA (i.e. both filter-bound and free, radioactive, DNA from the same strain) gives a measure of fidelity of hybridisation of DNA of the two organisms. The melting experiment should be performed in formamide-containing buffers so that lower temperatures can be used, which minimises nonspecific elution of DNA from filters.

The great advantage of the filter hybridisation system is its convenience, in that DNA-containing filters can be stored for use when required. It is probably best used for 'all or none' experiments on genetic relatedness, while questions of partial relatedness are better investigated by the liquid hybridisation system.

The procedure for liquid hybridisation involves incubating a mixture of sheared, denatured DNA from two strains, allowing reannealing to take place, and then analysing the products on columns of hydroxyapatite. DNA from one strain is radioactive, but the nonradioactive heterologous DNA is present in vast excess (e.g. 1,000-fold) so essentially all double-stranded structures containing radioactivity will be hybrids of the two DNA species. Incubation conditions described by Aulakh *et al.* (1979) should be followed, and at the end of the incubation the mixture is passed through a column of hydroxyapatite equilibrated with 0.14M phosphate buffer at 60°C. Material not sticking to the column is unhybridised single-stranded DNA. Double-stranded molecules are then eluted with 0.48M phosphate. If thermal analysis is to be undertaken the column should be eluted with portions of 0.14M buffer at increasing temperatures, and the radioactivity eluted at each temperature is determined. Again, a graph of cumulative eluted radioactivity against temperature gives a 'melting curve' enabling one to compare the fidelity of homologous and heterologous duplexes.

An alternative procedure for analysing hybrids formed in solution, which is much simpler than hydroxyapatite fractionation, was used by Lee and Davis (1980) to investigate DNA homology among spiroplasma serogroups. After reassociation had taken place the reaction mixture was treated with S_1 nuclease (from *Aspergillus oryzae*), which at pH 4.5 in the presence of Zn^{++} degrades single-stranded DNA. Thus any radioactivity in acid-insoluble material after digestion represents duplex material.

Carefully performed hybridisation experiments can yield two numerical estimates of genetic relatedness of two strains: (1) the proportion of the total genomes which are homologous and (2) the extent to which base sequences are conserved within the homologous regions. The meaning of these findings in terms of the evolution of the two organisms is a matter for the experimenter's judgement.

References

Allen, R.C. and Maurer, H.R. (1974). *Electrophoresis and Isoelectric Focusing in Polyacrylamide Gel.* New York: Walter de Gruyter.

Alexander, A.G. and Kenny, G.E. (1977). Characterisation of membrane and cytoplasmic antigens of *Mycoplasma arginini* by two dimensional (crossed) immunoelectrophoresis. *Infection and Immunology 15*, 313–21.

Aluotto, B.B., Wittler, R.G., Williams, C.O. and Faber, J.E. (1970). Standardised bacteriologic techniques for the characterisation of *Mycoplasma* species. *International Journal of Systematic Bacteriology 20*, 35–58.

Ames, G.F-L. and Nikaido, K. (1976). Two-dimensional gel electrophoresis of membrane proteins. *Biochemistry 15*, 616–23.

Arbuthnot, J.P. and Beeley, J.A. (1975). *Isoelectric Focusing.* London: Butterworths.

Archer, D.B. and Best, J. (1980). Serological relatedness of spiroplasmas estimated by enzyme-linked immunosorbent assay and crossed immunoelectrophoresis. *Journal of General Microbiology 119*, 413–22.

Archer, D.B., Rodwell, A.W. and Rodwell, E.S. (1978). The nature and location of *Acholeplasma laidlawii* membrane proteins investigated by two dimensional electrophoresis. *Biochimica et biophysica Acta 513*, 268–83.

Archer, D.B. and Townsend, R. (1981). Immunoelectrophoretic separation of spiroplasma antigens. *Journal of General Microbiology 123*, 61-8.

Aulakh, G.S., Tully, J.G. and Barile, M.F. (1979). Differentiation among some acholeplasmas by nucleic acid homology. *Current Microbiology 2*, 91–4.

Bak, A.L., Black, F.T., Christiansen, C. and Freundt, E.A. (1969). Genome size of mycoplasmal DNA. *Nature 224*, 1209–10.

Bjerrum, O.J. and Bøg-Hansen, T.C. (1976). The immunochemical approach to the characterisation of membrane proteins. Human erythrocyte membranes analysed as a model system. *Biochimica et biophysica Acta 455*, 66–89.

Bode, H.R. and Morowitz, H.J. (1967). Size and structure of the *Mycoplasma hominis* H39 chromosome. *Journal of Molecular Biology 23*, 191–9.

Bonner, M. and Laskey, R.A. (1974). A film detection method for tritium-labelled proteins and nucleic acids in polyacrylamide gels. *European Journal of Biochemistry 46*, 83–8.

Bové, J.M. and Saillard, C. (1979). Cell biology of spiroplasmas. In *The Mycoplasmas*, Vol. III, pp. 85–149, R.F. Whitcomb and J.G. Tully (eds). New York: Academic Press.

Chamberlain, J.P. (1979). Fluorographic determination of radioactivity in polyacrylamide gels with the water-soluble fluor, sodium salicylate. *Analytical Biochemistry 98*, 132–5.

Chau, N-H. and Blomberg, G. (1979). Immunochemical studies of thylakoid membrane polypeptides from spinach and *Chlamydomonas reinhardtii. Journal of Biological Chemistry 254*, 215–23.

Cirillo, V.P. and Razin, S. (1973). Distribution of phosphoenolpyruvate-dependent sugar phosphotransferase system in mycoplasmas. *Journal of Bacteriology 113*, 212–17.

Clark, H.G.M. and Freeman, T.A. (1967). A quantitative immunoelectrophoresis method (Laurell electrophoresis). In *Protides of the Biological Fluids*, XIV

Colloquium Bruges 1966, pp. 503–9, H. Peeters (ed). Amsterdam: Elsevier.

Crowle, A.J. (1961). *Immunodiffusion*. New York: Academic Press.

Daniels, M.J., Archer, D.B., Stephens, M.A., Townsend, R., Longland, J.M. and Best, J. (1980). Comparison of spiroplasmas by polyacrylamide gel electrophoresis of cell proteins. *Current Microbiology 4*, 377–80.

Daniels, M.J. and Johnson, M.W. (1978). Computer assisted identification of mycoplasmas. *Zentralblatt für Bakteriologie Parasitunkunde Infectionskrankheiten und Hygiene. Erste Abteilung Originale 241*, 174.

Daniels, M.J. and Meddins, B.M. (1973). Polyacrylamide gel electrophoresis of mycoplasma proteins in sodium dodecyl sulphate. *Journal of General Microbiology 76*, 239–42.

Davis, B.J. (1964). Disc electrophoresis II. Method and application to human serum proteins. *Annals of the New York Academy of Sciences 121*, 404-27.

Davis, R.E., Dupont, G., Saglio, P., Roy, B., Vignault, J.C. and Bové, J.M. (1974). Spiroplasmas: studies on the microorganisms associated with corn stunt disease. *Les Mycoplasmes/Mycoplasmas. Les Colloques de l'Institut National de la Santé et de la Recherche Médicale 33*, 187–94.

Davis, R.E., Lee, I.M. and Basciano, L.K. (1979). Spiroplasmas: serological grouping of strains associated with plants and insects. *Canadian Journal of Microbiology 25*, 861–6.

Denhardt, D.T. (1966). A membrane filter technique for the detection of complementary DNA. *Biochemical and Biophysical Research Communications 23*, 641–6.

Diezel, W., Kopperschläger, G. and Hofmann, E. (1972). An improved procedure for protein staining in polyacrylamide gels with a new type of Coomassie Brilliant Blue. *Analytical Biochemistry 48*, 617–20.

Doty, P., Marmur, J., Eigner, J. and Schildkraut, C.L. (1960). Strand separation and specific recombination in deoxyribonucleic acids: physical chemical studies. *Proceedings of the National Academy of Sciences of the United States of America 46*, 461–76.

Edward, D.G. (1971). Determination of sterol requirements for Mycoplasmatales. *Journal of General Microbiology 69*, 205–10.

Edward, D.G. and Moore, W.B. (1973). Determination of utilisation of glucose by mycoplasmas. In *Reports Presented at the Conferences on Taxonomy and Physiology of Mycoplasmas*, Brno 1970 & 1972. *In vitro v. CSSR 2(i)*, 148–55.

Ernø, H. and Stipkovits, L. (1973). Bovine mycoplasmas: cultural and biochemical studies II. *Acta Veterinaria Scandinavica 14*, 450–63.

Fabricant, J. and Freundt, E.A. (1967). Importance of extension and standardisation of laboratory tests for the identification and classification of mycoplasmas. *Annals of the New York Academy of Sciences 143*, 50–8.

Fairbanks, G., Levinthal, C. and Reeder, R.H. (1965). Analysis of C^{14}-labelled proteins by disc electrophoresis. *Biochemical and Biophysical Research Communications 20*, 393–9.

Fairbanks, F., Steck, T.L. and Wallach, D.F.H. (1971). Electrophoretic analysis of the major polypeptides of the human erythrocyte membrane. *Biochemistry 10*, 2606–17.

Flavell, R.A., Birfelder, E.J., Sanders, J.P.M. and Borst, P. (1974). DNA-DNA hybridisation on nitrocellulose filters 1. General considerations and non-ideal kinetics. *European Journal of Biochemistry 47*, 535–43.

Fowler, R.C., Coble, D.W., Kramer, N.C. and Brown, T.McP. (1963). Starch gel electrophoresis of a fraction of certain of the pleuropneumonia-like group of organisms. *Journal of Bacteriology 86*, 1145–51.

Freundt, E.A., Andrews, B.E., Ernø, H., Kunze, M. and Black, F.T. (1973). The sensitivity of *Mycoplasmatales* to sodium-polyanetholsulfonate and digitonin.

Zentralblatt für Bakteriologie, Parasitenkunde Infektionskrankheiten und Hygiene. Erste Abteilung Originale 225, 104–12.

Garrels, J.I. (1979). Two-dimensional gel electrophoresis and computer analysis of proteins synthesised by clonal cell lines. *Journal of Biological Chemistry 254*, 7961–77.

Garrels, J.I. and Gibson, W. (1976). Identification and characterisation of multiple forms of actin. *Cell 9*, 793–805.

Gillespie, D. and Spiegelman, S. (1965). A quantitative assay for DNA-RNA hybrids with DNA immobilised on a membrane. *Journal of Molecular Biology 12*, 829–42.

Gordon, A.H. (1969). Electrophoresis of proteins in polyacrylamide and starch gels. In *Laboratory Techniques in Biochemistry and Molecular Biology*, T.S. Work and E. Work (eds). Amsterdam: North Holland.

Grabar, P. and Williams, C.A. (1953). Méthode permettant l'étude conjuguée des propriétés électrophorétiques et immunochimiques d'un mélange de protéines. Application au sérum sanguin. *Biochimica et biophysica Acta 10*, 193–4.

Gross-Bellard, M., Oudet, P. and Chambon, P. (1973). Isolation of high-molecular-weight DNA from mammalian cells. *European Journal of Biochemistry 36*, 32–8.

Groth, S.F. de St., Webster, R.G. and Datyner, A. (1963). Two new staining procedures for quantitative estimation of proteins on electrophoretic strips. *Biochimica et biophysica Acta 71*, 377–91.

Harris-Warrick, R.M., Elkana, Y., Ehrlich, S.D. and Lederberg, J. (1975). Electrophoretic separation of *Bacillus subtilis* genes. *Proceedings of the National Academy of Sciences of the United States of America 72*, 2207–11.

Huggett, A. St. G. and Nixon, D.A. (1957). Use of glucose oxidase, peroxidase and o-dianisidine in determination of blood and urinary glucose. *Lancet ii*, 368–70.

Hull, R. (1971). Examination of alfalfa mosaic virus protein on polyacrylamide gels. *Virology 45*, 767–72.

Ifft, J.B., Voet, D.H. and Vinograd, J. (1961). The determination of density distributions and density gradients in binary solutions at equilibrium in the ultracentrifuge. *Journal of Physical Chemistry 65*, 1138.

Johansson, K-E., Blomqvist, I. and Hjertén, S. (1975). Purification of membrane proteins from *Acholeplasma laidlawii* by agarose suspension electrophoresis in Tween 20 and polyacrylamide and dextran gel electrophoresis in detergent-free media. *Journal of Biological Chemistry 250*, 2463–9.

Johansson, K-E. and Hjertén, S. (1974). Localisation of the Tween 20-soluble membrane proteins of *Acholeplasma laidlawii* by crossed immunoelectrophoresis. *Journal of Molecular Biology 86*, 341–8.

Johansson, K-E. and Wróblewski, H. (1978). Crossed immunoelectrophoresis in the presence of Tween 20 or Sodium Deoxycholate, or purified membrane proteins from *Acholeplasma laidlawii*. *Journal of Bacteriology 136*, 324–30.

Junca, P., Saillard, C., Tully, J., Garcia-Jurado, O., Degorce-Dumas, J.R., Mouches, C., Vignault, J.C., Vogel, R., McCoy, R., Whitcomb, R., Williamson, D., Latrille, J. and Bové, J.M. (1980). Characterisation de spiroplasmes isolés d'insectes et de fleurs de France continentale, de Corse et du Maroc: proposition pour une classification de spiroplasmes. *Comptes Rendus Hebdomadaires des Séances de l'Académie des Sciences, Paris, Série D 209*, 1209–12.

Kahane, I. and Razin, S. (1969). Immunological analysis of mycoplasma membranes. *Journal of Bacteriology 100*, 187–94.

Kieser, T., Hintermann, G., Crameri, R. and Hütter, R. (1981). Restriction analysis of Streptomyces DNA. In *Proceedings of Colloquium on Genetics of Actinomycetales* 1979 (in press).

Kirby, K.S. (1965). Isolation and characterisation of ribosomal RNA. *Biochemical Journal 96*, 266-9.
— (1968). Isolation of nucleic acids with phenolic solvents. In *Advances in Enzymology*, Vol. XII, part B, pp. 87-99, L. Grossman and K. Modave (eds). New York: Academic Press.
Laemmli, U.K. (1970). Cleavage of structural proteins during the assembly of the head of bacteriophage T4. *Nature (London) 227*, 680-5.
Laemmli, U.K. and Favre, M. (1973). Maturation of the head of bacteriophage T4, I. DNA packaging events. *Journal of Molecular Biology 80*, 575-99.
Laskey, R.A. and Mills, A.D. (1975). Quantitative film detection of ^{3}H and ^{14}C in polyacrylamide gels by fluorography. *European Journal of Biochemistry 56*, 335-41.
Laurell, C-B. (1965). Antigen-antibody crossed immunoelectrophoresis. *Analytical Biochemistry 10*, 358-61.
Leach, R.H. (1976). The inhibiting effect of arginine on growth of some mycoplasmas. *Journal of Applied Bacteriology 41*, 259-64.
Lee, I-M. and Davis, R.E. (1980). DNA homology among diverse spiroplasma strains representing several serological groups. *Canadian Journal of Microbiology 26*, 1356-63.
Lowry, O.H., Rosebrough, N.J., Farr, A.L. and Randall, R.J. (1951). Protein measurement with the Folin phenol reagent. *Journal of Biological Chemistry 193*, 265-75.
Mandel, M., Igambi, L., Bergendahl, J., Dodson, M.L. and Scheltgen, E. (1970). Correlation of melting temperature and caesium chloride buoyant density of bacterial deoxyribonucleic acid. *Journal of Bacteriology 101*, 333-8.
Mandel, M. and Marmur, J. (1968). Use of ultraviolet absorbance-temperature profile for determining the guanine plus cytosine content of DNA. In *Methods in Enzymology*, Vol. XII, part B, pp. 195-206, L. Grossman and K. Moldave (eds). New York: Academic Press.
Maniatis, T., Jeffrey, A. and Kleid, D.G. (1975). Nucleotide sequence of the rightward operator of phage. *Proceedings of the National Academy of Sciences of the United States of America 72*, 1184-8.
Marmur, J. (1961). A procedure for the isolation of deoxyribonucleic acid from micro-organisms. *Journal of Molecular Biology 3*, 208-18.
Marmur, J. and Doty, P. (1962). Determination of the base composition of deoxyribonucleic acid from its thermal denaturation temperature. *Journal of Molecular Biology 5*, 109-18.
Marmur, J. and Lane, D. (1960). Strand separation and specific recombination in deoxyribonucleic acids: biological studies. *Proceedings of the National Academy of Sciences of the United States of America 46*, 453-61.
Masover, G.K., Razin, S. and Hayflick, L. (1977). Effects of carbon dioxide, urea and ammonia on growth of *Ureaplasma urealyticum* (T-strain mycoplasma). *Journal of Bacteriology 130*, 292-6.
Masover, G.K., Sawyer, J.E. and Hayflick, L. (1976). Urea-hydrolysing activity of a T-strain mycoplasma: *Ureaplasma urealyticum*. *Journal of Bacteriology 125*, 581-7.
Maurer, H.R. (1971). *Disc Electrophoresis and Related Techniques of Polyacrylamide Gel Electrophoresis*. Berlin & New York: De Guyter.
McCarthy, B.J. and Church, R.B. (1970). The specificity of molecular hybridisation reactions. *Annual Review of Biochemistry 39*, 131-50.
McConaughy, B.L., Laird, C.D. and McCarthy, B.J. (1969). Nucleic acid reassociation in formamide. *Biochemistry 8*, 3289-95.
Mouches, C., Vignault, J.C., Tully, J.G., Whitcomb, R.F. and Bové, J.M. (1979). Characterisation of spiroplasmas by one and two dimensional protein analysis on polyacrylamide gel slabs. *Current Microbiology 2*, 69-74.

Ne'eman, Z., Kahane, I., Kovartovsky, J. and Razin, S. (1972). Characterisation of the mycoplasma membrane proteins. III, Gel filtration and immunological characterisation of *Acholeplasma laidlawii* membrane proteins. *Biochimica et biophysica Acta 266*, 255–68.

Neimark, H.C. (1979a). Extraction of an actin-like protein from the prokaryote *Mycoplasma pneumoniae*. *Proceedings of the National Academy of Sciences of the USA 74*, 4041–5.

— (1979b). Phylogenetic relationships between mycoplasmas and other pro-karyotes. In *The Mycoplasmas*, Vol. 1, pp. 43–61, M.F. Barile and S. Razin (eds). New York: Academic Press.

Nygaard, A.P. and Hall, B.D. (1963). A method for the detection of RNA-DNA complexes. *Biochemical and Biophysical Research Communications 12*, 98–104.

O'Farrell, P.Z. (1975). High resolution two dimensional electrophoresis of proteins. *Journal of Biological Chemistry 250*, 4007–21.

O'Farrell, P.Z., Goodman, H.M. and O'Farrell, P.H. (1977). High resolution two-dimensional electrophoresis of basic as well as acidic proteins. *Cell 12*, 1133–41.

Ornstein, L. (1964). Disc electrophoresis I. Background and theory. *Annals of the New York Academy of Sciences 121*, 321.

Razin, S. and Cleverdon, R.C. (1965). Carotenoids and cholesterol in membranes of *Mycoplasma laidlawii*. *Journal of General Microbiology 41*, 409–15.

Razin, S., Ne'eman, Z. and Ohad, I. (1969). Selective reaggregation of solubilised mycoplasma membrane proteins and the kinetics of membrane reformation. *Biochimica et biophysica Acta 193*, 277–93.

Razin, A. and Razin, S. (1980). Methylated bases in mycoplasmal DNA. *Nucleic Acids Research 8*, 1383–90.

Razin, S. and Rottem, S. (1967). Identification of *Mycoplasma* and other micro-organisms by polyacrylamide gel electrophoresis of cell proteins. *Journal of Bacteriology 94*, 1807–10.

Razin, S. and Tully, J.G. (1970). Cholesterol requirements of mycoplasmas. *Journal of Bacteriology 102*, 306–10.

Reid, M.S. and Bieleski, R.L. (1968). A simple apparatus for vertical flat-sheet polyacrylamide gel electrophoresis. *Analytical Biochemistry 22*, 374–81.

Reynolds, J.A. and Tanford, C. (1970). The gross conformation of protein-sodium dodecyl sulfate complexes. *Journal of Biological Chemistry 245*, 5161–5.

Rhoades, K.R., Phillips, M. and Yoder, H.W. (1974). Comparison of strains of *Mycoplasma gallisepticum* by polyacrylamide gel electrophoresis. *Avian Diseases 18*, 91–6.

Righetti, P.G. and Drysdale, J.W. (1976). Isoelectric focusing. In *Laboratory Techniques in Biochemistry and Molecular Biology*, T.S. Work and E. Work (eds). Amsterdam: North Holland.

Rodwell, A.W. and Rodwell, E.S. (1978). Phylogenetic relationships between strains of *Mycoplasma mycoides* subspp. *mycoides* and *capri* studied by two dimensional electrophoresis. *Journal of General Microbiology 109*, 259–63.

Rodwell, A.W., Rodwell, E.S. and Archer, D.B. (1979). Mycoplasmas lack a protein which resembles α-actin. *FEMS Microbiology Letters 5*, 235–8.

Rottem, S. and Markowitz, O. (1979). Carotenoids act as reinforcers of the *Acholeplasma laidlawii* lipid bilayer. *Journal of Bacteriology 140*, 944–8.

Rottem, S. and Razin, S. (1967). Uptake and utilisation of acetate by mycoplas-mas. *Journal of General Microbiology 48*, 53–63.

Saglio, P., L'Hospital, M., Laflèche, D., Dupont, G., Bové, J.M., Tully, J.G. and Freundt, E.A. (1973). *Spiroplasma çitri* gen. and sp. n: a mycoplasma-like organism associated with 'stubborn' disease of citrus. *International Journal of Systematic Bacteriology 23*, 191–204.

Sayed, I.A. and Hatten, B.A. (1976). Isoelectric focusing of mycoplasma proteins. *Applied and Environmental Microbiology 32*, 603–9.

Sayed, I.A. and Kenny, G.E. (1980). Comparison of the proteins and polypeptides of the eight serotypes of *Ureaplasma urealyticum* by isoelectric focusing and sodium dodecyl sulphate-polyacrylamide gel electrophoresis. *International Journal of Systematic Bacteriology 30*, 33–41.

Schildkraut, C.L., Marmur, J. and Doty, P. (1962). Determination of the base composition of deoxyribonucleic acid from its buoyant density in CsCl. *Journal of Molecular Biology 4*, 430–43.

Schimke, R.T. and Barile, M.F. (1963). Arginine metabolism in the pleuropneumonia-like organisms isolated from mammalian cell culture. *Journal of Bacteriology 86*, 195–206.

Shapiro, A.L., Vinuela, E. and Maizel, J.V. (1967). Molecular weight estimation of polypeptide chains by electrophoresis in SDS-polyacrylamide gels. *Biochemical and Biophysical Research Communications 28*, 815–20.

Shepard, M.C. and Howard, D.R. (1970). Identification of 'T' mycoplasmas in primary agar cultures by means of a direct test for urease. *Annals of the New York Academy of Sciences 174*, 809–19.

Smith, P.F. (1979). Membrane lipids and lipopolysaccharides. In *The Mycoplasmas*, Vol. I, pp. 231–58, M.F. Barile and S. Razin (eds). New York: Academic Press.

Smith, P.F. and Langworthy, T.A. (1979). Existence of carotenoids in *Acholeplasma axanthum*. *Journal of Bacteriology 137*, 185–8.

Stanbridge, E.J. and Reff, M.E. (1979). The molecular biology of mycoplasmas. In *The Mycoplasmas*, Vol. I, pp. 157–85, M.F. Barile and S. Razin (eds). New York: Academic Press.

Studier, F.W. (1965). Sedimentation studies on the size and shape of DNA. *Journal of Molecular Biology 11*, 373–90.

— (1973). Analysis of Bacteriophage T7 early RNAs and proteins on slab gels. *Journal of Molecular Biology 79*, 237–48.

Subcommittee on the Taxonomy of Mycoplasmatales (1979). Proposal for minimal standards for description of new species of the class Mollicutes. *International Journal of Systematic Bacteriology 29*, 172–80.

Tanford, C. and Reynolds, J.A. (1976). Characterisation of membrane proteins in detergent solutions. *Biochimica et biophysica Acta 457*, 133–70.

Teplitz, M. (1977). Isolation of folded chromosomes from *Mycoplasma hyorhinis*. *Nucleic Acids Research 4*, 1505–12.

Thirkill, C.E. and Kenny, G.E. (1974). Serological comparison of five arginine-utilising *Mycoplasma* species by two-dimensional immunoelectrophoresis. *Infection and Immunity 10*, 624–32.

Townsend, R. (1976). Arginine metabolism by *Spiroplasma citri*. *Journal of General Microbiology 94*, 417–20.

Townsend, R., Archer, D.B. and Plaskitt, K.A. (1980). Purification and preliminary characterisation of spiroplasma fibrils. *Journal of Bacteriology 142*, 694–700.

Tully, J.G. (1979). Special features of the Acholeplasmas. In *The Mycoplasmas*, Vol. I, pp. 431–49, M.F. Barile and S. Razin (eds). New York: Academic Press.

Tully, J.G. and Razin, S. (1969). Characteristics of a new sterol nonrequiring Mycoplasma. *Journal of Bacteriology 98*, 970–8.

Ulitzur, S. (1972). Rapid determination of DNA base composition by ultraviolet spectroscopy. *Biochimica et biophysica Acta 272*, 1–11.

Weber, K. and Osborn, M. (1969). The reliability of molecular weight determination by dodecyl sulphate-polyacrylamide gel electrophoresis. *Journal of*

Biological Chemistry 244, 4406-12.

Weickmann, J.L., Himmel, M.E., Squire, P.G. and Fahrney, D.E. (1978). Arginine deiminase from *Mycoplasma arthritidis*. Properties of the enzyme from log phase culture. *Journal of Biological Chemistry 253*, 6010-15.

Wetmur, J.G. and Davidson, N. (1968). Kinetics of renaturation of DNA. *Journal of Molecular Biology 31*, 349-70.

Williams, D.E. and Reisfeld, R.A. (1964). Disc electrophoresis in polyacrylamide gels: extension to new conditions of pH and buffer. *Annals of the New York Academy of Sciences 121*, 373-7.

Williams, C.O. and Wittler, R.G. (1971). Hydrolysis of aesculin and phosphatase production by members of the order Mycoplasmatales which do not require sterol. *International Journal of Systematic Bacteriology 21*, 73-7.

Wreghitt, T.G., Windsor, G.D. and Butler, M. (1974). Flat gel polyacrylamide gel electrophoresis of porcine mycoplasmas. *Applied Microbiology 28*, 530-3.

Wróblewski, H., Johansson, K-E. and Burlot, R. (1977). Crossed immunoelectrophoresis of membrane proteins from *Acholeplasma laidlawii* and *Spiroplasma citri*. *International Journal of Systematic Bacteriology 27*, 97-103.

Wróblewski, H., Johansson, K-E. and Hjertén, S. (1977). Purification and characterisation of spiralin, the main protein of the *Spiroplasma citri* membrane. *Biochimica et biophysica Acta 465*, 275-89.

Wróblewski, H. and Ratanasavanh, D. (1976). Etude par immunoeléctrophorèse bidimensionelle de la composition antigénique de la membrane de quelques souches de mycoplasmes. *Canadian Journal of Microbiology 22*, 1048-53.

10 INSECT VECTORS

P.G. Markham

1. Introduction

The prokaryotic plant pathogens which are associated with yellows
type diseases are found only in the vascular tissue of infected plants
(see Chapter 3). This confers a need for specialised methods of transmission such as grafting, dodder (Chapter 3) and insects. Most insect
vectors of plant diseases occur in two taxonomic groups, the Stern-
orrhyncha (aphids and psyllids) and the Auchenorrhyncha (leafhoppers, planthoppers, froghoppers). The aphids transmit most of the
insect-transmitted viruses, with over 200 species transmitting some 250
viruses. More than 150 species of 'hoppers' transmit some 120 diseases
of which most are associated with prokaryotic pathogens. Vectors
are known for more than half the 100 mycoplasma-associated diseases
of plants (Tsai, 1979) and in most cases these are leafhoppers
(Cicadellids); but froghoppers (Cercopids), planthoppers (Fulgorids)
and psyllids have also been implicated (Nielson, 1979). There is a single
unconfirmed report of an aphid acting as a vector of an MLO associated
with a rosette disease of Easter Lily (Wang and Hughes, 1976). Although
the number of vector species represents only about 2% of the known
species of leafhoppers, the majority of vectors are in the most

phylogenetically advanced subfamilies (Nielson, 1979). In fact 76 species out of the 130 leafhopper vector-species occur in one of the most phylogenetically advanced subfamilies, the Deltocephalinae. Furthermore these vectors occur in only five tribes, of which the Euscelini, considered to be one of the most advanced of these tribes, contains 48 of the 76 vector species. This marked phylogenetic grouping largely reflects the feeding behaviour of these insects, although the biology, morphology and physiology may also have some relevance (Tsai, 1979). For example, Pierce's disease of grapes, which is caused by a xylem-restricted bacterium or rickettsia-like organism (RLO) is transmitted by 28 species of xylem-feeding leafhoppers and froghoppers. Aster yellows, which is associated with a phloem-restricted MLO, is transmitted by 31 species of phloem-feeding leafhoppers. Just as some diseases have many vectors, some vectors can transmit several diseases. In fact, only 17 species transmit a disease not transmitted by any other species (Nielson, 1979) and this may only reflect a lack of research.

2. Feeding Behaviour and the Vector-pathogen Relationship

All the Auchenorrhyncha have mouthparts which are adapted for piercing and sucking. For a species to be a good vector it must be able to penetrate the plant tissues, causing minimal damage. It must also feed most of the time in tissues containing a high titre of infectious organisms (Day *et al.*, 1952). The majority of leafhoppers feed in the phloem (Forbes and McCarthy, 1969; Putman, 1941), but others feed mainly in the mesophyll or in the xylem. It is likely that the insects feed in any tissue for short periods but that they will feed the longest in the preferred tissue (Saxena, 1954; Carter, 1962). Leafhoppers usually transmit diseases most efficiently to those plants preferred for feeding (Lehmann and Claus, 1970). They also have a well-developed sensory system which enables them to reject most of the unsuitable host plants without having to sample the sap. There exists a complex relationship between vector, pathogen and plant.

As the vector penetrates the plant tissue two types of saliva are produced (Miles, 1972). One solidifies and produces the flange and salivary sheath (Figure 10.1), the other is 'watery' and may contain enzymes to help in penetration and ingestion. Phloem-feeding insects are able to detect the vascular tissue and alter the direction of the stylets, in order to reach it (Pollard, 1969).

The infectious agent is acquired during feeding, passes through the

Figure 10.1: Feeding Track of *Euscelis plebejus* in Leaf of White Clover (a) Penetration between Cells to Reach the Phloem, (b) Enlargement of Entry Point Showing Flange of Saliva on Surface

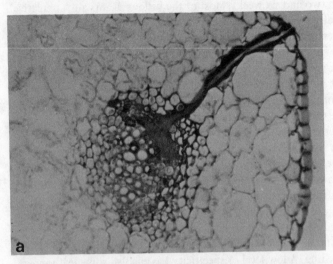

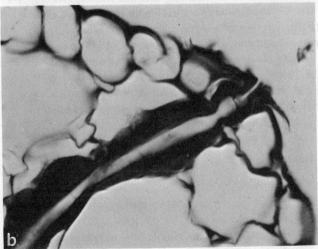

gut wall into the blood or hemolymph in which it can then circulate to all parts of the body. The MLOs are known to multiply in the blood and in many organs (Maramorosch, 1963; Townsend *et al.*, 1977; Tsai, 1979) including the salivary glands. From the salivary glands the agents can be passed back into the plant during feeding. The time lapse between acquiring and transmitting the agent is called the 'incubation period'. The length of the incubation period varies, depending on the agent, the vector, the temperature and many other factors; it is usually between two and six weeks. Most of the yellows agents are 'circulative', 'propagative' and 'persistent'; this implies that they not only multiply in the vector and survive a moult, but often render the insect infective for life (Harris, 1979). Some leafhoppers and froghoppers may regurgitate or egest during feeding which makes it possible for them to transmit 'noncirculative' agents which may be 'persistent', 'semi-persistent' or 'nonpersistent' (Harris, 1977, 1979). This may be the case with the transmission of some viruses and some of the RLOs.

The criteria that contribute to the phenomenon of specificity between vector and pathogen are not fully understood, but have been extensively reviewed (Day and Bennets, 1954; Black, 1959; Maramorosch 1963; Bawden, 1964; Sinha, 1968; Oman, 1969). It is likely that the vector, the pathogen and the host plant all contribute to specificity. Much of our understanding of the vector-pathogen relationship comes from studying both the natural acquisition and transmission processes, and from the experimental procedures of micro-injection and membrane feeding. A low level of specificity has enabled some leafhoppers such as *Euscelidius variegatus* (Kirsch) (Figure 10.2) and *Euscelis plebejus* (Fallén) to be used as experimental (artificial) vectors (Markham and Townsend, 1979; Markham *et al.*, 1977). Leafhoppers may have limited plant host ranges but often a common plant host enables one disease to be transmitted by several vectors to a wide range of plants. The feeding behaviour of an insect may be significantly affected not only by the host plant on which it is feeding but also by the previous host plant.

3. Insect Transmission

A. Natural Acquisition and Transmission

Although some MLOs may be acquired by leafhoppers after as little as 8 hr access to infected plants (Tsai, 1979) it is usual to use periods of more than 24 hr. Insects are often caged for 1-2 weeks, or even reared on infected plants to ensure maximum infectivity. The incubation period, under ideal conditions, is not likely to be less than 10 days, and more usually 2-6 weeks. The incubation period should be spent on a favoured food plant and ideally one which is not susceptible to the pathogen. Following the incubation period the insects are then able to transmit during feeds of a few hours on a test plant. However test

Figure 10.2: The Leafhopper, *Euscelidius variegatus*: Male, Left; Female, Right

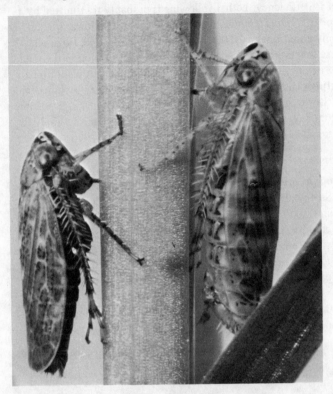

feeding (access) periods of 1–7 days are more likely to give successful results. Measured in terms of daily tests, individual insects may transmit continuously or intermittently. When determining minimum acquisition and transmission periods, the major problem is assessing when an insect actually reaches the phloem and begins to feed. Factors such as the previous food plant, the species and age of the test plant and the age of the insects should all be considered, especially during short access periods.

The proportion of the population which becomes infective varies considerably between various disease-vector combinations. One of the most efficient vectors is *Dalbulus maidis* D & W which can acquire and transmit corn stunt spiroplasmas with 100% efficiency. Conversely diseases such as citrus stubborn and lethal yellowing of palms are apparently very inefficiently transmitted. Citrus stubborn is transmitted in California by a leafhopper, *Circulifer tenellus* Baker, probably with less than 1% efficiency. Lethal yellowing is probably transmitted by a planthopper *Myndus (Haplaxius) crudus* Van Duzee (Howard, 1980), where only about one in 20,000 insects may be infective. However even these low rates of transmission can cause devastation in the field.

The efficiency of a colony (or race) of leafhoppers or planthoppers, transmitting plant viruses, is at least partially determined by inheritable factors (Storey, 1932; Timian and Alm, 1973) which makes it possible to breed more efficient races. Whether the same mechanisms apply to the transmission of MLOs is still to be established.

B. Experimental Methods

(1) Micro-injection Technique. The micro-injection technique was first used by Storey (1933) to infect leafhoppers with a virus and has become an important technique in plant pathology. The development of the technique has been extensively reviewed and described (Markham and Townsend, 1979), and only the most commonly used methods, useful for the transmission of MLOs, will be discussed below.

The apparatus is shown in Figure 10.3. The insects must be

Figure 10.3: The Apparatus used for Injecting Insects using Multiple Holder and Pump

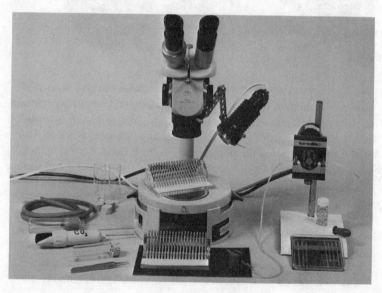

restrained during the injection process and where large numbers are to be inoculated it is most convenient to use a multiple insect holder (Maramorosch and Jernberg, 1970) or stretched Parafilm (Caudwell *et al.*, 1977). A convenient multiple insect holder has been developed (Figure 10.4), which will restrain 20 insects. It is adjustable for tension and can be quickly altered to accommodate species which differ widely

Figure 10.4: Insects in a Multiple Holder (a) and Held by the Tips (b)

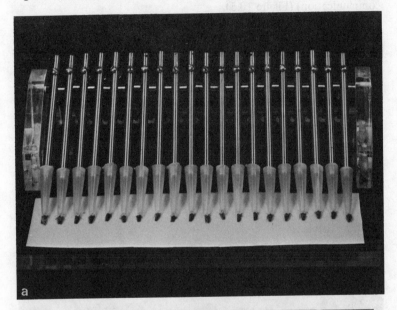

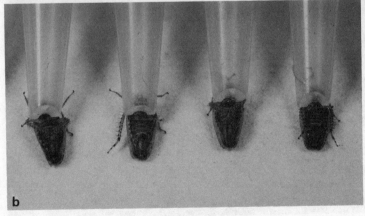

in size by changing the tip of each holder. An insect, anaesthetised by exposure to CO_2 for a few seconds, is placed on its back and restrained around the thorax by the shaped tip of a holder (Figure 10.4). The insects are injected, from the posterior, between a pair of abdominal sclerites. Another method is to place anaesthetised insects on to the base of an inverted (5 cm) Petri dish, over which a piece of Parafilm has been stretched; they are covered by another piece of stretched Parafilm, and injected through the Parafilm (Ms A.J. Smith, personal communication) (Figure 10.5).

The needles are usually made from glass tubing which is either hand-drawn or pulled in a commercial micro-forge to give a capillary needle with a tapering point which is 10-15 mm long (Markham and Townsend, 1979). The point is broken, to give a capillary about 10-20 μm in diameter.

The needle is filled with inoculum, then connected to a rubber or polythene tube and the dose ejected by pressure (Markham and Townsend, 1979). For example the operator may blow down the tube (through a Millipore filter if required), or the tube may be connected to a peristaltic pump. The accuracy with which the dose is estimated depends on the type of experiment (Markham and Townsend, 1979).

Figure 10.5: The Apparatus used for Injecting Insects, Held between Parafilm Membranes

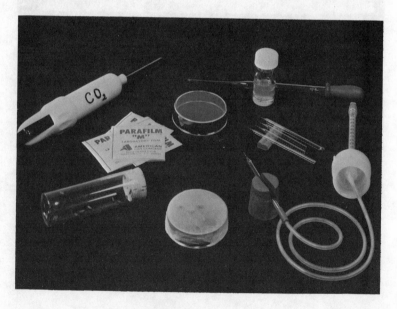

Sampling a proportion of the insects to ascertain the number of viable organisms is possible when using culturable agents, such as *S. citri*. For most plant pathological work it is more important to have a quick and efficient method of infecting all the inoculated insects, and such a method was used by Markham *et al.* (1974). CO_2-anaesthetised insects were held in a multiple insect holder. A hand-drawn glass needle was connected to a peristaltic pump and adjusted to give a continuous flow of inoculum at the rate of about 0.5 ml per min. The dose given to each insect was sufficient to induce a slight swelling in the abdomen. This method enables two people to inject 400–500 insects per hour, with 100% of the insects becoming infected. Mortality due to the injection process should be less than 5%.

(2) Membrane Feeding. Feeding leafhoppers through membranes was first attempted in 1927 by Carter to study the acquisition of a plant virus. Early workers used animal membranes but the advent of Parafilm M in the mid 1950s (Bradley, 1956) contributed to a wider use of the membrane feeding techniques, not only in plant pathology, but for rearing aphids (Kunkel, 1977) and leafhoppers (Mitsuhashi, 1979) on artificial diets. The technique is now proving useful in the study of the pathogen-vector relationship of spiroplasmas and leafhoppers, enabling both acquisition and transmission to be investigated *in vitro*.

The various types of apparatus which have been devised by many workers over the years have been reviewed by Mitsuhashi (1979). The apparatus is essentially two vessels, one in which to cage the insect and the other to contain the feeding solution. The insects must be able to feed through the membrane into the solution. To study individual insects we have found it convenient to contain the feeding solution in a sachet of Parafilm membrane (Mitsuhashi, 1970; Mitsuhashi and Koyama, 1971; Kunkel, 1977) using, as a frame, a drilled polypropylene top from a scintillation vial (Figure 10.6). This ensures that the solution is under a slight pressure. The insect is anaesthetised and placed in a glass scintillation vial which contains a moistened, glass fibre 'paper' disc in the base. The drilled top with the feeding sachet is screwed to the vial. The vial is then placed under a yellow light, in a suitable environment. Leafhoppers secrete typical feeding sheaths when feeding through membranes (Figure 10.7).

It is important for the contents of the feeding sachets to be aseptic. The surface of the membranes can be sterilised using UV light (Kunkel, 1977) or 70% ethanol for 1–2 min. The solutions can be sterilised by autoclaving or by passing them through appropriate Millipore filters. Although diets have been devised for leafhoppers

Figure 10.6: Diagram of Apparatus for Feeding Insects through Membranes

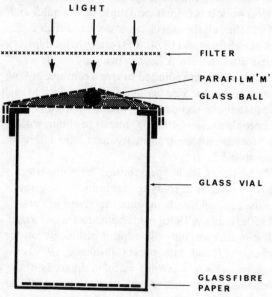

LIGHT

FILTER

PARAFILM 'M'

GLASS BALL

GLASS VIAL

GLASSFIBRE PAPER

Figure 10.7: Feeding Track Produced by a Leafhopper while Feeding through a Membrane. Note flange of saliva on surface.

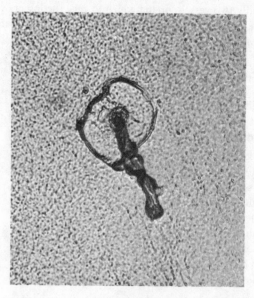

(Mitsuhashi, 1979) such complex solutions are not necessary for the experimental acquisition and transmission of plant pathogens. Leaf-hoppers feed well on 5-10% sucrose solutions but a compromise may have to be established between adequate feeding by the insect and viability of the pathogen. Consequently buffers and stabilising agents may have to be incorporated, together with antibiotics. The antibiotics must be assessed for their effect on the insect, the pathogenic agent and any symbionts that may occur in the leafhoppers. For most of the work with leafhopper acquisition and transmission of mycoplasmas and spiroplasmas a simple feeding solution is used — phosphate buffered sucrose with added antibiotic and serum (Table 10.1).

Table 10.1: A Feeding Solution for *Euscelidius variegatus*

1 ml of the following sterile, stock solutions:
  50% w/v sucrose in water
  Phosphate buffer*
  Penicillin G (1 mg/ml) aqueous soln
  [^{3}H] glycerol (100 μCi/ml)
Then add:
  Fetal calf serum 0.1 ml
  Sterile distilled water to 10 ml
  Adjust to pH 7.4

* 0.5M KH_2PO_4/0.5M $NaHPO_4$ in distilled water, I = 0.6.

Where acquisition is required imbibition may be stimulated by chemical additives, such as sucrose or amino acids (Sakai and Sagawa, 1976), or by alcohols (Alivizatos, 1981), or by a suitable pH, ionic balance and ionic strength of the medium.

The balance of K^+, Na^+, Mg^+, $SO_4^=$ and Cl^- are particularly important but the feeding response may vary from one vector species to another (Alivizatos, 1981).

Radioactive isotopes may also be incorporated and can be used as a measure of feeding activity (Kloft, 1977; Markham and Townsend, 1979). Individual insects, having fed on the isotope, may be ground with scintillant or Soluene and the activity counted to give a measure of internal radioactivity. The contents of the feeding chamber may be monitored for radioactivity, which would indicate those insects which had excreted excess feeding solution. Those which have excreted the largest volume are most likely to acquire the pathogen.

Environmental conditions, such as temperature and humidity, may play an important role, especially during extended feeding periods. Since leafhoppers are attracted to yellow, insects can be encouraged to collect on the feeding surface by either illuminating the solutions with yellow light or in some diets the concentration of riboflavin is sufficient to colour the solution yellow.

4. Survival and Pathogenicity

The pathogenicity of mycoplasmas to arthropods has been reviewed by Whitcomb and Williamson (1979) but the mechanics are poorly understood. The relationship of the yellows plant pathogens can be described by examples of pathogenicity, of tolerance and even of benefit to the vector. There is no general correlation between pathogenicity and the ability to transmit. The microorganism may experimentally affect other species, other orders of insects or even other taxa in various ways. Spiroplasmas, which seem to exhibit extreme adaptiveness, may become more pathogenic if passed from insect to insect (Whitcomb *et al.*, 1974). Strains of an organism may affect the same insect species in different ways.

In practice the easiest method of determining pathogenicity is by survival of the insects, providing suitable controls are maintained. Some of the factors which determine survival under experimental conditions are: the age of the insect; environmental conditions, particularly temperature and humidity; the host plant; a change in host plant, either to the same species or different species; the age and physiological state of the host plant; the experimental treatment and handling of the insect; and the disease agent.

5. Analysis of Results

The analysis of the type of work described in this chapter is made more complex by the interaction of three biological entities (insect, plant and pathogen) with each other and the environment. The experimental design is usually a compromise between the desirable theoretical requirements and practical limitations (such as numbers of insects and plants, and the space available). Therefore it is essential to obtain not only the maximum efficiency of estimation from these laborious procedures but also any other information that may be incidentally available (Whitcomb *et al.*, 1966).

It is essential to maintain appropriate controls and to understand the 'normal' state or the state where only one factor is variable. Lehmann and Claus (1970) used biometrics as a basis for studying the longevity of a vector on various host plants, which could then be extended to study the effect of the pathogen.

The analysis of transmission tests have been discussed by a number of authors (Caudwell *et al.*, 1977; Gibbs and Gower, 1960; Whitcomb, 1972; Whitcomb *et al.*, 1966). Analysis may be made on data collected from insects transferred singly (Whitcomb *et al.*, 1966) or in groups (Gibbs and Gower, 1960). Data, such as incubation periods, are often given as a range of values or a minimum value; however Sylvester (1965) advocates the use of a median, e.g. median latent period (LP_{50}), as a more accurate statistic.

Simple statistical analysis (Bailey, 1959) may often be preferable, especially where the variation is considerable; procedures such as transformation of data should be used with caution.

6. Leafhoppers and their Culture

A. Life Cycle

The biology and life history of many leafhopper vectors has been summarised by DeLong (1971), Nielson (1968) and Tsai (1979). The following summary may apply to many species but there may also be considerable variation in detail from species to species, particularly in their behaviour. Leafhoppers are usually bisexual and eggs are laid 2-10 days after mating. Eggs are often deposited singly in the leaves and stems of plants, but some species lay in organic material on the soil. A female may lay eggs for several weeks and produce about 300 eggs, although females laying more than 1,000 eggs have been recorded. Eggs may take from 2 days to 3 weeks to hatch, or several months in those species which diapause in the egg stage. There are normally five nymphal instars but the number of these stages may be reduced or increased by environmental conditions. The nymphal development varies and may take from 7-66 days. Adults often live for 1-4 months but some species can hibernate and may live up to 10 months. Certain species, particularly those which have only one generation per year, may overwinter as eggs, nymphs or adults; in which case that particular stage may be extended by several months. There may also be a facultative or an obligate diapause. Other species may have 2-5 generations per year and under appropriate conditions will breed continuously.

The duration of each stage of the life cycle is determined by factors such as temperature, humidity and light. Other factors such as the host plant species, the physiological state of the plant and the degree of crowding in the colony are also important.

B. Culturing

It has been possible to rear some leafhoppers on artificial diets, and even under aseptic conditions, but both methods are tedious and fecundity is usually poor (Mitsuhashi, 1979). Where large numbers are required insects are usually reared on plants under controlled environmental conditions.

(1) Host Plants. It is important to find a host plant that is both convenient to grow and handle experimentally, and on which the leafhoppers not only feed well but maintain a high fecundity. The adult lifespan has been used as a measure of the suitability of a host plant species (Lehmann and Claus, 1970). This may be useful in assessing the likelihood of MLO transmission but not as a criterion for the suitability of a plant on which breeding can take place. *D. maidis* adults will feed on at least 33 plant species but the eggs will hatch from only 16 species of Gramineae, and the nymphs develop to adults only on teosinte, maize (Pitre, 1967) or gamma grass (Pitre, 1970). *E. variegatus* showed poor survival and poor fecundity on *Zea mays*; good survival and better fecundity on *Lolium perenne* L; but good survival and high fecundity on *L. multiflorum. M. crudus*, a cixid which probably transmits lethal yellowing of coconuts, feeds on the stems and leaves of several plants when adult but will only breed on the roots of a few grass species (e.g. *Stenotaphum secundatum*) (Eden-Green, 1978; Tsai *et al.*, 1976). However leafhoppers may adapt to a nonpreferred host and establish colonies under experimental conditions.

(2) Pests of Host Plants. Stock plants should be maintained under pest-free conditions, and sprayed regularly with nonpersistent pesticides (e.g. Mevinphos). Small traces of substances such as nicotine may not kill a colony immediately but can either reduce fecundity or induce sterility. When breeding leafhoppers under glasshouse conditions the most common pests are aphids, whiteflies and red spider mites. When it is not possible or desirable to re-establish a mass culture of leafhoppers then biological control methods are successful by removing the specific pest which is in competition with the leafhoppers. Many species of aphids can be controlled by *Aphelinus varipes* Vorster, a parasitic wasp, whiteflies by another wasp, *Encarsia formosa* Gahan, and red

spider mites, *Tetranychus urticae* (Koch), by a predatory mite *Phytoseiulus persimilis*. None of these predators affects the leafhoppers.

C. Conditions

The three most important environmental parameters to control when culturing leafhoppers are temperature, humidity and light. Many workers use a glasshouse as in insectary and although often adequate, the main disadvantages are poor control of temperature and light, and difficulty in excluding seasonal influences. Controlled environment rooms or cabinets are therefore preferable.

A leafhopper species may have unique optimal requirements and these will have to be determined.

(1) Temperature. Temperature influences the duration of all stages of the life cycle. Many species of leafhoppers can be successfully cultured at 24°C. Some tropical species, e.g. *D. maidis*, may have a higher temperature requirement (27-30°C). *D. maidis* fails to lay eggs at temperatures below 18°C. Consideration must be given to the temperature within a rearing cage. The proximity to a high wattage light source and poor circulation of air through a cage may raise the temperature excessively.

(2) Humidity. Leafhoppers will breed over wide ranges of humidity. The egg is the stage most susceptible to desiccation and this is usually laid within the moist plant tissue. Humidities about 75% RH are preferable but where condensation occurs on the internal surfaces of cages insects become trapped and drown. Condensation is most likely to occur when the sun shines directly on to plants within cages causing excessive transpiration, and is a disadvantage associated with glasshouse rearing facilities.

More accurate control can be achieved by forcing air through each cage. The conditioned air may also be filtered to remove fungal spores and reduce infections such as *Beauveria bassiana* (Bals.) Viull., an entomophagous fungus.

(3) Light. Most leafhoppers are cultured under a 16-24 hr photoperiod. Shorter photoperiods may give rise to diapausing stages. It may be possible to maintain cultures under light intensities below 6,000-8,000 lux. However it is recommended by the author that intensities suitable for maintaining actively growing plants be used, i.e. 20,000 lux and above, or more accurately, from the plant growth aspect, illumination above 500 $\mu Ecm^{-2}s^{-1}$. Any suitable light source may be used e.g. high pressure sodium or mercury vapour, fluorescent tubes, metal halide or tungsten filaments. A spectrum comparable to normal

daylight would be ideal, and in practice a mixture of light sources may give the best results, for example warm white fluorescent tubes with some tungsten filament bulbs to provide extra wavelengths at the red end of the visible spectrum. It is also important to measure the light intensity at plant level within the cage, since there will be loss of light due to the distance from the source and due to materials from which the cage is constructed. It should also be remembered that the output of many light sources deteriorates after a certain number of hours of use.

D. Cages

The construction of cages (Figure 10.8) is a matter for the individual researcher. Ease of access and adequate ventilation are two major considerations. Materials such as Xylonite (cellulose nitrate sheet), polystyrene, perspex and glass are useful and non-toxic materials. Xylonite however becomes brittle especially under conditions used for rearing insects (warm temperatures and light sources which produce ultra-violet light in their emission). Perspex TX, which has been

Figure 10.8: Some Cages used for Rearing Insects and Transmission Work. Large rectangular cage is fitted with drip-feed watering system, and connector for air ventilation pipe.

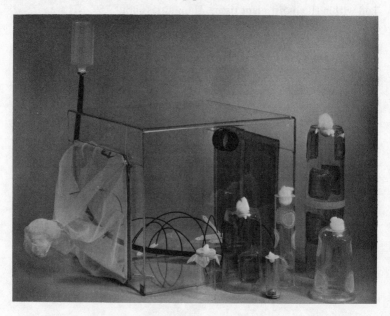

developed for use in areas with UV radiation, is preferable.

Ventilation holes are best covered with fine nylon mesh or stainless steel gauze. For ease of maintenance a drip-feed watering system is the most convenient in large cages (Figure 10.8).

E. Handling

Leafhoppers are often collected, under culture conditions, using mouth-operated aspirators (pooters). However, the author finds an electrically-driven vacuum pump most satisfactory, as the air flow can be controlled by a valve or a variac to give the required constant suction, which will ensure the least damage to insects. The apparatus for handling insects is shown in Figure 10.9. A 'transfer-cage', with sleeved access ports and a sliding front, is most convenient. Many insects are attracted to light and can be induced to collect at a convenient place by shining a light through the cage and covering other areas with a black cloth, enclosing the operator if necessary. A vacuum cleaner with disposable bags is

Figure 10.9: The Apparatus for Handling Insects

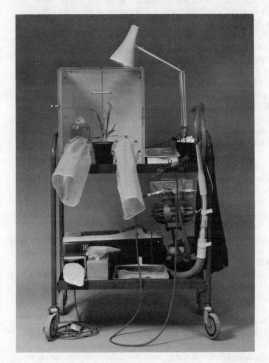

useful for collecting unwanted insects. Methods using CO_2 to anaesthetise insects within a cage (Maramorosch, 1953) are not widely used.

References

Alivizatos, A.S. (1981). Studies on two plant pathogenic spiroplasmas. PhD Thesis, University of East Anglia.

Bailey, N.T.J. (1959). *Statistical Methods in Biology*. London: English Universities Press Ltd.

Bawden, F.C. (1964). *Plant Viruses and Virus Diseases*, 4th edn. New York: Ronald Press.

Black, L.M. (1959). Biological cycles of plant viruses in insect vectors. In *The Viruses*, Vol. 2, pp. 157–85, F.M. Burnet and W.M. Stanley (eds). New York: Academic Press.

Bradley, R.H.E. (1956). Effect of depth of stylet penetration on aphid transmission of PVY1. *Canadian Journal of Microbiology 2*, 539–47.

Carter, W. (1927). A technic for use with Homopterous vectors of plant diseases, with special reference to the sugar-beet leafhopper, *Eutettix tenellus* (Baker). *Journal of Agricultural Research 34*, 449–51.

— (1962). *Insects in Relation to Plant Diseases*. New York: Wiley Interscience.

Caudwell, A. (1972). Aspects statistiques des épreuves d'infectivité chez les Jaunisses (Yellows) des plantes et chez les viroses transmises selon le mode persistant. Intérêt de la Fève (*Vicia faba*) comme plante-test pour les Jaunisses. *Annales des Phytopathologie 9, 141–59*.

Caudwell, A., Bachalier, J.C., Kuszala, C. and Larrue, J. (1977). Un appareil permettant d'immobiliser les insectes à injecter dans les épreuves d'infectivité des Jaunisses. *Annales des Phytopathologie 9, 521–3*.

Day, M.F. and Bennets, M.J. (1954). *A Review of Problems of Specificity in Arthropod Vectors of Plant and Animal Viruses*. Canberra, Australia: Commonwealth Scientific Research Organisation.

Day, M.F., Irzykiewicz, M. and McKinnon, A. (1952). Observations on the feeding of the virus vector *Orosium argentatus* (Evans) and comparisons with certain other Jassids. *Australian Journal of Scientific Research B5*, 128–42.

DeLong, D.M. (1971). The bionomics of leafhoppers. *Annual Review of Entomology 162*, 179–82.

Eden-Green, S.J. (1978). Rearing and transmission techniques for *Haplaxius* sp. (Hom:Cixiidae), a suspected vector of lethal yellowing disease of coconuts. *Annals of Applied Biology 89*, 173–6.

Forbes, A.R. and McCarthy, M.R. (1969). Morphology of the Homoptera with emphasis on virus vectors. In *Viruses, Vectors and Vegetation*, pp. 211–35, K. Maramorosch (ed). New York: Wiley Interscience.

Gibbs, A.J. and Gower, J.C. (1960). The use of a multiple-transfer method in plant virus transmission studies – some statistical points arising in the analysis of results. *Annals of Applied Biology 48*, 75–83.

Harris, K.F. (1977). An ingestion-egestion hypothesis of noncirculative virus transmission. In *Aphids as Virus Vectors*, pp. 165–220, K.F. Harris and K. Maramorosch (eds). New York: Academic Press.

— (1979). Leafhoppers and aphids as biological vectors: vector-virus relationships. In *Leafhopper Vectors and Plant Diseases Agents*, pp. 216–308, K. Maramorosch and K.F. Harris (eds). New York: Academic Press.

Howard, F.W. (1980). Population densities of *Myndus crudus* van Duzee (Homoptera:Cixiidae) in relation to coconut lethal yellowing distribution in

Florida. *Principes 24*, 174-8.

Kloft, W.J. (1977). Radioisotopes in aphid research. In *Aphids as Virus Vectors*, pp. 292-310, K.F. Harris and K. Maramorosch (eds). New York: Academic Press.

Kunkel, H. (1977). Membrane feeding systems in aphid research. In *Aphids as Virus Vectors*, pp. 311-38, K. Maramorosch and K.F. Harris (eds). New York: Academic Press.

Lehmann, W. and Claus, S. (1970). Die eignung von pflanzenarten für die ernährung von *Euscelis plebejus* Fall. in beziehung zu ihrer bedeutung als viruswirte. *Biologisches Zentralblatt 89*, 9-21.

Maramorosch, K. (1963). Arthropod transmission of plant viruses. *Annual Review of Entomology 8*, 369-416.

— (1953). A new leafhopper-borne plant disease from Western Europe. *Plant Disease Reporter 37*, 612-13.

Maramorosch, K. and Jernberg, N. (1970). An adjustable multiple-insect holder for microinjection. *Journal of Economic Entomology 63*, 1216-18.

Markham, P.G. and Townsend, R. (1979). Experimental vectors of spiroplasmas. In *Leafhopper Vectors and Plant Disease Agents*, pp. 413-45, K. Maramorosch and K.F. Harris (eds). New York: Academic Press.

Markham, P.G., Townsend, R., Bar-Joseph, M., Daniels, M.J., Plaskitt, A. and Meddins, B.M. (1974). Spiroplasmas are the causal agents of citrus little leaf disease. *Annals of Applied Biology 78*, 49-57.

Markham, P.G., Townsend, R., Plaskitt, K. and Saglio, P. (1977). Transmission of corn stunt to dicotyledonous plants. *Plant Disease Reporter 61*, 342-5.

Miles, P.W. (1972). The saliva of Hemiptera. *Advances in Insect Physiology 9*, 183-255.

Mitsuhashi, J. (1970). A device for collecting planthopper and leafhopper eggs (Hemiptera:Delphacidae and Deltocephalidae). *Applied Entomology and Zoology 5*, 47-9.

— (1979). Artificial rearing of leafhopper vectors. In *Leafhopper Vectors and Plant Disease Agents*, pp. 369-412, K. Maramorosch and K.F. Harris (eds). New York: Academic Press.

Mitsuhashi, J. and Koyama, K. (1971). Rearing of planthoppers on a holidic diet. *Entomologia Experimentalis et Applicata 14*, 93-8.

Nielson, M.W. (1968). The leafhopper vectors of phytopathogenic viruses (Homoptera, Cicadellidae) taxonomy, biology and virus transmission. *United States Department of Agriculture Technical Bulletin 1382*, 386.

— (1979). Taxonomic relationships of leafhopper vectors of plant pathogens. In *Leafhopper Vectors and Plant Disease Agents*, pp. 1-28, K. Maramorosch and K.F. Harris (eds). New York: Academic Press.

Oman, P.W. (1969). Criteria of specificity in virus-vector relationships. In *Viruses, Vectors and Vegetation*, pp. 1-22, K. Maramorosch (ed). New York: Wiley Interscience.

Pitre, H.N. (1967). Greenhouse studies on the host range of *Dalbulus maidis. Journal of Economic Entomology 60*, 417-21.

— (1970). Notes on the life history of *Dalbulus maidis* on gamma grass and plant susceptibility to the corn stunt disease agent. *Journal of Economic Entomology 63*, 1661-2.

Pollard, D.G. (1969). Directional control of the stylets in phytophagous Hemiptera. *Proceedings of the Royal Entomological Society (London) A44*, 173-85.

Putman, W.L. (1941). Feeding habits of certain leafhoppers. *Canadian Entomologist 73*, 39-53.

Sakai, T. and Sagawa, K. (1976). Effect of salicylic acid on probing and oviposition of the rice plant and leafhoppers (Homoptera:Delphacidae and Deltocephalidae). *Applied Entomology and Zoology 11*, 75–81.

Saxena, K.N. (1954). Feeding habits and physiology of digestion of certain leafhoppers Homoptera:Jassidae. *Experientia 10*, 383–4.

Sinha, R.C. (1968). Recent work on leafhopper transmitted viruses. *Advances in Virus Research 13*, 181–224.

Storey, H.H. (1932). The inheritance by an insect vector of the ability to transmit a plant virus. *Proceedings of the Royal Society (London) B112*, 46–60.

— (1933). Investigations of the mechanisms of the transmission of plant viruses by insect vectors. I. *Proceedings of the Royal Society (London) B113*, 463–85.

Sylvester, E.S. (1965). The latent period of pea-enation mosaic virus in the pea aphid *Acyrthosiphon pisum* (Harris) – An approach to its estimation. *Virology 25*, 62–7.

Timian, R.G. and Alm, K. (1973). Selective inbreeding of *Macrosteles fascifrons* for increased efficiency in virus transmission. *Phytopathology 63*, 109–12.

Townsend, R., Markham, P.G. and Plaskitt, K.A. (1977). Multiplication and morphology of *Spiroplasma citri* in the leafhopper *Euscelis plebejus. Annals of Applied Biology 87*, 307–13.

Tsai, J.H. (1979). Vector transmission of mycoplasmal agents of plant disease. In *The Mycoplasmas*, Vol. III, pp. 266–307, R.F. Whitcomb and J.F. Tully (eds). New York: Academic Press.

Tsai, J.H., Woodiel, N.L. and Kirsch, O.H. (1976). Rearing techniques for *Haplaxius crudus* (Homoptera:Cixiidae). *Florida Entomologist 59*, 41–3.

Wang, E.L.H. and Hughes, I.W. (1976). Development and association of mycoplasma-like organisms in vector aphid and Easter Lily infected with Rosette Disease. *Proceedings of Society for General Microbiology 3*, 153.

Whitcomb, R.F. (1972). Bioassay of clover wound tumour virus and the mycoplasma-like organisms of peach western X and aster yellows. *United States Department of Agriculture Technical Bulletin 1438*, 1–32.

Whitcomb, R.F., Jensen, D.D. and Richardson, J. (1966). The infection of leafhoppers by western X-disease virus. I. Frequency of transmission after injection or acquisition feeding. *Virology 28*, 448–53.

Whitcomb, R.F., Shapiro, M. and Richardson, J. (1966). An Erwinia-like bacterium pathogenic to leafhoppers. *Journal of Invertebrate Pathology 8*, 299–307.

Whitcomb, R.F. and Williamson, D.L. (1979). Pathogenicity of mycoplasmas for arthropods. *Zentralblatt für Bakteriologie, Parasitenkunde, Infektionskraukheiten und Hygiene. Erste Abteilung Originale 245*, 200–21.

Whitcomb, R.F., Williamson, D.L., Rosen, J. and Coan, M. (1974). Relationship of infection and pathogenicity in the infection of insects by wall-free prokaryotes. *Les Mycoplasmes/Mycoplasmas. Les Colloques de l'Institut National de la Santé et de la Recherche Médicale 33*, 274–82.

MISCELLANEOUS METHODS

M.A. Stephens and M.J. Daniels

1. Mycoplasma Viruses

A. Introduction

The presence of viruses in mycoplasmas was first suggested by observations of 'virus-like' particles in electron micrographs of mycoplasma
cells (Edwards and Fogh, 1960; Swartzendruber *et al.*, 1967). Extrachromosomal or satellite DNA in mycoplasmas was reported by Haller
and Lynn (1968) and Morowitz (1969) but there was no correlation
with the presence of virus particles.

Numerous 'virus-like' particles have been observed associated with
presumptive mycoplasmas in some diseased plants (Ploaie, 1971;
Gourret *et al.*, 1973; Cadilhac and Giannotti, 1975) but none of these
viruses has been isolated.

The first isolation of a mycoplasma virus was reported by Gourlay
(1970), using *Acholeplasma laidlawii* as host. Subsequently Gourlay
was able to isolate two more morphologically distinct viruses using
A. laidlawii indicator strains (Gourlay, 1971; Gourlay and Wyld, 1973).
These acholeplasma viruses (usually referred to as mycoplasma viruses)
were classified morphologically and serologically into three groups.

Table 11.1 summarises the general properties of the viruses in these groups.

Electron microscopic studies (Horne, 1972; Robertson *et al.*, 1972; Rahman and Sethi, 1979) have suggested that *Mycoplasma* species may be infected with viruses and recently Howard *et al.* (1980) have propagated a virus in a *Mycoplasma* host (*M. bovirhinis*). *A. laidlawii* strains have in the past been used to propagate viruses originating possibly from *Mycoplasma* species, but since the acholeplasma hosts themselves carry viruses, the propagated virus could not unequivocally be said to originate from a *Mycoplasma* species. The mycoplasma viruses have been extensively reviewed by Gourlay (1974), Maniloff *et al.* (1977), Razin (1978), Cole (1979) and Maniloff *et al.* (1979).

Virus-like particles were first observed in a plant pathogenic mycoplasma during the original ultrastructural characterisation of *Spiroplasma citri* (Cole *et al.*, 1973a, b). Subsequently three morphologically distinct types of particle were distinguished and named SVC1, SVC2 and SVC3 (for *Spiroplasma* virus *citri* 1, etc.) (Cole *et al.*, 1974). Detection of these types of virus in other spiroplasma strains suggests that a more suitable nomenclature may be SpV1, SpV2 and SpV3 respectively (*Spiroplasma* virus 1, etc.). Some of the main characteristics of the spiroplasma viruses are summarised in Table 11.2.

Electron microscopic studies have revealed SpV1 and SpV3 virus particles in *S. citri*, corn stunt spiroplasmas, tick spiroplasmas and spiroplasmas associated with sex-ratio phenotype in *Drosophila*. The SpV1 virus has also been found in spiroplasmas isolated from honey bees. The SpV2 virus has so far only been observed in *S. citri* strains.

The first spiroplasma viruses to be propagated were the SVC3 (SpV3) viruses from *S. citri* and the suckling mouse cataract agent (SMCA) (Cole *et al.*, 1977). The viruses were propagated to high titres and purified, permitting characterisation of the viral nucleic acid and proteins. Subsequent investigations of the SpV3 viruses (Cole, 1978; Cole *et al.*, 1978; Stephens, 1978, 1980) have examined the molecular biology of the particles and their mode of interaction with their host cells. Recently, the isolation and preliminary characterisation of the SVC1 (SpV1) virus has been reported (Liss and Cole, 1979).

B. Isolation of Mycoplasma Viruses

The isolation of viruses from mycoplasmas has followed the standard procedures used for the isolation of bacteriophages from bacterial cultures. Samples from culture filtrates or supernatants have been added to test host organisms. The clearing of broth cultures or the appearance

Table 11.1: Properties of Mycoplasma Viruses

	Morphology	Size (nm)	Buoyant Density (g cm^{-3})	Sensitivity to Non-ionic Detergent	Plaque Size (diam.) (mm)	Nucleic Acid Type	Nucleic Acid M.Wt	Protein Composition (M.Wts)
Group 1 (MVL 1)	naked, rod-shaped particles	14-16 $\times$ 70-90	1.37 in CsCl	–	usually turbid (0.5-0.6)	single-stranded circular DNA	2×10^6	4 proteins 70,000 53,000 30,000 19,000
Group 2 (MVL 2)	enveloped, roughly spherical particles	52-125 in diameter (mean = 80)	1.19 in sucrose 1.26 in CsCl	+	turbid (1-2)	super-helical covalently closed circular DNA	7.4×10^6 to 7.8×10^6	4-5 (7?) proteins
Group 3 (MVL 3)	polyhedron with short tail and collar	head: 57 $\times$ 61 tail: 25 $\times$ 9	1.32 & 1.26 in K tartrate 1.48 in CsCl	–	clear (0.5-2)	linear double-stranded DNA	25.8×10^6	5 proteins 172,000 81,000 73,000 68,000 43,000
MVBrI	polyhedron with tail	head: 72 tail: 71 $\times$ 19	?	?	?	?	?	?

Table 11.2: Properties of Spiroplasma Viruses

	Morphology	Size (nm)	Buoyant Density (g cm^{-3})	Plaque Characteristics (diameter, mm)	Nucleic Acid	Proteins
SpV1 (SVC1)	rod-shaped	230-280 x 10-15	1.21 in metrizamide 1.39 in CsCl	Turbid (2)	DNA	7 proteins 72,000-142,000
SpV2 (SVC2)	polyhedron with a long non-tractile tail	48-51 (flat side to flat side) tail: 75-83 x 6-8	–	–	–	–
SpV3 (SVC3)	polyhedron with short tail	35-37 (flat side to flat side) tail: 13-18 x 8-10	1.26 in metrizamide 1.45 in CsCl	Clear with ring of enriched growth of lawn (1.5)	linear, double-stranded, circularly permuted, terminally redundant DNA M.Wt: 13.4 x 10^6	5 proteins 130,000 110,000 67,000 48,000 38,000

of zones of inhibition of growth (plaques) on plates, seeded with the
test organisms, usually indicates phage activity.

Infected cells for virus isolation can be grown in solid or liquid
medium. Viruses can be removed from solid medium by washing
plates with buffer or broth for a few hours at room temperature or
overnight at 4°C.

A variety of methods has been used to separate viruses from suspensions of mycoplasmas. A large proportion of spiroplasma cells can be
removed by filtration through a membrane filter (0.2 μm pores). Fewer
cells pass through the filter if external pressure is applied than if the
liquid passes through under gravity (Saglio, 1979). Spiroplasmas can
also be removed by centrifugation (12000 g, 4°C, 15 min). If the
viruses are resistant to chloroform, remaining cells can be destroyed by
the addition of 1/10 volume chloroform. A method used in the isolation
of viruses from *Acholeplasma* species involved centrifugation of the
mycoplasma cells through a layer of 30% sucrose. The cells pelleted,
while the viruses were left in the sucrose layer, perhaps stripped from
the surface of the cells (Maniloff, 1972).

A number of methods have been used to prepare 'lawns' of spiroplasma cells suitable for the detection of virus plaques. For SVC3
viruses Cole *et al.* (1977) prepared lawns of *S. citri* by flooding Petri
dishes (6 cm diameter), containing 8 ml of solid medium (1.5% agar),
with 0.2 ml of a late exponential phase culture of cells. After drying,
the lawns were incubated at 32° for 6 hr, and inoculated with viruses
by allowing 20 μl samples to soak into the agar. The plates were
incubated in an atmosphere of 95% N_2/5%CO_2 for 4-5 days at 32°C
before being examined for plaques. The enriched atmosphere of CO_2
was not essential for plaque development but increased the growth of
the lawn and therefore improved the visibility of the plaques.

SVC3 virus plaques are more distinct if host lawns are prepared by
pouring a soft-agar (0.6% agar) top layer, containing *S. citri* cells into
Petri dishes containing a bottom layer of solid medium (1 or 5% agar).
Viruses and cells can be mixed either by placing portions of virus
suspension on the lawns, as described above, or by incorporating viruses
and cells in the soft-agar top layers. SVC3 plaques are clear, suggesting
that the viruses are lytic. The clear plaques are surrounded by a region
of enriched growth of the lawn, possibly due to growth-promoting
substances released from lysed cells. Visualisation of the plaques is
improved by staining the colonies with Dienes' stain (Scriba, 1968) and
by using an indirect light source with a dark background. Plaques can
be photographed directly or magnified using either a photomicroscope

or by inserting the Petri dish into the negative holder of a photographic enlarger and recording the images on reproduction film. Stephens (1980) noted that using the soft-agar top layer method, the diameters of the plaques depended on the number of colony-forming units (cfu) in the top layer. As the number of cfus were decreased the diameters of the plaques increased.

Figure 11.1: Plaques Produced on a Lawn of *S. citri* Strain ASP2 by 25 μl Drops of Serial Tenfold Dilutions of a Suspension of SpV3 Viruses. Since 12 plaques were produced at a dilution of 10^6, the suspension contained about 4.8×10^8 pfu ml^{-1}.

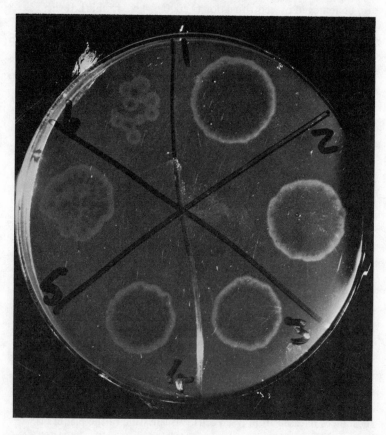

The titre of infectious virus particles in a suspension can be found by inoculating lawns with serial tenfold dilutions of the virus suspension (Figure 11.1).

Confirmation that the spiroplasma lawn has grown can be obtained by placing a disc of filter paper impregnated with digitonin at the edge of the seeded plate before incubation. A clear area around the disc confirms that the lawn has grown.

The existence of infectious virus particles can usually be assumed if individual plaques arise on lawns of a suitable indicator host strain, but confirmation of the viral nature of the agent can only be obtained if large numbers of virus particles are observed and if the agent can be propagated in the presence of the host. Discrete zones of inhibition can occur as a result of the release of growth inhibitors, e.g. bacteriocins, from colonies. Addition of chloroform should destroy the cells but may not destroy infectious virus particles. Plaque-forming agents should be cloned by picking single plaques into buffer or broth with the aid of a sterile needle and inoculating serial dilutions of this suspension on to lawns of the host. The procedure should be repeated at least twice to reduce the chance of isolating a mixture of virus strains.

C. Propagation of Mycoplasma Viruses

Spiroplasma viruses can be propagated to high titres in liquid or solid medium. In liquid medium, an exponentially growing culture (10^8 cfu ml^{-1}) should be infected with virus at a multiplicity of infection of 1-5 and incubated at $32°C$ to allow multiplication of the virus. Unpublished observations by R.M. Cole (personal communication) suggest that the latent period for SVC3 infection of *S. citri* cells is very long (approx 20 hr). The highest titre of the SVC3 viruses is reached 4-5 days after infection. Very few intact cells remain, and a 100-500-fold increase in virus titre can be achieved.

High titres of SVC3/AV9 viruses have been produced in soft-agar top layers. Sufficient viruses are incorporated into the top layer to give almost confluent lysis of the lawn. The appearance of large numbers of plaques confirms that the infection has been successful. Viruses can be recovered by scraping off the top layer and extracting the viruses with buffer or broth. Agar and cells can be removed by centrifugation.

The demonstration of viruses associated with the uncultivable sex-ratio spiroplasma (SRO) was made possible by the development of a bioassay (Oishi and Poulson, 1970) which involved injecting extracts from a *Drosophila* fly carrying one particular strain of SRO into flies carrying a different SRO. The ability of these extracts to destroy the sex-ratio phenotype provided an assay of the titre of virus.

D. Purification of Mycoplasma Viruses

Characterisation of the nucleic acid and protein composition of viruses requires sufficient purification of the viruses to remove contaminating material originating from the host cells and medium constituents. A high proportion of the intact mycoplasma cells can be removed by filtration or centrifugation. Viruses can be concentrated by ultra-centrifugation or by 'precipitation' with polyethylene glycol (PEG) 6000, but large amounts of medium constituents may co-sediment with the viruses when the PEG precipitate is collected by centrifugation. Contaminating membraneous material can be disrupted by addition of nonionic detergents, e.g. Triton X-100, Nonidet P40, if the viruses are resistant. Repeated cycles of low-speed centrifugation and ultracentrifugation will remove most of the nonviral contaminants. Further purification of the SVC3 viruses has been achieved by isopycnic centrifugation in metrizamide, a nonionic iodinated compound, followed, if necessary, by rate-zonal centrifugation in sucrose or fructose.

Cole *et al.* (1977) purified the SVC3 virus by isopycnic centrifugation in CsC1. The virus particles were, however, severely disrupted. Gradients of metrizamide were subsequently used to obtain SVC3 viruses from various spiroplasmas relatively free of contaminants. The SVC3/ASP9 virus can also be banded by rate-zonal centrifugation in linear gradients of sucrose or fructose. Fructose is preferable to sucrose since solutions can be applied directly to the carbon-coated grids used in electron microscopy and the sugar does not interfere with the visualisation of virus particles by negative staining.

A preliminary report (Liss and Cole, 1979) indicated that the SVC1 virus can also be purified using isopycnic centrifugation in metrizamide.

E. Characterisation of Mycoplasma Viruses

Morphology. Some information about virus structure can be obtained by examination of purified virus particles or infected cells in the electron microscope. Ammonium molybdate (2-6%), potassium phosphotungstate (0.75%) and methylamine tungstate (2%) have been used as negative stains for SVC3 virus particles. A useful method for detecting viruses carried by spiroplasma strains is to examine negatively-stained cells, for virus particles are often seen adsorbed on to the surface of cells. The SVC3 viruses have been observed apparently budding through the cell membrane and sometimes surrounded by an envelope which eventually disappears and is not essential for infection.

Plaques. The plaques produced by the SVC1 and SVC3 viruses appear to be distinct in size and morphology. The SVC1 plaques (2 mm diameter) are usually larger than the SVC3 plaques (1.5 mm diameter) although, as previously noted, the conditions used to prepare the host lawns are important. The SVC3 plaques are clear, while the SVC1 plaques are turbid due to growth of colonies within the plaques. In addition, the SVC1 plaques lack the ring of enriched growth usually found around the SVC3 plaques. The temperature range at which plaques develop will depend, to a certain extent, on the optimum temperature of growth of the host. *S. citri* has a rather narrow temperature range, centred around 32°C and therefore SVC3 plaques on *S. citri* lawns develop at about 32°C. The SVC1 viruses however, will multiply in lawns of bee spiroplasmas which grow over a wider temperature range and consequently the virus will produce plaques at temperatures between 22°C and 40°C. The temperature sensitivity of the virus may also be a limiting factor, since it has been observed that the MVL2 virus has a narrower temperature range for growth than the MVL1 virus on the same *A. laidlawii* host.

Serology. Comparison of viral antigens provides a relatively simple method of establishing the relationships between viruses. The use of purified viruses, free of cell contaminants, is important since antibodies raised against the contaminants will inhibit the growth of the host lawns.

Using relatively low titres of viruses (10^6-10^8) the neutralisation antigens of mycoplasma viruses have been compared by measuring the inactivation of virus infectivity when incubated with antisera. Static tests, in which infectivity is measured after incubation with dilutions of antiserum for a certain period of time, have been used to distinguish the group 1, 2 and 3 acholeplasma viruses (Gourlay, 1972, 1974; Clyde, 1974).

A comparison of the kinetics of neutralisation of different viruses with the same antiserum, however, provides a more sensitive serological comparison. Maniloff and Liss (1974) observed a threefold range of neutralisation rates among four group 1 acholeplasma virus isolates suggesting some degree of serological heterogenicity among the group 1 viruses.

Very little information is available on the serological comparison of spiroplasma viruses. Cole *et al.* (1978) reported that the SVC3/608 and SVC3/SMCA viruses were both inactivated by antiserum raised against the SVC3/608 virus, while Stephens (1980) reported that unmodified and modified AV9/3 viruses were serologically very similar (see below). Analysis of the kinetics of virus neutralisation only provides information about the neutralisation antigens on the virus particles. *Miscellaneous Tests.* Relatively simple experiments can be carried out to characterise virus particles. Filtration through membrane filters of varying pore size can provide an approximate estimate of the physical dimensions of a virus particle. Pre-coating the filters with serum reduces the likelihood of nonspecific absorption of the viruses on to the nitro-cellulose filters. Sensitivity of the virus infectivity to the action of nonionic detergents usually suggests that a lipid-containing envelope surrounds the virus. The acholeplasma virus, MLV2, can be distinguished from the MVL1 and MVL3 viruses by its increased sensitivity to heat. *Viral Proteins.* Mycoplasma virus proteins have been studied by electro-phoretic analysis in polyacrylamide gels containing sodium dodecyl sulphate (SDS). As shown in Table 11.1 the three acholeplasma virus groups contain polypeptides which vary considerably in molecular weight. The SVC3/608 and SVC3/SMCA virus proteins were found to be identical in mobility on 7.5% polyacrylamide gels by Cole *et al.* (1977), while the AVq/3 virus proteins were analysed on 15% poly-acrylamide slab gels by Stephens (1980). Virus proteins can be solubi-lised by heating (90°C) for a few minutes in a neutral solution containing 0.1% (w/v) SDS.

The molecular weights of the polypeptides can be interpolated from a graph of electrophoretic mobility against logarithm of the molecular weights of standard proteins. Care must be taken to purify the virus particles sufficiently to reduce contamination by proteins from the medium and the host cells. It should be noted that although, originally, it was believed that the mobility of proteins in SDS-polyacrylamide gels was relatively independent of amino-acid compo-sition, subsequent studies have shown that differences in the electro-phoretic mobility of proteins can sometimes be due to single amino-acid substitutions (Noel *et al.*, 1979). Anomalous mobilities can also occur due to the presence of carbohydrate moieties attached to proteins (Bretscher, 1971). Although there is no evidence for the existence of glycoproteins in mycoplasma viruses, Rottem and Greenberg (1978) noted that some MVL2 virus preparations appeared to adsorb serum glycoproteins. Additional bands may arise due to degradation of virus proteins during solubilisation procedures.

Viral Nucleic Acids. All the mycoplasma viruses examined have been shown to contain DNA. A commonly used procedure for the disruption of virus particles is heating to 60°C for 3-5 min in the presence of 1-2% (w/v) SDS. Viruses resistant to this treatment can usually be disrupted using the procedure introduced by Shepherd *et al.* (1970) in the isolation of DNA from plant viruses, involving proteolytic hydrolysis of the virus particles in the presence of SDS. If the virus particles are resistant to nucleases, contaminating RNA and DNA can be removed by preliminary digestion with nucleases. The aqueous phenol method (Kirby, 1965) has been routinely used to deproteinise samples. The nucleic acids which partition into the aqueous layer can be concentrated by ethanol precipitation and residual phenol can be removed either by extraction with ether or by extensive dialysis. Addition of a chelating agent, e.g. EDTA, reduces degradation due to nuclease activity. DNA samples should be stored in a buffer, in the presence of EDTA and 0.05-0.15M NaCl at 4°C or -20°C. Freeze-thawing of DNA samples will introduce single-stranded breaks in the DNA, while DNA stored at 4°C is more susceptible to nuclease action and contamination by bacterial growth. Characterisation of the DNA can be achieved by rate-zonal centrifugation in neutral or alkaline sucrose gradients, isopycnic centrifugation in CsCl gradients in the presence of ethidium bromide, electrophoretic analyses in agarose gels and observations of the DNA in the electron microscope. By studying the buoyant density in CsCl-ethidium bromide gradients and sedimentation characteristics in neutral and alkaline sucrose gradients Lombardi and Cole (1979) showed that the MVL2 virus DNA was double-stranded and supercoiled. Nowark and Maniloff (1979) reached similar conclusions by electron microscopy. The contour length of the DNA suggested a molecular weight of about 7.8×10^6, similar to that estimated by a sedimentation analysis.

Electron microscopic studies have shown that the SVC3 viruses isolated by Cole *et al.* (1977) and Stephens (1980) contain linear, double-stranded DNA of molecular weight about 13.4×10^6. The usual method employed for electron microscopy of DNA involves the spreading of a mixture of protein (usually cytochrome c) and DNA as a monolayer on the surface of a liquid. The monolayer is picked up on to a grid, negatively stained and shadowed to provide contrast (Kleinschmidt, 1968). The micromethod of Lang and Mitani (1970) was used by Stephens (1980) to spread DNA molecules extracted from the SVC3/AV9 virus particles.

The existence of terminal redundancy at the ends of phage double-stranded DNA molecules can be determined by partial digestion of exonuclease III, which removes nucleotides progressively from the DNA in the 3' to 5' direction. After denaturation and reannealing, linear DNA molecules with terminal duplications tend to form circular molecules as a result of the complementarity of regions of single-stranded DNA at opposite ends of the molecule (MacHattie *et al.*, 1967). Cole (1978) reported that 5-7% of the SVC3 virus DNA was terminally redundant. In addition, circular permutation of linear DNA should be suspected if, after denaturation and reannealing, circular molecules are detected (Thomas and MacHattie, 1964). Cole (1978) reported that the SVC3 DNA was circularly permuted.

The base composition of the viral DNA can be determined by the method of Bendich (1957) which involves acid hydrolysis of the DNA followed by paper chromatography. Bases, located on the chromatograms by UV illumination, can be identified by comparing their R_f values with those of standards. The base composition of the MVL3 virus DNA was established using this method (Garwes *et al.*, 1975). A method recently introduced by Davies *et al.* (1979) which involves radioactive labelling of nucleotides *in vitro* may prove useful, in the future, for the base composition analyses of mycoplasma virus DNA.

The guanine plus cytosine (G + C) content of mycoplasma virus DNA has been determined using two physical methods, which have been discussed in detail in Chapter 9. The G + C contents of the MVL3, SVC3/608 and SVC3/AV9 virus DNAs have been determined by measuring the buoyant density of the DNA in CsCl (Garwes *et al.*, 1975; Cole, 1978; Stephens, 1980).

The G + C contents of the MVL3 and SVC3/608 virus DNA have also been determined from the midpoint of the melting curve (T_m) of the DNA. While similar G + C values were obtained for the SVC3 virus, using both methods, there was a discrepancy between the values obtained for the MVL3 virus DNA, which suggested that the MVL3 virus DNA might contain modified bases. Base compositional analysis, however, did not reveal the existence of any modified bases.

The double-stranded DNA from the MVL2 and SVC3 viruses has been cleaved by site-specified endonucleases. Nowak and Maniloff (1979) used a number of endonucleases of known specificity to cleave the MVL2 virus DNA and produce an endonuclease map of the MVL2 virus genome. Stephens (1980) used cleavage with the enzyme *Taq*I to show that the DNAs from three separate spiroplasma viruses were different from each other, while two SVC3 viruses, suspected to be identical, were shown to produce fragments of identical molecular weights when cleaved separately with the site-specific endonucleases *Alu*I, *Mbo*I and *Taq*I. Only endonucleases which recognised A + T rich hexanucleotide sequences or tetranucleotide sequences cleaved the SVC3 DNA. This correlated well with the A + T rich composition (G + C content = 27%) of the virus DNA.

F. Methods of Investigating the Interaction of Mycoplasma Viruses with their Hosts

The interaction of mycoplasma viruses with their hosts can be studied using suitable adaptations of standard bacteriophage techniques. Variable results are obtained if the condition of the host cells is not controlled and spiroplasmas, especially *S. citri* and corn stunt strains, are particularly sensitive to physical manipulation. Cell lysis frequently occurs when cells are resuspended after centrifugation.

Adsorption. The adsorption of phages on to bacteria follows the kinetics of a first-order reaction (Adams, 1959). Over a limited range of concentration of cells and virus particles, the rate of adsorption should be constant for given strains of virus and bacteria. It is necessary to use concentrations of viruses and cells such that there is a high probability of cells and viruses colliding. Selection of a suitable ratio of cells to virus particles ensures that the adsorption is not limited by the number of available adsorption sites.

Adsorption rates are usually measured using one of two basic methods: (i) the titre of unadsorbed viruses can be determined either after removal of the cells by centrifugation or filtration or after killing the cells, e.g. by the addition of chloroform; (ii) the titre of adsorbed viruses can be measured by estimating the number of infected cells.

If the titre of unadsorbed viruses is measured the adsorption rate can be calculated using the equation:

$$K = \frac{2.3B}{t} \cdot \log_{10} \frac{P_0}{P}$$

Where K = adsorption rate constant (cm^{-3} min^{-1})
  B = concentration of cells (cfu ml^{-1})
  P_0 = concentration of unadsorbed viruses at time 0
  P = concentration of unadsorbed viruses at time t

Fraser and Fleischman (1974) measured the adsorption rate of MVL1 viruses on to *A. laidlawii* cells by titration of the infectivity remaining in the culture after removal of the cells by filtration. Filtration of unadsorbed viruses, either after removal of the cells by centrifugation or after lysis of the cells by osmotic shock was used by Putzrath and Maniloff (1977) to measure the adsorption rate of the MVL2 virus. Similar adsorption rates were obtained using both methods.

Stephens (1980) investigated the adsorption of the AV9/3 virus on to *S. citri* cells by centrifugation, either by assaying infectivity or radioactivity (when labelled viruses were used). The adsorption rate constant was 1.16-1.89 x 10^{-9} cm^{-3} min^{-1}.

Little is known about the mechanisms involved in the adsorption of viruses on to mycoplasmas. Fraser and Fleischman (1974) showed that there was relatively little effect of temperature, over the range 0-42°C, on the adsorption rate. Primary adsorption of the MVL1 virus appeared to be ionic in mechanism, with an optimum pH of approximately 6.
Multiplication. No data have been published on the multiplication of spiroplasma viruses. One-step growth kinetics of the MVL1, MVL2 and MVL3 acholeplasma viruses have, however, been determined. Cells were infected at a multiplicity of about 1 and after allowing time for adsorption at room temperature the infection mixtures were diluted (10^4-10^5 fold) to prevent further adsorption and incubated at the optimum temperature for virus multiplication. A gradual increase in virus titre over several hours suggested that MVL1 and MVL2 infections were nonlytic, there being a gradual release of viruses from the cells (Liss and Maniloff, 1971, 1973). Artificial lysis of infected cells, using nonionic detergents, showed that the numbers of infectious virus particles on the lysed samples never exceeded the numbers in the unlysed samples suggesting that there was no intracellular pool of completed viruses. In contrast studies by Liss (1977) and Haberer (1978) have shown that there is an intracellular accumulation of mature virus particles during infection by MVL3 viruses, suggesting that infection is lytic.

The molecular details of virus replication have only been published for MVL1, which is a single-stranded DNA virus (Das and Maniloff, 1975, 1976a, b, c). The steps in DNA replication were investigated using radioactively-labelled virus DNA. Viral DNA replicative intermediates were released by lysing the cells with nonionic detergent and studied using sedimentation and buoyant density analysis. Using rifampicin-resistant host cells, it was shown that early steps in the multiplication are resistant to rifampicin and therefore depend upon host-coded RNA polymerase(s). Later steps during the assembly of the virions required virus-coded RNA polymerase since these steps were sensitive to rifampicin. The detection of virus-specific proteins *in vivo* was enhanced by ultra-violet irradiation of the host cells prior to infection (Das and Maniloff, 1978).
Host Range. Many bacteriophages have been shown to exhibit a host range which depends on the last host in which the virus was propagated (Arber, 1974). The growth of a virus may be reduced or restricted on one particular host strain. The viruses that do grow, however, are

sometimes no longer restricted on that host. This host-induced alteration in the host range differs from mutational change in that it is not heritable. Restriction of virus growth in a number of bacterial species has been shown to be due to the action of site-specific endonucleases in the host which cleave invading, foreign DNA. Modification enzymes, usually methylases (methyl transferases), protect the host DNA against cleavage and also protect a low percentage of the invading virus DNA molecules. The plating efficiencies of the MVL2 viruses on various *Acholeplasma* hosts, suggested that these viruses are subject to host-controlled restriction and modification (Das and Maniloff, 1975; Phillpotts *et al.*, 1977).

Host-controlled restriction and modification of spiroplasma viruses were observed by Stephens (1978, 1980). The *S. citri* virus AV9/3, last propagated in *S. citri* strain ASP2, produced nearly 300 times fewer plaques on lawns of *S. citri* strain SP4 than on lawns of ASP2, i.e. the virus was restricted on SP4. Viruses isolated from individual plaques which appeared on the SP4 lawns plated with equal efficiency on ASP2 and SP4. The viruses were, therefore, modified in SP4. Repeated propagation of the viruses in ASP2 and SP4 showed that the alteration in plating efficiency depended on the previous host. One cycle of growth in ASP2 removed the modification so that the virus was again restricted on SP4. Since the host-range of the virus depended on the host, host-range variation due to the selection of mutant viruses was ruled out. The unmodified and modified viruses were morphologically identical and cleavage of the virus DNAs with commercially available endonucleases of known cleavage specificity produced identical fragmentation patterns suggesting that the unmodified and modified viruses were identical. The adsorption kinetics of the unmodified and modified viruses on to the restricting strain, SP4, were identical, confirming that the restriction did not occur at adsorption. Using viruses radioactively labelled in the DNA, it was shown that the unmodified, but not the modified, virus DNA was broken down during the infection of the restricting strain. The degradation of the virus DNA was determined by measuring the radioactivity which was converted to acid soluble material. Neither of the virus DNAs were broken down upon infection of the nonrestricting strain ASP2, as expected, since the growth of the viruses was not restricted on ASP2. The restriction nuclease responsible for the restriction of the AV9 virus in SP4 has not been isolated. The only nuclease detected degraded both modified and unmodified virus DNAs.

A site-specific endonuclease has, however, been isolated from the

S. citri strain ASP2. Cells harvested by centrifugation were disrupted by sonication and fractionated by chromatography on heparin bound to agarose following the procedure of Bickle *et al.* (1977). Fractions were screened for nuclease activities which increased the electrophoretic mobility of DNA from *E. coli* plasmid pBR322 or lambda phage on agarose (1–1.2%) or polyacrylamide (5 or 10%) gels. Lambda phage DNA has been shown to be cleaved by a large number of site-specific endonucleases (Roberts, 1976) and therefore is likely to be cleaved by any spiroplasma endonuclease. pBR322 is a low molecular weight recombinant DNA plasmid. Since its complete base sequence has been determined (Sutcliffe, 1978), the site-specificity of an endonuclease can often be predicted by comparison of DNA fragment sizes with the base sequence. The site-specific endonuclease isolated from ASP2, called *Sci* NI, cleaved pBR322 DNA to produce more than 30 discrete bands. The fragmentation pattern was identical to that produced by cleavage of the pBR322 DNA with the site-specific endonuclease *Hha*I which recognises and cleaves within the tetranucleotide 5′ GCGC 3′. Confirmation of the recognition site of *Sci* NI was achieved by cleaving a specific portion of the pBR322 molecule with *Sci* NI and aligning the fragments produced with the published base sequence of that portion of the DNA molecule. Determination of the exact cleavage specificity of the enzyme has been determined using the method of Brown and Smith (1976). The enzyme cleaves the 5′ GCGC 3′ sequence between the first guanine and cytosine residues. *Sci* NI did not cleave the virus DNAs, as expected, since the viruses are not restricted *in vivo* by ASP2. In addition the enzyme did not cleave ASP2 chromosomal DNA suggesting that a corresponding *Sci* NI modification enzyme also exists in ASP2.

2. Motility and Chemotaxis of Spiroplasmas

A. Introduction

Motility among the mycoplasmas was first described by Andrewes and Welch (1946) but despite recent work, described by Bredt (1979), it remains one of the least understood aspects of mycoplasmology. Mycoplasmas do not have flagella (with the exception of *Thermoplasma*) and cannot therefore use the means of locomotion available to the majority of motile eubacteria. *Mycoplasma* species which have been found capable of motility (*M. pneumoniae, M. gallisepticum* and *M. pulmonis*) glide along surfaces (of glass microscope slides, for example) at speeds up to $2 \mu m \ s^{-1}$, but they are unable to swim freely through liquid media. All these species appear to be polarised, having filaments or specialised structures at the anterior end of the cell. These structures have been suggested to be responsible for adhesion to membranes of host cells, but some role in motility seems equally possible. Motion of mycoplasmas over surfaces is reminiscent of gliding motility displayed by organisms such as myxobacteria. Very little is known about the mechanisms involved.

Turning to the spiroplasmas, their striking motile behaviour was one of the first properties to be described. Davis and Worley (1973) coined the trivial name 'spiroplasma' to describe the helical organisms they observed in juice expressed from corn stunt-infected plants, and their description and illustration of the movements of the organisms gives a graphic introduction to the topic. They noted that in liquid media of low viscosity the spiroplasmas seemed to make little headway, but if soft agar was incorporated the organisms progressed rapidly through the medium, appearing to wriggle around the agar particles (Davis and Worley, 1974). Cole *et al.* (1973b) observed that cultured *S. citri* displayed similar motile behaviour.

The ability of spiroplasmas to penetrate agar is illustrated by the appearance of colonies on plates containing agar (c. 1%) which are not too dry. The colonies have a 'rough' appearance which close inspection shows to be due to the presence of large numbers of satellite micro-colonies established by spiroplasmas migrating radially from the parent colony (Figure 11.2). Townsend *et al.* (1977) isolated *S. citri* variants from diseased *Citrus* material which produced 'smooth' colonies without satellites, and these variants proved to have lost both helicity and motility. The strains were identical to normal helical forms by all criteria tested, save that a single membrane protein was missing or greatly reduced in amount.

The motility of spiroplasmas was exploited by Saglio (1979) as the basis of a selective isolation technique. It has been mentioned earlier (Chapter 1) that the lack of a cell wall confers a degree of deformability on mycoplasmas enabling them to be forced through pores of a smaller diameter than the cell, and this property can often be used to free mycoplasma cultures of contaminating bacteria or fungi. Passing the culture through a membrane filter (e.g. Millipore filter of diameter 0.45 or 0.22 μm) allows a proportion of the mycoplasmas to pass into the filtrate, but the contaminants are usually retained quantitatively. Saglio found that if a spiroplasma culture was allowed to drip slowly (under gravity alone) through a 0.22 μm pore membrane filter a much higher proportion of the spiroplasmas emerged in the filtrate than if the

Figure 11.2: Colonies of *S. citri* (a) A motile strain showing peripheral satellite colonies initiated by migrating cells. (b) A nonmotile strain showing absence of satellite colonies.

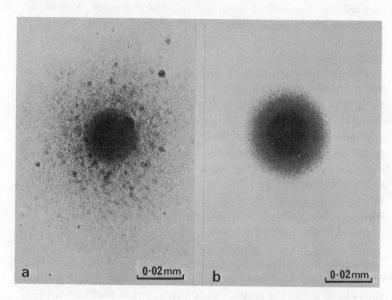

culture was forced through under pressure. Motility was apparently responsible for this phenomenon, because filtration at 3°C or addition of the inhibitor iodoacetate abolished the differential recovery. Lee (1977) undertook similar experiments and showed that motility was optimal at pH 7.

Daniels *et al.* (1980) studied the motility of spiroplasmas in media rendered viscous by addition of inert polymers and found that the speed at which spiroplasmas swim increases with viscosity. This property is also possessed by leptospiras, and is to be contrasted with the effect on flagellated bacteria which swim more slowly as the viscosity increases. In consequence of this behaviour spiroplasmas move 'up' a viscosity gradient, a phenomenon called 'viscotaxis' by Petrino and Doetsch (1978). Motility was optimal at pH 7 and was inhibited by the glycolysis inhibitors iodoacetate, fluoride and arsenate, and by dicyclohexylcarbodiimide (which inhibits membrane-bound ATPases). However cyanide (an inhibitor of aerobic respiration) and dinitrophenol (an uncoupler of oxidative phosphorylation) had no effect on motility. Motility was also lost if spiroplasmas were suspended in a medium lacking a fermentable substrate. None of the treatments affected the helical shape of the cells.

Little can yet be said about the mechanism of spiroplasma motility. Attention has recently focused on the possibility that mycoplasma membranes contain contractile proteins, perhaps actin-like, but the situation is still to be clarified (cf. Chapter 1).

Motile microorganisms have usually, when studied, been found to be capable of chemotaxis, that is motion towards or away from specific chemical substances. Microbial chemotaxis was first described by Pfeffer (1888), and modern work was initiated by Adler and his associates in the 1960s, interestingly using basically similar methods to Pfeffer's. Chemotaxis implies that a microorganism can sense changes in concentrations of specific chemicals and can in consequence direct its motility in preferred directions; it can be regarded as a sensory-response system analogous perhaps to systems in higher organisms. Since microorganisms (and in particular members of the Enterobacteriaceae) offer such favourable experimental material, chemotaxis has been extensively studied in the hope that principles discovered will be applicable to higher organisms which are more difficult to study. Reviews by Adler (1975, 1978), Parkinson (1977) and Springer *et al*. (1979) describe recent work in detail. The essential features are as follows. (1) Substances which act as attractants or repellents bind to receptor proteins at the cell surface. (2) Binding of the effector substance to the cell receptor initiates a signal. Changes in transmembrane potential can be detected, although their significance is a matter of controversy. (3) Transduction of the signal involves reversible enzymatic methylation reactions of specific proteins located in the cell membrane. (4) In a manner which is not yet understood, the signal can affect the direction of rotation of the flagellar 'motor'. Rotation of the flagellum in one direction gives smooth swimming ('runs' in a straight line) whereas contra-rotation generates 'tumbles' (Berg and Brown, 1972; Larsen *et al*., 1974). The chemotaxis system acts by suppressing tumbles when the concentration of attractants is perceived to be increasing (or, for repellents, decreasing). Reciprocal changes give more tumbling. Since tumbling generates directional randomness, the effect of tumble suppression is to bias random motion in the direction of increasing attractant concentrations (or decreasing repellent concentrations).

Until recently chemotaxis by mycoplasmas had not been studied, as Bredt (1979) pointed out, because suitable experimental systems had not been devised, but Cirillo (1979) suggested that spiroplasmas would be found to be capable of chemotaxis. This prediction was fulfilled by Daniels *et al*. (1980). Using a capillary assay for chemotaxis similar to

Figure 11.3: Migration of *S. citri* through Soft (0.6%) Agar. The cells were initially confined to the central circular area of the 10 cm diameter plate, but migrated radially over a period of 4–5 days to occupy an annular region. (Stained with Diene's stain.)

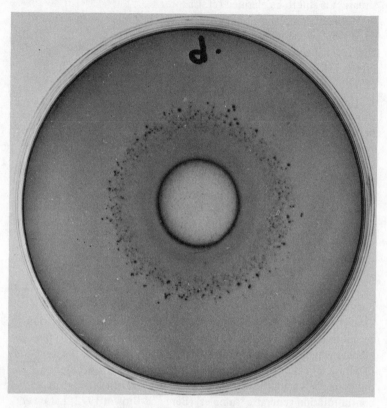

that introduced by Adler (1969) they found that spiroplasmas are attracted to many amino acids and sugars (including some which cannot be metabolised), and repelled by hydrophobic amino acids, aromatic compounds, acids and heavy metals. Chemotaxis could also be demonstrated by radial migration of spiroplasmas through soft-agar plates following inoculation in the centre of the plate (Figure 11.3). Accumulation of metabolites and depletion of nutrients generated gradients of chemoeffector substances. The effect of chemoeffectors on random motility can be graphically shown by photographs of 'motility tracks' in diffusion-generated effector gradients (Figure 11.4), in which the 'random walk' tracks seen when no concentration gradients are

Figure 11.4: Spiroplasma Chemotaxis. Spiroplasmas were suspended in 0.01M sodium phosphate, 10% sorbitol, 0.1% fructose, 0.25% methyl-cellulose, and photographed with a Zeiss Photomicroscope 2 with dark-field optics. (400 ASA film, 10 s exposure.) Motility tracks indicated random swimming in the unstimulated state (a), but when a diffusion-generated concentration gradient of an attractant is applied, the cells swim 'up' the gradient (b). Bar = 10 μm.

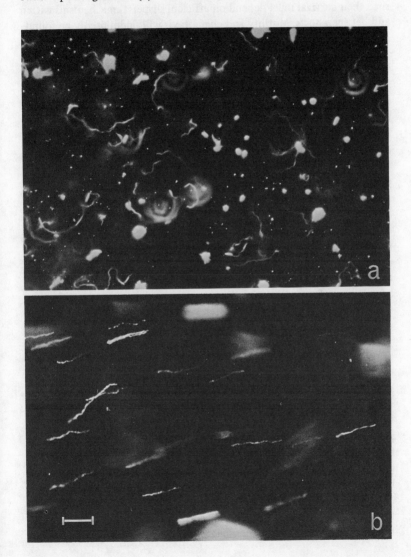

applied are converted into almost straight lines parallel with the gradient. Little is known about the mechanisms governing suppression of randomness. It may be that spinning of the cells about the helix axis generates 'runs' whereas periodic flexing of the cell body produces a situation analogous to 'tumbling' in bacteria. If so we might expect that flexing of the cell body is under the control of the chemotaxis system. Spiroplasmas are parasites (in most cases, pathogens) and as such their survival must depend on efficient dispersal mechanisms within and between hosts. Motility and chemotaxis will undoubtedly be found to be important factors in this respect.

B. Methods for Studying Spiroplasma Motility and Chemotaxis

Microscopy. Most of the studies of mycoplasma motility reported to date have depended on observations of living cells with the light microscope. The small size of mycoplasmas makes demands which can be satisfied only by instruments of high quality (and price). Phase-contrast systems have often been used, but excellent results can also be obtained using dark-field optical arrangements, particularly for spiro-plasmas (Cole *et al.*, 1973b).

The selection of microscope slides and the design of observation chambers requires care. We have noticed that certain batches of slides cause a large proportion of spiroplasmas to adhere firmly to the surface, which is unacceptable in motility experiments, while other batches may completely eliminate helical morphology to give a population composed of round bodies, leading to the erroneous conclusion that cultures have been contaminated. Sometimes such slides may be rendered usable by scrupulous cleaning in acid and detergent solutions.

Good optical contrast requires that as thin a layer of liquid as possible be used, but the thinner the layer the higher is the proportion of cells likely to attach to the glass. Moreover pressing down on the cover-slip to express surplus liquid may distort spiroplasmas (Cole *et al.*, 1973b). It is therefore necessary to compromise by sacrificing some optical quality. Various types of observation chamber may be used. For observations lasting a short time it may be enough simply to place a cover-slip over a drop of culture on a slide. Bredt and collaborators used chambers prepared by sandwiching thin rings of glass or plastic between cover-slips and slides, and in our laboratory we have successfully used chambers prepared very simply by attaching two cover-slips to a slide with grease, side by side and about 1 cm apart, and then bridging the gap with a third cover-slip. The culture is allowed to run into the gap and the open sides sealed with 'Vaseline' petroleum jelly to prevent evaporation which causes streaming of the fluid and renders observation impossible.

Cultures for motility experiments should be in early exponential growth. Media should be filtered before use to eliminate particulate matter and all batches of serum should be pre-tested, because some can cause clumping of spiroplasmas or promote attachment to glass. Fetal calf serum or PPLO Serum Fraction (Difco) may be substituted for horse serum if necessary.

As noted above, the viscosity of liquid media must be increased if translational motility of spiroplasma is to be observed. Davis and Worley (1974) incorporated 0.25% agar to give a semi-solid medium in which they cultured *S. citri* for cinematographic experiments. Daniels *et al.* (1980) found that methylcellulose gave excellent results. This polymer is manufactured by Dow Chemicals and is known as Methocel. The grade giving a viscosity of 4000 cp (2% solution) is suitable. Stock solutions can be dissolved in media by standing the mixture at 4°C for several days with occasional mixing, and the stock can be added to cultures to give final polymer concentrations up to 1% (w/v). Above this concentration the viscosity becomes inconveniently high. Two methods of measuring speed of swimming have been used (Daniels *et al.*, 1980). In the first method, an eyepiece graticule is fitted to the microscope and the time taken for individual organisms to cover a certain distance is measured with a stopwatch. This method is tedious because many organisms alter course before completing the distance, and those which do travel in a straight line enabling them to be measured may constitute a distinct subpopulation, unrepresentative of the majority of spiroplasmas. In the second method, photomicrographs are made using 10 second time exposures (400 ASA film). In this time the spiroplasmas travel up to 50 μm, so 'motility tracks' appear on the photographs and can be measured with a map-measuring device. Conversion factors to give true distances are calculated from the known magnification of the optical systems and checked with a stage micrometer. A possible source of error with this method is vertical migration of spiroplasmas out of focus, thus causing tracks to be shorter. However, both methods give very similar values for speed of swimming (Daniels *et al.*, 1980).

The 'motility track' techniques can be adapted to permit observation of chemotaxis (Daniels and Longland, 1980). The 'three cover-slip' chamber described above is partially filled with molten agar containing a suitable buffer and the attractant or repellent. When the agar has set, the remainder of the chamber is filled with a spiroplasma suspension in the same buffer containing methylcellulose but lacking the chemo-effector. Diffusion from the agar generates a concentration gradient from the interface through the medium, and motility tracks are found to be oriented parallel to the gradient (perpendicular to the agar interface) (see Figure 11.4).

Cinematographic systems have been used in conjunction with microscopes to record motility of mycoplasmas (Bredt *et al.*, 1970) and spiroplasmas (Davis and Worley, 1974), but the complexity of the apparatus required places the method beyond the reach of most experimenters.

Capillary Techniques. A capillary method was used by Daniels *et al.* (1980) to study spiroplasma viscotaxis and chemotaxis. The arrangement which they adopted was essentially the same as that employed by Petrino and Doetsch (1978) for leptospira viscotaxis. Sealed capillaries made from 10 μl disposable micropipettes were partially filled with attractant, repellent or viscous solutions by gently heating the tubes and plunging the open ends under the solution. They were then dipped into suspensions of spiroplasmas in buffered sorbitol containing fructose. The tubes were incubated at 32°C for 30–60 min and the capillaries were then withdrawn, broken, and the contents ejected into 0.2 ml of growth medium. The number of viable organisms which had entered the capillaries was determined by plating dilutions of the suspensions. The experiments were all performed using the spiroplasma strain BC3 isolated from diseased bees (Clark, 1977) because of the rapid growth and relative robustness of this strain. Nevertheless careful attention to plating conditions was found to be necessary to obtain reproducible, accurate viable counts. Plates were poured freshly each day and after the agar had set surface moisture was dried by exposure for 20–30 min to the sterile air stream in a laminar flow cabinet. Use of wet plates gave large spreading coalescent colonies, whereas excessive drying gave tiny colonies. Plates were sealed in polyethylene bags during incubation.

Membrane Filter Methods. Saglio (1979) allowed spiroplasma cultures to pass under gravity through 0.22 μm Millipore filters clamped in syringe adaptors and showed that spiroplasmas can 'swim' through the pores of filters. He proposed that this phenomenon can be used as a selective isolation method for spiroplasmas. This behaviour was not seen when the operation was performed at 3°C, or when the spiroplasmas were treated with iodoacetate, an inhibitor of glycolysis and motility (Daniels *et al.*, 1980). In principle the method could be used to study aspects of motility, but early attempts to demonstrate spiroplasma chemotaxis with similar apparatus met with failure (M.J. Daniels and S.A. Field, unpublished experiments). Lee (1977) also used passage through membrane filters as an index of spiroplasma motility, and showed that motility is optimal around pH 7, and is temperature-dependent.

3. Detection and Assay of Spiroplasma Toxins

A. *Introduction*

Disease symptoms constitute the most obvious manifestations of spiroplasma infections of plants and insects. The mode of action of the pathogen, that is the biochemical basis of symptom production, is an important subject of enquiry because any information gained may give some guidance in attempts to control or cure disease. It must be pointed out that a comprehensive picture is available for few, if any, diseases and this applies to both plant and animal disease.

Of the large number of plant mycoplasma diseases, the spiroplasma diseases citrus stubborn and corn stunt offer the most favourable experimental material because the pathogens can be cultured *in vitro* so that it is possible to study independently three systems: (1) the healthy plant; (2) the diseased plant, differing from the healthy plant as a result of the interaction of the metabolic activities of the plant and spiroplasmas; and (3) the isolated spiroplasmas. It must not be assumed that the spiroplasmas in plants necessarily behave in the same way as those in culture — for example factors in the plant may induce or repress synthesis of substances. An example of such a phenomenon occurs with the fungus *Helminthosporium sacchari* in which toxin production is induced by serinol, a compound found in sugar cane plants (Pinkerton and Strobel, 1976).

The symptoms of spiroplasma infection of plants have been described by Calavan and Oldfield (1979) and by Markham (Chapter 3), and the implications for the biochemical pathologist have been discussed by Daniels (1979a). It is sufficient to recall here that *S. citri* produces symptoms in herbaceous hosts suggestive of the production of a phytotoxin which damages cells, particularly those in the roots, resulting in impaired water uptake and wilting. The majority of plant mycoplasma diseases do not however show such symptoms, but for these the corn stunt spiroplasma may be a good model, possibly affecting plants by interfering with some aspects of hormone metabolism.

When embarking upon an investigation of a hypothetical biologically-active natural product such as a microbial toxin it is almost always necessary to use a bioassay to monitor extraction and purification attempts. Bioassays are notoriously unreliable because the response of the test organism to the toxin if often obscured by nonspecific effects caused by other components of crude preparations. The aim of the experimenter is to use the bioassay to assemble sufficient information to permit its replacement by a more specific chemical or biochemical assay. In the case of the toxin(s) of *S. citri* the problem is particularly acute because the normal growth medium is toxic to plant tissues and moreover the toxin in a semi-purified state is unstable. To circumvent these problems two approaches have been tried: (1) the use of alternative complex or semi-defined growth media which might be less toxic and (2) the development of bioassays which are less sensitive to growth medium components. The first approach has been unsuccessful, but the bean leaf assay described below was a reasonably satisfactory solution to the second problem. In any case it is essential to test control preparations from uninoculated medium to guard against being misled by nonspecific effects. An area of great potential interest concerns the mode of action of spiroplasmas on insects. Some spiroplasmas (e.g. the bee and some flower strains) rapidly kill insects into which they are introduced and may therefore synthesise insecticidal compounds. So far, there are no reports of experiments designed to detect such substances.

B. Assay Procedures

Microbial Test Organisms. A number of cases have been reported where microbial cells have been used to assay phytotoxins, an example being provided by the work of Braun (1955) who used the alga *Chlorella vulgaris* to study the tobacco wildfire toxin produced by *Pseudomonas tabaci*. In other cases bacteria have been used (see for example, Gasson, 1976).

Daniels and Meddins (1974) used the green alga *Chlorogonium euchlorum* as a test organism for *S. citri* toxin. The algae were sensitive to the spiroplasma growth medium, so harvested spiroplasma cells were used as a source of toxin, it being reasoned that even if the bulk of the toxin was excreted into the medium, a detectable amount should be within the cells. The procedure was to set up cultures of algae in a minimal salts medium containing a range of dilutions of the extract to be tested and to incubate them in the light for 16 hr. Growth was measured either by cell counts or by measuring incorporation of a radioactive amino acid into cell protein. It was found that *S. citri* produced a toxin of low M. Wt which killed algae, and which appeared to be a polar, uncharged, hydrophilic compound, possibly a polyol derivative. The assay was sensitive and convenient, but suffered from the disadvantage of not being usable with crude culture fluids. To overcome this problem the following assay was devised.

Broad Bean Leaf Test. Daniels (1979b) exploited a property of *Vicia faba* leaf tissue to develop a toxin assay which was relatively insensitive to nonspecific interference and could be used for crude unfractionated *S. citri* cultures. The tissue contains a latent polyphenoloxidase which is activated by protein denaturing agents, and which then oxidises endogenous polyphenol substrates to polymeric black pigments. Exposure of leaf tissue to *S. citri* toxins causes rupture of cells and the latent enzyme is activated by proteolytic enzymes or other agents released from organelles with subsequent blackening of the tissue. Thus the final product (the black pigment) depends on the presence of the toxin, and by dilution of the latter to a point where blackening no longer occurs the titre can be estimated. In practice the youngest fully expanded leaves are removed from a broad bean plant, the lower epidermis is removed and pieces of the stripped tissue are floated on dilutions of the toxin-containing solution. Incubation overnight at 37°C is required to develop the black colour. Similar dilutions of inoculated spiroplasma growth medium give no blackening. Daniels (1979b) described the use of this assay to study the properties of a low M. Wt acidic, polar toxin, which unfortunately was too unstable to permit detailed characterisation.

One of the merits of this assay is that, since it is possible to test cultures directly without fractionation, a large number of spiroplasma strains may be easily surveyed. On the other hand, the blackening reaction is given by relatively few plant species, so that it is not possible to study the effect of the toxin on other plants by this method. The next test can be used for almost any plant.

Inhibition of Seed Germination. Partially purified preparations of *S. citri* toxins were found to inhibit germination of seeds (Daniels and Niven, 1977). For routine work lettuce seeds (*Lactuca sativa*) were convenient. Four to five seeds were placed on small filter paper bridges in multi-well plastic plates containing the test solutions, the wells were sealed with transparent tape and the plates incubated at room temperature for three days. Germination was scored visually and the toxin titre recorded as the highest dilution preventing germination. Inhibited seeds imbibed and the radicle began to emerge, but further development ceased, even when the seeds were washed free of toxins. Undiluted spiroplasma growth medium inhibited seed germination by virtue of its high osmotic pressure and of the toxicity of the PPLO broth component

— a dilution factor of about ten was necessary to allow germination in the presence of unfractionated medium.

Other Assays. Many other bioassays have been used for phytotoxins. Some have been tested in this laboratory for their suitability for *S. citri* toxin study, but results have either been inconclusive or toxin activity has been masked by nonspecific effects of growth media. The tests include inhibition of seedling growth, inhibition of tissue culture growth, inhibition of pollen germination, induction of wilting of cuttings, induction of chlorosis of leaves and leakage of electrolytes from tissues (i.e. destruction of permeability barriers). So far insufficient information is at hand concerning the mode of action of spiroplasma toxins to enable one to devise specific biochemical assays.

References

Adams, M.H. (1959). *Bacteriophages*. New York: Interscience Publishers.

Adler, J. (1969). Chemoreceptors in bacteria. *Science 166*, 1588–97.

— (1975). Chemotaxis in bacteria. *Annual Review of Biochemistry 44*, 341–56.

— (1978). Chemotaxis in bacteria. *Harvey Lectures Series 72*, 195–320.

Andrewes, C.H. and Welch, F.V. (1946). A motile organism of the pleuropneumonia group. *Journal of Pathology and Bacteriology 58*, 578–80.

Arber, W. (1974). DNA modification and restriction. *Progress in Nucleic Acid Research and Molecular Biology 14*, 1–37.

Bendich, A. (1957). Methods for characterisation of nucleic acids by base composition. In *Methods in Enzymology*, Vol. III, pp. 715–23, S.P. Colowick and N.O. Kaplan (eds). New York: Academic Press.

Berg, H.C. and Brown, D.A. (1972). Chemotaxis in *Escherichia coli* analysed by three-dimensional tracking. *Nature 239*, 500–4.

Bickle, T.A., Pirrotta, V. and Imber, R. (1977). A simple general procedure for purifying restriction endonucleases. *Nucleic Acids Research 4*, 2561–72.

Braun, A.C. (1955). A study on the mode of action of the wildfire toxin. *Phytopathology 45*, 659–64.

Bredt, W. (1979). Motility. In *The Mycoplasmas*, Vol. I, pp. 141–55, M.F. Barile a and S. Razin (eds). New York: Academic Press.

Bredt, W., Höfling, K.H., Heunert, H.H. and Milthaler, B. (1970). Measurements on motile cells of *Mycoplasma pneumoniae*. *Zeitschrift für Medizinische Mikrobiologie und Immunologie 156*, 39–43.

Bretscher, M.S. (1971). Major human erythrocyte glycoprotein spans the cell membrane. *Nature, New Biology 231*, 229–32.

Brown, N.L. and Smith, M. (1976). The mapping and sequence determination of the single site in ϕX174 am 3 replicative form DNA cleaved by restriction endonuclease PstI. *FEBS Letters 65*, 284–87.

Cadilhac, B. and Giannotti, J. (1975). Sur la présence d'elements à structure hélicoidale dans le phloème de *Vinca rosea* atteinte de stolbur. *Comptes Rendus Hebdomadaires des Séances de l'Académie des Sciences. Paris, Série D. 281*, 539–42.

Calavan, E.C. and Oldfield, G.N. (1979). Symptomatology of spiroplasmal plant diseases. In *The Mycoplasmas*, Vol. III, pp. 37–64, J.G. Tully and

R.F. Whitcomb (eds). New York: Academic Press.

Cirillo, V.P. (1979). Transport systems. In *The Mycoplasmas*, Vol. I, pp. 323–49, M.F. Barile and S. Razin (eds). New York: Academic Press.

Clark, T.B. (1977). *Spiroplasma* sp., a new pathogen in honey bees. *Journal of Invertebrate Pathology 29*, 112–13.

Clyde, W.A. (1974). Studies on Mycoplasmatales viruses and mycoplasma pathogenicity. *Les Mycoplasmes/Mycoplasmas. Les Colloques de l'Institut National de la Santé et de la Recherche Médicale 33*, 109–16.

Cole, R.M. (1978). Spiroplasma viruses: recent developments. *Zentralblatt für Bakteriologie, Parasitenkunde, Infektionskrankheiten und Hygiene. Erste Abteilung Originale 241*, 187–8.

— (1979). Mycoplasma and spiroplasma viruses: ultrastructure. In *The Mycoplasmas*, Vol. I, pp. 385–410, M.F. Barile and S. Razin (eds). New York: Academic Press.

Cole, R.M., Garon, C.F., Mitchell, W.O., Jabonska, E. and Ranhand, J.M. (1978). Spiroplasma viruses: current status. *Abstracts of the Fourth International Congress of Virology*, 175.

Cole, R.M., Mitchell, W.O. and Garon, C.F. (1977). *Spiroplasma* virus *citri* 3: propagation, purification, proteins and nucleic acid. *Science 198*, 1262–3.

Cole, R.M., Tully, J.G. and Popkin, T.J. (1974). Virus-like particles in *Spiroplasma citri. Les Mycoplasmes/Mycoplasmas. Les Colloques de l'Institut National de la Santé et de la Recherche Médicale 33*, 125–32.

Cole, R.M., Tully, J.G., Popkin, T.J. and Bové, J.M. (1973a). Ultrastructure of the agent of citrus 'stubborn' disease. *Annals of the New York Academy of Sciences 225*, 471–93.

— (1973b). Morphology, ultrastructure and bacteriophage infection of the helical mycoplasma-like organism (*Spiroplasma citri* gen. nov., sp. nov.) cultured from stubborn disease of citrus. *Journal of Bacteriology 115*, 367–86.

Daniels, M.J. (1979a). Mechanisms of spiroplasma pathogenicity. In *The Mycoplasmas*, Vol III, pp. 209–27, R.F. Whitcomb and J.G. Tully (eds). New York: Academic Press.

— (1979b). A simple technique for assaying certain microbial phytotoxins and its application to the study of toxins produced by *Spiroplasma citri. Journal of General Microbiology 114*, 323–8.

Daniels, M.J. and Longland, J.M. (1980). Chemotaxis by spiroplasmas. *Society for General Microbiology Quarterly 7*, 85.

Daniels, M.J., Longland, J.M. and Gilbart, J. (1980). Aspects of motility and chemotaxis in spiroplasmas. *Journal of General Microbiology 118*, 429–36.

Daniels, M.J. and Meddins, B.M. (1974). The pathogenicity of *Spiroplasma citri. Les Mycoplasmes/Mycoplasmas. Les Colloques de l'Institut National de la Santé et de la Recherche Médicale 33*, 195–200.

Daniels, M.J. and Niven, C.F. (1977). Sensitivity of plants to *Spiroplasma citri* toxins. *Sixty Eighth Annual Report of the John Innes Institute*, 105.

Das, J. and Maniloff, J. (1975). Replication of mycoplasmavirus MVL51: I. Replicative intermediates. *Biochemical and Biophysical Research Communication 66*, 599–605.

— (1976a). Replication of mycoplasma-virus MVL51: II. Attachment of MVL51 parental DNA to host membrane. *Proceedings of the National Academy of Sciences of the United States of America 73*, 1489–93.

— (1976b). Replication of mycoplasmavirus MVL51: III. Identification of progeny viral DNA-protein intermediates. *Microbios 15*, 127–34.

— (1976c). Replication of mycoplasma-virus MVL51: IV. Inhibition of viral synthesis by rifampin. *Journal of Virology 18*, 969–76.

— (1978). Replication of mycoplasmavirus MVL51: V. *In vivo* synthesis of virus-specific proteins. *Virology 86*, 186-92.

Davies, P.L., Van de Sande, J.H. and Dixon, G.H. (1979). Base compositional analysis of nanogram quantities of unlabelled nucleic acids. *Analytical Biochemistry 93*, 26-30.

Davis, R.E. and Worley, J.F. (1973). Spiroplasma: motile, helical microorganism associated with corn stunt disease. *Phytopathology 63*, 403-8.

— (1974). Spiroplasma motility: translational movement in semi-solid media. *Abstracts of the International Congress on Mycoplasmas of Man, Animals, Plants and Insects*, 15-16.

Edwards, G.A. and Fogh, J. (1960). Fine structure of pleuropneumonia-like organisms in pure culture and in infected tissue culture cells. *Journal of Bacteriology 79*, 267-76.

Fraser, D. and Fleischman, C. (1974). Interaction of mycoplasma with viruses. I. Primary adsorption of virus is ionic in mechanism. *Journal of Virology 13*, 1067-74.

Garwes, D.J., Pike, B.V., Wyld, S.G., Pocock, D.H. and Gourlay, R.N. (1975). Characterization of *Mycoplasmatales* virus – *laidlawii* 3. *Journal of General Virology 29*, 11-24.

Gasson, M.J. (1976). Phytotoxins produced by plant pathogenic pseudomonads. *Sixty Seventh Annual Report of the John Innes Institute*, 94-6.

Gourlay, R.N. (1970). Isolation of a virus infecting a strain of *Mycoplasma laidlawii*. *Nature 225*, 1165.

— (1971). *Mycoplasmatales* virus – *laidlawii* 2, a new virus isolated from *Acholeplasma laidlawii*. *Journal of General Virology 12*, 65-7.

— (1972). Isolation and characterization of mycoplasma viruses. In *Pathogenic Mycoplasmas. Ciba Foundation Symposium*, pp. 145-64, K. Elliott and J. Birch (eds). Amsterdam: Associated Scientific Publishers.

— (1974). Mycoplasma viruses: isolation, physicochemical and biological properties. *Critical Reviews in Microbiology 3*, 315-31.

Gourlay, R.N. and Wyld, S.G. (1973). Isolation of *Mycoplasmatales* virus – laidlawii 3, a new virus infecting *Acholeplasma laidlawii*. *Journal of General Virology 19*, 279-83.

Gourret, J.P., Maillet, P.L. and Gouranton, J. (1973). Virus-like particles associated with the mycoplasmas of clover phyllody in the plant and in the insect vector. *Journal of General Microbiology 74*, 241-9.

Haberer, K. (1978). Mycoplasma virus L3: biological properties and molecular weight of DNA. *Abstracts of the Fourth International Congress of Virology*, 173.

Haller, G.J. and Lynn, R.J. (1968). Satellite DNAs in *Mycoplasma arthritidis* and a stable bacterial L-form. *Bacteriological Proceedings*, 68.

Horne, R.W. (1972). Comparison between the structure of animal and plant mycoplasmas: extracellular and intracellular morphology. In *Pathogenic Mycoplasmas. Ciba Foundation Symposium*, pp. 39-66, K. Elliott and J. Birch (eds). Amsterdam: Associated Scientific Publishers.

Howard, C.J., Gourlay, R.N. and Wyld, S.G. (1980). Isolation of a virus, MVBRI, from *Mycoplasma bovirhinis*. *FEMS Microbiology Letters 7*, 163-5.

Kirby, K.S. (1965). Isolation and characterization of ribosomal RNA. *Biochemical Journal 96*, 266-9.

Kleinschmidt, A.K. (1968). Monolayer techniques in electron microscopy of nucleic acid molecules. In *Methods in Enzymology*, Vol. XIIB, pp. 361-77, L. Grossman and K. Moldave (eds). New York: Academic Press.

Lang, D. and Mitani, M. (1970). Simplified quantitative electron microscopy of biopolymers. *Biopolymers 9*, 373-9.

Larsen, S.H., Reader, R.W., Kort, E.N., Tso, W.-W. and Adler, J. (1974). Change in direction of flagellar rotation is the basis of the chemotactic response in *Escherichia coli. Nature 249*, 74–7.

Lee, I.-M. (1977). The *in vitro* life cycle, morphology and ultrastructure of the citrus stubborn organism, *Spiroplasma citri.* PhD Dissertation, University of California, Riverside, Calif.

Liss, A. (1977). *Acholeplasma laidlawii* infection by group 3 mycoplasmavirus. *Virology 77*, 433–6.

Liss, A. and Cole, R.M. (1979). *Spiroplasmavirus* group 1: isolation and preliminary characterization. *Abstracts of the Annual Meeting of the American Society for Microbiology*, G22.

Liss, A. and Maniloff, J. (1971). Isolation of Mycoplasmatales viruses and characterization of MVL1, MVL51, MVL52. *Science 173*, 725–7.

— (1973). Infection of *Acholeplasma laidlawii* by MVL51 virus. *Virology 55*, 118–26.

Lombardi, P.S. and Cole, B.C. (1979). Characterization of mycoplasmavirus MVL2 DNA. *Journal of Virology 29*, 381–4.

MacHattie, L.A., Ritchie, D.A., Thomas, C.A.Jr. and Richardson, C.C. (1967). Terminal repetition in permuted T2 bacteriophage DNA molecules. *Journal of Molecular Biology 23*, 355–63.

Maniloff, J. (1972). In discussion of paper by Gourlay, R.N., Isolation and characterisation of mycoplasma viruses. In *Pathogenic Mycoplasmas. Ciba Foundation Symposium*, pp. 156–64, K. Elliott and J. Birch (eds). Amsterdam: Associated Scientific Publishers.

Maniloff, J., Das, J. and Christensen, J.R. (1977). Viruses of mycoplasmas and spiroplasmas. *Advances in Virus Research 21*, 343–80

Maniloff, J., Das, J., Putzrath, R.M. and Nowak, J.A. (1979). Mycoplasma and spiroplasma viruses: molecular biology. In *The Mycoplasmas*, Vol. I, pp. 411–30, M.F. Barile and S. Razin (eds). New York: Academic Press.

Maniloff, J. and Liss, A. (1974). Comparative structure, chemistry and evolution of mycoplasmaviruses. In *Viruses, Evolution and Cancer*, pp. 583–604, E. Kurstak and K. Maramorosch (eds). New York: Academic Press.

Morowitz, H.J. (1969). The genome of mycoplasmas. In *The Mycoplasmatales and the L-Phase of Bacteria*, pp. 405–12, L. Hayflick (ed). Amsterdam: North Holland.

Noel, D., Nikaido, K. and Ames, G.F.L. (1979). A single amino-acid substitution in a histidine transport protein drastically alters its mobility in sodium dodecyl sulphate–polyacrylamide gel electrophoresis. *Biochemistry 18*, 4159–65.

Nowak, J.A. and Maniloff, J. (1979). Physical characterization of the superhelical DNA genome of an enveloped mycoplasma virus. *Journal of Virology 29*, 374–80.

Oishi, K. and Poulson, D.F. (1970). A virus associated with SR-spirochaetes of *Drosophila nebulosa. Proceedings of the National Academy of Sciences of the United States of America 67*, 1565–72.

Parkinson, J.S. (1977). Behavioural genetics in bacteria. *Annual Review of Genetics 11*, 397–414.

Petrino, M.G. and Doetsch, R.N. (1978). 'Viscotaxis', a new behavioural response of *Leptospira interrogans (biflexa)* strain B16. *Journal of General Microbiology 109*, 113–17.

Pfeffer, W. (1888). Uber chemotaktische Bewegungen von Bacterien, Flagellaten und Volvocineen. *Untersuchungen aus dem Botanischen Institut in Tubingen 2*, 582–661.

Philpotts, R.J., Patel, K.K.T. and Edward, D.G. ff. (1977). Heterogeneity among strains of *Mycoplasmatales* virus *laidlawii 2. Journal of General Virology 36*,

211–15.

Pinkerton, F. and Strobel, G.A. (1976). Serinol as an activator of toxin production in attenuated cultures of *Helminthosporium sacchari. Proceedings of the National Academy of Sciences of the United States of America 73*, 4007–11.

Ploaie, P.G. (1971). Particles resembling virus associated with mycoplasma-like organisms in plants. *Revue Roumaine de Biologie. Série de Botanie 16*, 3–6.

Putzrath, R.M. and Maniloff, J. (1977). Growth of an enveloped mycoplasma-virus and establishment of a carrier state. *Journal of Virology 22*, 308–14.

Rahmann, A.A. and Sethi, K.K. (1979). Presence of viruses in a strain of *Mycoplasma pulmonis. Experientia 35*, 1029–30.

Razin, S. (1978). The mycoplasmas. *Microbiological Reviews 42*, 14–70.

Roberts, R.J. (1976). Restriction endonucleases. *Critical Reviews in Biochemistry 4*, 123–64.

Robertson, J., Gomersall, M. and Gill, P. (1972). Virus-like particles in *Mycoplasma hominis. Canadian Journal of Microbiology 18*, 1971–2.

Rottem, S. and Greenberg, N. (1978). Membrane structure of the enveloped MVL-2 virus. *Zentralblatt für Bakteriologie, Parasitenkunde, Infektionskrankheiten und Hygiene. Erste Abteilung Originale 241*, 172–3.

Saglio, P.H.M. (1979). Motility and improvement in selective isolation of spiroplasmas. *Plant Disease Reporter 63*, 293–6.

Scriba, M. (1968). Experiments to eliminate mycoplasmas from tissue cultures by means of antibiotics. *Zeitschrift für Medizinische Mikrobiologie und Immunologie 154*, 267–76.

Shepherd, R.J., Bruening, G.E. and Wakeman, R.J. (1970). Double-stranded DNA from cauliflower mosaic virus. *Virology 41*, 339–47.

Springer, M.S., Goy, M.F. and Adler, J. (1979). Protein methylation in behavioural control mechanisms and in signal transduction. *Nature 280*, 279–84.

Stephens, M.A. (1978). Restriction and modification of viruses in *Spiroplasma citri. Zentralblatt für Bakteriologie, Parasitenkunde, Infektionskrankheiten und Hygiene. Erste Abteilung Originale 241*, 187–8.

— (1980). Studies of spiroplasma viruses. PhD Thesis, University of East Anglia, Norwich.

Sutcliffe, J.G. (1978). pRB322 restriction map derived from the DNA sequence: accurate DNA size markers up to 4361 nucleotide pairs long. *Nucleic Acids Research 5*, 2721–8.

Swartzendruber, D.C., Clark, J. and Murphy, W.H. (1967). Detection of phage-like particles by electron microscopy in a human strain of mycoplasma. *Bacteriological Proceedings*, 151.

Thomas, C.A.Jr. and MacHattie, L.A. (1964). Circular T2 DNA molecules. *Proceedings of the National Academy of Sciences of the United States of America 52*, 1297–301.

Townsend, R., Markham, P.G., Plaskitt, K.A. and Daniels, M.J. (1977). Isolation and characterization of a non-helical strain of *Spiroplasma citri. Journal of General Microbiology 100*, 15–21.

CONTRIBUTORS

D.B. Archer: John Innes Institute, Colney Lane, Norwich NR4 7UH, England.

L.M. Black: Department of Genetics and Development, University of Illinois, Urbana, Illinois 61801, USA.

T.A. Chen: Department of Plant Pathology, Rutgers University, The State University of New Jersey, New Brunswick, New Jersey 08903, USA.

M.J. Daniels: John Innes Institute, Colney Lane, Norwich NR4 7UH, England.

S.J. Eden-Green: Rothamsted Experimental Station, Harpenden AL5 2JQ, England.

C.H. Liao: Department of Plant Pathology, Rutgers University, The State University of New Jersey, New Brunswick, New Jersey 08903, USA.

P.G. Markham: John Innes Institute, Colney Lane, Norwich NR4 7UH, England.

R.E. McCoy: University of Florida, Agricultural Research Center, 3205 S.W. College Avenue, Fort Lauderdale, Florida 33314, USA.

M.A. Stephens: John Innes Institute, Colney Lane, Norwich NR4 7UH, England.

R. Townsend: John Innes Institute, Colney Lane, Norwich NR4 7UH, England.

H. Waters: UK Overseas Development Lethal Yellowing Research Team, Coconut Industry Board, Box 204, Kingston 10, Jamaica.

R.F. Whitcomb: US Department of Agriculture, Science and Education Administration, Agricultural Research, Insect Pathology Laboratory, Beltsville, Maryland 20705, USA.

D.S. Williams: University of Florida, Agricultural Research Center, 3205 S.W. College Avenue, Fort Lauderdale, Florida 33314, USA.

D.L. Williamson: Department of Anatomical Sciences, State University of New York at Stony Brook, Stony Brook, New York 11794, USA.

359

INDEX